THE PRICE OF PROPHECY

FR. ALEXANDER F. C. WEBSTER is academic dean and associate professor of moral theology at St. Sophia Ukrainian Orthodox Theological Seminary in South Bound Brook, New Jersey. He has an
M.T.S. from Harvard Divinity School and a Ph.D. from the University of Pittsburgh. Fr. Webster serves concurrently as parish
priest of a small English-language congregation in Falls Church,
Virginia (Orthodox Church in America–Romanian Episcopate),
lecturer in religious studies at George Mason University, and assistant division chaplain for the 29th Infantry Division (Light) of
the Virginia Army National Guard. His articles have appeared in
numerous publications, including the *Journal of Ecumenical Studies*,
East European Quarterly, *Strategic Review*, *Army of Ukraine*, *Modern Age*,
Greek Orthodox Theological Review, *St. Vladimir's Theological Quarterly*,
The Christian Century, the *Wall Street Journal*, the *Washington Post*, and
the *Christian Science Monitor*.

THE PRICE
OF PROPHECY

*Orthodox Churches on
Peace, Freedom, and Security*

SECOND EDITION

by
Alexander F. C. Webster

Foreword by
George Huntston Williams

ETHICS AND PUBLIC POLICY CENTER
WASHINGTON, D.C.

WILLIAM B. EERDMANS PUBLISHING COMPANY
GRAND RAPIDS, MICHIGAN

First edition 1993
Second edition published jointly 1995 by the
Ethics and Public Policy Center and
Wm. B. Eerdmans Publishing Co.
255 Jefferson Ave. S.E., Grand Rapids, Michigan 49503

00 99 98 97 96 95   7 6 5 4 3 2 1

Library of Congress Cataloging-in-Publication Data

Webster, Alexander F. C.
The price of prophecy: Orthodox churches on peace, freedom, and security /
by Alexander F. C. Webster; foreword by
George Hunston Williams. — 2nd ed.
p.   cm.
Includes index.
ISBN 0-8028-0836-0 (pbk.)
1. Christian ethics — Orthodox Eastern authors. 2. Peace — Religious aspects —
Orthodox Eastern Church. 3. Liberty — Religious aspects — Orthodox Eastern
Church. 4. National security — Religious aspects — Orthodox Eastern Church.
5. Orthodox Eastern Church — Doctrines.
I. Title.
BJ1250.W432   1995
241'.62'088219 — dc20   94-43977
CIP

To those spiritual and academic mentors
whose personal loyalty is itself a prophetic witness:
Bishop Maximos Aghiourgoussis
Father Stanley S. Harakas
Metropolitan Christopher Kovacevich
Dr. Ernest W. Lefever
Bishop Nathaniel Popp
Archbishop Antoniy Scharba
The Rev. Dr. George Huntston Williams

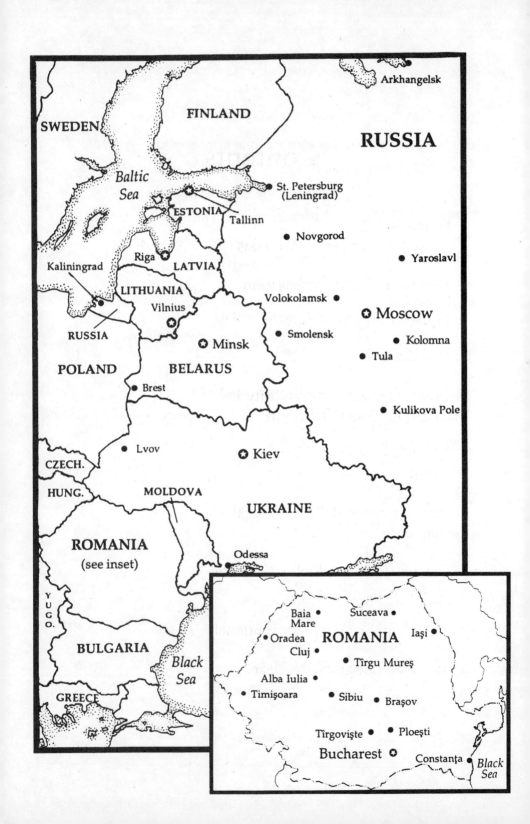

Contents

Foreword

GEORGE HUNTSTON WILLIAMS

Patriarch Pavle of Belgrade was in the United States during most of October 1992 to visit the Serbian Orthodox churches so long divided on political lines and now rejoined, partly under his conciliatory suasion. Two years earlier, at age seventy-six, he had been chosen by lot, on apostolic precedent, to succeed to the Serbian patriarchal throne amid ethnic and confessional turbulence in what was once Croat Marshal Josip Broz Tito's federal republic of Yugoslavia. On May 27, 1992, the new Serbian patriarch had presided over the Holy Synod of Bishops, which in the midst of the Croatian campaign issued a statement distancing the Orthodox faithful from the residual Communist nationalist regimes of Serbia and Montenegro.

The bishops' statement deplored the resort to violence following the dissolution of Yugoslavia (which in 1918, as an Orthodox kingdom, had been enlarged with Catholic and Muslim ethnic pieces from the Hapsburg Empire, in fulfillment of one of Woodrow Wilson's Fourteen Points). It protested also, in solidarity with Serbs throughout the stricken federal republic, the abuses of the Croats in their war of secession from the federation. Bishop Pavle had long since taken as his Christian ideal the all-forgiving Zossima of Dostoevsky's *Brothers Karamazov*. As patriarch he had led several demonstrations in the streets of Belgrade against the ethnic war, one of priests and seminarians, one of students in general, another of workers sympathetic to his prophetic Christian protest. Americans who were privileged to

---

George Huntston Williams is Hollis Professor of Divinity *emeritus*, Harvard University.

meet with Pavle during his visit encountered a prelate who embodies the best in the Orthodox moral tradition.

The Serbs constitute one of the five major groupings of the Orthodox in the United States that figure prominently in the present volume. (1) The Greeks are under an archbishop who oversees the faithful in the whole of the Western Hemisphere. The four others are organized for North America only (Canada, the United States, and most commonly also Mexico): (2) the Orthodox Church in America, which includes within it a Romanian diocese, (3) the Antiochians in the United States and Canada, who are mostly of Lebanese, Syrian, and Palestinian origin, (4) the autocephalous Ukrainian Church, centered in South Bound Brook, New Jersey, and (5) the newly conjoined Serbs. Two of these jurisdictions are mildly competitive for recognition as the preeminent representation of ecumenical Orthodoxy in the country: the Greek Archdiocese, ethnically and culturally closest to the Ecumenical Patriarch in the Phanar (in modern Istanbul, Turkey) and headquartered in New York City; and the Orthodox Church in America, taking historic precedence through bonds with the Orthodox mission in Alaska and as far south as California, and now headquartered in the nation's capital. The latter, whose ranking hierarch bears the title Archbishop of Washington and Metropolitan of All America and Canada, is a daughter Church of the Moscow Patriarchate.

Father Alexander Webster, author of the present volume, is a convert to Orthodoxy and a priest of the Romanian diocese of the Orthodox Church in America. He holds a degree from the Harvard Divinity School (1977) and is a long-time friend of this writer, who co-authored the article on Russian Orthodoxy that launched his publishing career in 1976. Fr. Webster has also served as a chaplain on active duty in the armed services of his country and has written on military service in the Orthodox tradition. Along with other Orthodox social ethicists, like Fr. Stanley Harakas of Hellenic College in Brookline, Massachusetts, Father Webster has long been at work helping to evolve a distinctive voice for all the Orthodox faith communities in the United States on moral issues such as civil and ethnic rights, abortion, family values, and the growing separation and alienation of classes on the basis of income and ethnicity—issues that transcend confessional and even religious groupings and involve the commonweal.

Fr. Webster has in mind the development of what he tentatively calls a neo-Byzantine vision of American society, in which all Orthodox groups, out of their Eastern Christian roots and particularly their belief in the symphonic ideal of a "church-state dyarchy" or of a "virtuous commonwealth of peoples," can help to clarify, in an age of acute pluralism, the role of religion in the American public square, in the halls of legislation, and in the media of public communication. The Byzantine Empire, at its creative height and depth, encouraged —both within and without the far-flung realm of Christian Hellenist speech, culture, law, and liturgy—the closeness of priest and parishioners, of liturgy and mother tongue, of disciplined monasteries and the episcopate. Fr. Webster intends to bring to bear the Orthodox Christian perspective in America and to lay the foundation for eventual works on the maturing role of Orthodox thought and praxis amid the pluralistic variety of piety and principle.

Orthodoxy fits well into the American scheme of allowing for diverse religious groupings, none of which enjoys the monopoly of establishment. Indeed, it might well be argued that American citizens of Orthodox fealty may all the more readily function in this way, in that they have chosen to live within ethnic religious jurisdictions and cultural traditions that extend beyond the borders of the United States to embrace kinsmen in Canada and also (for most) in Mexico and even beyond. In this way they have, perhaps providentially, broken with Old World practice by transcending, in their loyalties and cohesion, political and national boundaries. For these Christians, the originating nation determines their jurisdictional contours in a way true of no other state-church tradition, not even of Episcopalians/Anglicans.

Fr. Webster's lifetime program may make his eventual ethico-political contribution something akin to that of James Viscount Bryce in his two-volume *The American Commonwealth* (1888), wherein the British lord suggested that the interconnected local and regional jurisdictions and judicatories in the United States and the vitality of innumerable voluntary associations, including the churches, had come to exhibit something of the vigorous pluralism of medieval (Latin) Christendom before the rise of the absolute monarchies and national states. This observation about Fr. Webster's program, though it refers to a possible lifetime achievement and not solely to the work before us, nevertheless suggests the scope, mastered detail, texture, and critical judgment in *The Price of Prophecy*. Fr. Webster here deals with Orthodox "prophecy" at home and abroad, that is, with social and political utterances in the line of the prophets in the former Soviet Union, Romania, and the United States. Many of these utterances, alas, have been more like those of the sycophantic court prophets in the Old Testament who proclaimed support for any Hebrew rulership regardless of merit, than like those of the revered and canonized risk-taking prophets such as Amos and Jeremiah, or like the dramatic public moral witness of Patriarch Pavle in Belgrade today.

The public issues Fr. Webster here examines do not, by intention, cover the whole spectrum of Christian concern for the commonweal. They are, however, issues that for several of the Orthodox jurisdictions in the United States were, until recently, uppermost in their homelands, and issues on which the Orthodox in their American home and abroad have most often gone on public record: namely, international peace, corporate and individual religious freedom, and national security, and, to that end, the proper use of conventional and especially nuclear weapons. In chapter 4, where he deals thematically and comparatively with the public issues addressed by selected Orthodox jurisdictions headquartered in the United States, Fr. Webster correctly notes that these proclamations and appeals regarding governmental policy in their homelands have often alerted the American public as a whole to pressing problems for their spiritual kinsmen abroad. The author has thus chosen as his major themes the official utterances of greatest moment to Orthodox Christians who for seventy-four years in Russia and Ukraine attempted to function under a dictatorial Communist superpower, or, in Romania, for forty-two years under a Stalinist-nationalist regime that eventually was headed by a grotesquely, even morbidly self-aggrandizing dictatorial couple who perverted even the originally classless and raceless Marxist ideal. Fr. Webster is well aware of the historic anomaly in Russia that the dyarchy of patriarch and ruler was destroyed by Tsar Peter the Great in 1721 and not restored until 1917 under the Communist regime, and that the tradition of independent judgment by the Church on public issues therefore lacked appropriate precedent in that vast land.

As an Orthodox ethicist, Fr. Webster feels constrained to regard as normatively Christian the Byzantine period rather than the sixteenth century (which brought forth Protestantism and fully reshaped Catholicism). Orthodoxy is indeed most clearly linked with the achievements of the age of the Ecumenical Councils, when Byzantium was the chief capital of the Roman Empire, eventually to become the religio-political center of the gradually receding Byzantine Empire—that is, from A.D. 330 to 1453. The author declines to take as normative the ante-Nicene, pre-Constantinian era (as did much of the sectarian Protestantism that shaped the American republic). He does, however, assimilate the norms of that quite different era, primarily in the pacifism and martyrdom-readiness that lives on in the clergy of the Church and in the ideal of the Church Fathers, ante-Nicene no less than post-Nicene.

Fr. Webster is fully aware that the experience of Orthodox peoples under different Orthodox rulers, notably under tsars and various national patriarchs, especially after 1453 (when the fall of Constantinople brought the Byzantine Empire to an end), cannot be equally normative for all Orthodox jurisdictions. Yet what has over the generations been achieved and handed down from national synods and the other theological and ethical enterprises of Orthodox churchmen since then must be taken into account in the clarification of an appropriately Orthodox stance in today's religiously pluralistic world. And by the very title of his work, Fr. Webster is suggesting as highly relevant the experience of the Hebrew/Jewish people as recorded in the Old Testament, holding up the socially critical role of the ancient prophets as an ideal for hierarchs and synods of today—public "prophecy" with its "price."

By setting forth in extensive detail the prevailingly deplorable accommodation of hierarchs abroad in forced but also sometimes obsequious public utterances under oppressive regimes, Fr. Webster makes the case that Orthodox leadership has all too often sacrificed true Orthodox ethical principles in failing to act forthrightly (prophetically) under ideologically oppressive, or indifferently secular, governments. His painstaking and comprehensive analysis of the public moral witness of the various Churches on the selected issues, set against his identification of the whole range of possible utterances—from courageous prophecy, through prudential evasion, to ignoble propaganda—reveals, alas, that the record of the Orthodox in the twentieth century has been far, far below expectations.

Fr. Webster identifies as "cosmocracy" any polity that is wholly worldly, recognizing that this is a strain in the Byzantine tradition that has been pilloried by Catholics in particular as Caesaropapism. This, of course, he deplores, wherever and whenever it has been manifest in the history of Christianity in Eastern lands. In his view and that of all modern interpreters of the Orthodox tradition (e.g., Frs. Georges Florovsky and John Meyendorff), this is a perversion or secularization of what was ideally the dyarchy, the symphony of church and state, organically related whenever possible. But when a harmonious cooperation is no longer possible, as in modern states of diverse religious loyalties or none, Fr. Webster is critical of any over-accommodation to such a constitutional separation, whether wholehearted or merely pragmatic on the part of the Orthodox. His ideal remains the always precarious stance of prophecy and moral guidance for the good of the whole society and polity of which Orthodox Christian citizens have become a part.

Preface to the Second Edition

The passage of twenty months would not normally warrant a second edition of a book pertaining to morality. But these are not, for the Orthodox Churches in Eastern Europe and the United States, normal times, if ever the turbulent moral and political world of Eastern Orthodox Christianity has been characterized by anything approaching "normalcy."

Since I completed the first edition of this book in October 1992, several events and trends have rocked the Orthodox world, with profound ramifications for the public moral witness of the various Orthodox Churches. Among these are the sudden rise of the ethno-nationalist right wing in Russian secular and ecclesial politics, the death of Patriarch Mstyslav of Kyyiv and All-Ukraine, rapprochement between the state of Israel and Yasir Arafat's Palestine Liberation Organization, and, of course, an escalation of the barbaric civil war in the former Yugoslavia. This new edition takes into account these and other recent developments.

The conclusions, however, have remained substantially the same. Perhaps the French slogan *"Plus ça change . . ."* applies with unusual force to the social ethics of the ancient, venerable, but struggling Orthodox Churches in the modern era. Names, places, and events may succeed one another with great rapidity or all deliberate speed. But the moral character of the Orthodox, forged in the Communist gulags and immigrant ghettoes, requires more than a few years of political liberation and social assimilation before it can image once again the glory of Byzantium or Holy Rus.

I wish to thank the William B. Eerdmans Publishing Company for its decision to co-publish this second edition with the Ethics and Public Policy Center. Although my tenure as a research fellow at the Center ended in June 1993, Center president George Weigel suggested the need for a second edition of this book and graciously provided the space and resources to accomplish the mission. I also wish to acknowledge several colleagues, in addition to those mentioned in the preface to the first edition, whose insights and assistance have enhanced the final product: Fr. Michael Bourdeaux, Fr. Frank Estocin, Fr. Remus Grama, Fr. George Rados, Fr. Roland Roberson, C.S.P., Randy Tift, Derek Mogck, Fr. Rastko Trbuhovich, Fr. Eugen Vasilescu, and Alan Wisdom. Sole responsibility for errors in fact or judgment, however, resides, as always, with the author.

Washington, D.C.   Fr. Alexander F. C. Webster
June 9, 1994
Ascension of Our Lord

Preface to the First Edition

A work of this length is the product of many creative minds. I wish to thank Hrach Gregorian and Barry O'Connor at the United States Institute of Peace for a two-year grant that funded the research and writing of the book. The senior staff at the Ethics and Public Policy Center—particularly Ernest W. Lefever, Robert Royal, George Weigel, and, earlier, John Cooper—have provided a lively scholarly and ecumenical environment. A special team of consultants offered valuable critiques of the rough draft: Fr. Nicholas Apostola, Vigen Guroian, Fr. Stanley S. Harakas, Kent R. Hill, Fr. Leonid Kishkovsky, Fr. John Langan, S.J., Earl A. Pope, Gerry Powers, and the Rev. V. Bruce Rigdon.

Others who have furnished useful information or shared their own insights include my bishop, the Rt. Rev. Bishop Nathaniel Popp of the Romanian Orthodox Episcopate of America; my ordaining bishop, the Most Rev. Metropolitan Christopher Kovacevich of the Serbian Orthodox Metropolitanate of Midwest America; my long-time spiritual mentor, the Rt. Rev. Bishop Maximos Aghiourgoussis of the Greek Orthodox Diocese of Pittsburgh; the Most Rev. Archbishop Antony Scharba of the Ukrainian Orthodox Church of the U.S.A.; the Most Rev. Bishop Louis Puşcaş of the Romanian Catholic Diocese of Canton, Ohio; Alexandra Brkic; Fr. Gheorghe Calciu-Dumitreasa; Fr. George Corey; Fr. William Diakiw; Fr. Miltiades Efthimiou; Nicholas Gvosdev; James George Jatras; Fr. Rodion Kondratick; Alexis Liberovsky; Fr. Milan Markovina; Fr. Rade Merick; Eugenia Ordynsky; Dean Popps; Fr. Victor Potapov; Fr. Paul Schneirla; Fr. Anthony Ugolnik; Lawrence Uzzell; Sarah Vilankulu; Joyce Visnick; David Vuich; and George Huntston Williams.

I owe a special debt of gratitude to my gracious hosts in Romania: Bishop Nifon Ploieşteanul in Bucharest, Fr. Alexander Moraru in

Cluj, Emil Chiosa in Iaşi, and especially Fr. Deacon Ion Chivu, assistant professor of patristics at the Orthodox Theological Faculty of the University of Bucharest, whose generosity and hospitality displayed Romania at its best.

To my editor at the Ethics and Public Policy Center, Carol Griffith, I express my heartfelt thanks for her kind cuts and craftsmanship. Also at the Center, Christopher Ditzenberger and Ronald Rosenberger helped prepare the many revisions of the manuscript, and James Warner tended to the notes and produced the maps and the index.

Most of all, I rejoice at having such a supportive wife, Kathleen, and a family willing to endure my frequent absences at odd hours. But they are aware — more than most — of the remarkable times in which we live. Perhaps this volume will, albeit in a modest way, help my four Orthodox children (Kristen Mary, Beverly Ann, Andrew Patrick, and Colleen Elizabeth) grow up in a world with a little more peace, freedom, and security.

Introduction

On November 6, 1991, *New York Times* foreign correspondent Serge Schmemann chronicled the official passing of Soviet Communism in St. Petersburg (formerly Leningrad). Writing on the eve of the seventy-fourth anniversary of the revolution that brought Vladimir Ilych Lenin and his Bolsheviks to power, Schmemann—son of a fondly remembered Orthodox priest—said:

> It used to be the evening when Communist leaders gathered in the Kremlin for a solemn ceremony ushering in the premier feast day of their revolution. Today, a descendant of the Romanovs and the Patriarch of the Russian Orthodox Church celebrated the dropping of Lenin's name from this city and President Boris N. Yeltsin decreed a final ban on the Communist Party anywhere in the Russian republic.[1]

The sudden demise of Communism in Eastern Europe in 1989 and, since August 1991, in the Soviet Union is nothing less than a modern miracle, the unexpected fulfillment of the most fervent hopes of millions of people throughout the world.

The moral revitalization and democratic reforms that have graced this region in recent years should have vaulted its Eastern Orthodox Churches—Russian or otherwise—to the forefront of world history. This territory is, after all, the center of gravity for these venerable Christian communities. But the public moral witness of these Churches on issues of peace, freedom, and national security has been largely ignored by the media and intellectual elites in the United States.

That witness, to be sure, has not been morally consistent. Nor has it been evenly distributed among the fourteen to sixteen "autocephalous," or self-governing, Churches, particularly in Eastern

1

Europe, the Middle East, and North America, that constitute the Eastern Orthodox faith group—a distinctive Christian community that, contrary to popular misconception in the West, is neither Roman Catholic nor Protestant.[2] The Moscow Patriarchate of the huge Russian Orthodox Church, for example, has used its political leverage in ecumenical circles such as the Geneva-based World Council of Churches. But that Patriarchate's influence, at least prior to the failed coup in August 1991, was due in large measure to its close adherence to prevailing Soviet policies.

The public moral witness of the Romanian Orthodox Patriarchate is, even in the aftermath of the Communist regime, still tentative at best. At worst, it is needlessly deferential to the political authorities. In an interview in Bucharest in October 1990, for example, Bishop Nifon Mihăiţă, then assistant to the patriarch and head of the Patriarchate's department of external relations, tried to rationalize the questionable behavior of the bishops in the era of the despised dictator Nicolae Ceauşescu.[3] Responding to criticism of the Church's *modus vivendi* with the Communists, Bishop Nifon characterized that collaboration as empty rhetoric not to be taken seriously—merely the obligatory two or three pages in each issue of the Church's state-sponsored religious publications. That was the price to be paid for the "survival" of the Church. According to Nifon's moral calculus, if the intentions are good and the results generally favorable, an act may be deemed moral. For this young, well-educated bishop, what counts is ends; the question of proper means, particularly the proportionality of means to ends, is inconsequential.

In comparison to the giant Russian and Romanian Orthodox Churches, which claim some 70 million and 19 million members, respectively, the smaller, much younger, predominantly ethnic Orthodox bodies in North America have not been as well organized, as closely identified with the nation, or as willing to speak out either for or against government policies. Consequently, the public moral witness of the American Orthodox has been sporadic at best and generally ineffectual.

In all three countries the public moral witness of the Orthodox Church has lacked self-assurance and internal coherence. This has not served Orthodoxy well. These Churches can hardly blame the media entirely for the marginal role they seem to occupy in their societies.

Short-Lived Visibility

Several events provided unprecedented visibility for the Orthodox Churches on the American religious scene in recent years. First, the celebration in June 1988 of a millennium of Christianity in lands then under Soviet rule may, in retrospect, have marked a turning point in the bitter hostility between Church and state in that country. In the United States, this celebration enabled American Protestants and Roman Catholics to appreciate, perhaps for the first time, the distinctive, venerable religious traditions of Russian and Ukrainian Orthodoxy.

Second, the presidential candidacy of Governor Michael Dukakis of Massachusetts in 1988 embroiled the several Orthodox Churches in the United States in a year-long public debate. At issue were the repeated claims by the Democratic nominee that he was a "member" of the Greek Orthodox Archdiocese of North and South America.[4] For the first time in their two centuries on this continent, Orthodox Christians had to come to grips with whether and how they, as a minority religious community in a secular, pluralistic society, might exercise their moral and political rights to influence a national election and subsequent public-policy decisions.

Finally, in 1990 and 1992 three of the highest-ranking Orthodox patriarchs visited the United States in succession. Each occasion marked the first time a leading prelate from one of these three ancient Churches had crossed the Atlantic Ocean. Patriarch Dimitrios of Constantinople, Ecumenical Patriarch and "first among equals" in the worldwide Orthodox hierarchy until his death in 1991, conducted a whirlwind tour of eight American cities in July 1990 that concluded with meetings and photo sessions with President George Bush, Vice President Dan Quayle, the leaders of the U.S. Congress, state and local elected officials, and prominent religious figures. Yet despite considerable effort and expense on the part of the host Greek Orthodox Archdiocese of New York, and faithful reporting in the major media,[5] this extraordinary event in the life of the American Orthodox community quickly faded from view. Even less noted were the visits by Patriarch Aleksii II of Moscow in November 1991 and again in September 1993, neither of which made the first page of America's national newspapers. If Dimitrios and Aleksii suffered from benign neglect, the cold shoulder offered Patriarch Pavle of Serbia in October 1992 appears to have been a more calculated gesture by media elites who had, for the most part, already chosen sides in the violent conflicts raging in the former Yugoslavia.

In general, however, ignorance rather than overt hostility characterizes the popular American consciousness of Eastern Orthodoxy. The Orthodox still remain outside the accepted troika of faith groups: Protestant, Roman Catholic, and Jewish. Their virtual invisibility persists despite the international spotlight that has shone upon their homelands in the former Soviet Union and Eastern Europe for almost a decade. This ancient Christian family of 250 million equals or exceeds in number the worldwide Protestant community. In the United States there are roughly four million Orthodox Christians, distributed among a dozen or so independent jurisdictions; by comparison, there are six million Jews, including both the religiously observant and the non-religious.

The Public-Policy Arena

If the Orthodox, particularly those in America, wish to become more visible, they must first come to grips with their public moral witness, however checkered or disappointing they may find it. The most logical place to begin is in the realm of national and international security issues. This is the arena where, especially since the Vietnam War in the 1960s, the Roman Catholic and Protestant communions have, as bearers of venerable moral traditions, emerged as major players in the policymaking process. Their national assemblies and hierarchies, together with the leadership of the National Council of Churches, have generated a plethora of resolutions, messages, pronouncements, and encyclicals on an impressive array of social and moral issues.

The document that earned the mainline Christian religious organizations a prominent place in the national debate concerning peace, freedom, and security was the controversial 1983 pastoral letter of the National Conference of Catholic Bishops, *The Challenge of Peace*.[6] This cogently reasoned statement makes both moral and prudential judgments, most of which are critical of the main planks of U.S. defense policy. It has become a standard reference in any informed discussion of the morality of nuclear weaponry and deterrence. The Catholic bishops' letter inspired the United Methodist Council of Bishops to issue a more stringent denunciation of nuclear deterrence in a similar encyclical published in 1986 as *In Defense of Creation: The Nuclear Crisis and a Just Peace.*[7]

From a decidedly more conservative vantage, the National Association of Evangelicals (NAE) in 1987 launched a unique project called "Peace, Freedom, and Security Studies." Its goal is "to improve the skills of evangelical leadership in supporting religious liberty, promoting the security of free societies and encouraging progress toward the non-violent resolution of international conflict."[8]

While U.S. Catholics and Protestants, both mainline and evangelical, were joining these debates, what were the Orthodox Churches doing? The present study is intended to answer that question by focusing on the Orthodox Churches in the former Soviet Union, Romania, and the United States. Among the autocephalous Orthodox Churches in the world, the Russian and Romanian Patriarchates have been the most active in this arena, while the Orthodox Churches in the United States, however small and disorganized by comparison, are of particular interest to American readers. We shall examine the activities and proclamations of these three groups of Churches ostensibly intended to advance international peace, political and religious freedom, and national security.

The demise of the Soviet Union as a nuclear superpower affords the Orthodox Churches in the surviving independent republics of Russia and Ukraine unprecedented opportunities to exert a profound moral influence on the nuclear and conventional defense policies of their governments. The recent record of the Moscow Patriarchate, in particular, assumes a special import as a predictor of that Church's willingness and ability to criticize government policies in the new era of domestic *glasnost'* ("openness") and international good will toward the United States.

Chapter 1 will outline the Orthodox moral tradition relevant to these matters. Then the next three chapters will focus on issues of freedom and human rights in the four countries. Chapter 2 will describe how various factions within the Moscow Patriarchate advanced or hindered political and religious freedom in the Soviet Union and in the new republics of Russia and Ukraine. Chapter 3 will analyze the symbiosis of Church and nation in Romania that drove the Orthodox Patriarchate, based in Bucharest, to function as an arm of the Communist state in implementing its domestic and foreign policies. Chapter 4 will explore the disparate, generally parochial, primarily ethnic moral witness of the Orthodox Churches in the United States.

The study will then shift to peace and security issues pertaining to both "conventional" (that is, non-nuclear) and nuclear war. Chapter 5 will examine the public moral witness of the Orthodox Churches on conventional warfare in relation to the histories of each of the three countries (the former Soviet Union, Romania, and the United States). The problems of militarism and nationalism loom large, for example, in the legacy of the "Great Patriotic War" in the Moscow Patriarchate and in the surprisingly malleable responses to the Vietnam War of the Orthodox Churches in the United States. Chapter 6 will address the unique challenges posed by nuclear weapons and the prospects of nuclear war: it will chronicle the massive nuclear-disarmament campaign spearheaded by the Moscow Patriarchate (beginning in 1950) and the Romanian Orthodox Church (during the 1980s) and the occasional utterances of several of the Orthodox jurisdictions in the United States.

Throughout the discussion we shall also review the Orthodox contribution to the public moral witness of three historically significant ecumenical organizations: the Prague-based Christian Peace Conference, the World Council of Churches, and the National Council of Churches of Christ in the United States.

Chapter 7 will conclude the study by highlighting the moral, political, and ecclesial dilemmas in which the Orthodox Churches find themselves as a result of their effort to witness actively in unfriendly or, at best, "neutral" political milieus.

The primary sources relevant to this study are voluminous, even in English translation. In addition, I interviewed many of the bishops and other Church leaders—especially Romanians—who figure prominently in the book. I studiously tried to preserve the distinction between moral assessment of behavior and moral judgment of persons, and to avoid the latter.

THE PRICE OF PROPHECY

A recurring theme throughout this book is the importance of "prophecy" in the public moral witness of the Church. Prophecy in the biblical sense was not a simple foretelling of future events. The Old Testament prophet was instead someone anointed by God to criticize boldly and forthrightly the current religious, moral, and social ills of Israel in light of the covenant traditions established between God and Israel's patriarchs, Abraham and Moses. Sometimes this form of religiously motivated public moral witness required the prophet to warn that the wrath of God would be visited upon the people of Israel if they or their political leaders failed to mend their ways. Since people in power are likely to resent that kind of criticism, the life of a prophet was often short and unpleasant.

The prophetic task requires men and women of uncommon virtue who are willing to live heroic lives in conformity to ideal standards. In Orthodox moral tradition this means the higher, revealed, "transfigurative" morality of the New Testament Gospel epitomized in the Sermon on the Mount, especially the enduring formal norms expressed by the Beatitudes of Jesus Christ. Only this kind of moral perspective enables human beings and their communities to transcend, or "transfigure," their own limitations and self-interest and to advance toward spiritual perfection, a process that the Orthodox call *thēosis*—becoming more and more like God.

Most persons fall short of this transfigurative standard. They compromise their ideals and settle for something less than moral perfection, accepting a mixture of vice and virtue or altogether abandoning the pursuit of virtue in favor of more mundane values such as sheer survival or creature comforts. They are unwilling to pay the price of prophecy. That is not to say they are devoid of a moral sense. The ancient Church Fathers of the Orthodox Church also recognized another set of norms: a low-level one that they felt conformed to the "natural law" though it failed to express the moral plenitude of the Gospel. Epitomized in the Decalogue in the Old Testament, this "civilizing" morality—or, in Fr. Stanley S. Harakas's apt phrase, "a sort of common denominator ethic" for all humanity—can be perceived by all men and women of sound reason.[9] Such a natural-law ethic based on rational self-interest and a measure of cooperation among persons usually constitutes the only common ground of discourse between Christians and their non-Christian societies, nations, and governments. But this ethic is hardly the full expression of the Orthodox moral sense and, consequently, may not serve in the long run as an adequate ground of public and private moral witness.

The distinction between transfigurative and civilizing moralities, though useful, does not suffice to describe the lived experiences of Orthodox Christians in the former Soviet Union, Romania, and the United States. In their finest moments, many bishops, lower clergy, and laymen have courageously assumed the mantle of prophet and taken the moral high ground—willing to risk everything they hold dear, including their lives—in order to proclaim without compromise what they sincerely believe is the will of God for their societies, nations, or governments. Irrespective of the specific content of their positions on issues of public policy, their moral witness is clearly in accord with the spirit of the biblical prophets, the ancient Church Fathers, and the Orthodox martyrs and confessors in every age.

Propaganda vs. Prophecy

Far more common, however, are various alloys of virtue and vice, prophecy and propaganda. The term "propaganda" is used neutrally in Europe to denote the transmission of particular doctrines or principles, but in the United States it has a more negative meaning. Webster's Third New International Dictionary defines it secondly as the "dissemination of ideas, information, or rumor for the purpose of helping or injuring an institution, a cause, or a person." Americans tend to think of propaganda as information that is false, misleading, or designed to foster an ulterior end. This more peculiarly American usage has informed the present study.

Some Orthodox leaders, unfortunately far more numerous than most Orthodox may be prepared to admit, have functioned as propagandists. They have actively sought, or allowed themselves to be used, to promote the social values and political policies of their governments or ethnic groups. Whether consciously or not, these propagandists have abandoned their Orthodox birthright or simply set it aside; they have proceeded to witness not in harmony with the Orthodox moral tradition but in spite of it, and without due regard for the consequences of their actions for the Orthodox communities they ostensibly represent.

And yet a more charitable perspective might preclude summary judgment even of those leaders who have collaborated with hostile anti-Christian forces. Perhaps their behavior has been a sign of moral weakness, a conformity to perceived "realities," a falling short of the prophetic ideal more pathetic than sinister.

In truth, the majority of Orthodox spokesmen and representative bodies fall somewhere between the antipodes of prophecy and propaganda, valor and cowardice, purity and corruption. This is the considered judgment of Nobel laureate and former expatriate Aleksandr Solzhenitsyn, who is widely regarded as a Russian Orthodox prophet for our times. The motives and behavior of most men and women are unremarkably mixed and are not always clearly understood by the principals themselves. The present study will, therefore, attempt to sort out the genuine prophecy, ignoble propaganda, and ambiguous middle ground in the public moral witness of the Eastern Orthodox Churches.

"Collaboration" with antithetical political regimes is itself a more complex phenomenon than it may seem on its face. Considering only the activities of Orthodox moral agents in the former Soviet bloc, we may deduce the grounds of six modes of collaboration:

1. *Instrumental:* fear of personal punishment and/or an opportunistic seeking of personal privilege;

2. *Conventional:* automatic deference and obedience to existing authority, whatever its political and moral qualities;

3. *Ideological:* genuine Marxist-Leninist convictions together with a sincere profession of the Orthodox Christian faith;

4. *Covert:* calculated use of the moral authority and credibility of the Church to advance the program of the Communist Party;

5. *Interim:* reluctant, minimalistic support for the government until the political climate—and church-state relations in particular—changes for the benefit of the Church;

6. *Pragmatic:* willingness to cut deals with existing authority to curry favors for the Church.

Few Orthodox Church leaders fit perfectly into any of these distinct types, but in various combinations, and certainly in the aggregate, the types help to explain this widespread phenomenon of collaboration with hostile regimes.

The Past as Prologue

In light of the dramatic political trends in the former Soviet Union and Romania, the Orthodox leadership in these nations may at last be on the verge of breaking out of the politico-ethical patterns of the recent past. Younger, morally energized bishops such as Metropolitan Daniel of Moldova and Bukovina in Romania and, perhaps, Archbishop Khrizostom of Vilnius in the independent state of Lithuania may be the vanguard of a new generation of genuinely prophetic spiritual leaders. Positive signs of a dramatic, irrevocable change for the better continue to appear—not least of which were the dramatic interventions of Patriarch Aleksii II of Moscow in the failed coup by hard-line Soviet Communists in August 1991 and in the political showdown in October 1993 between President Boris Yeltsin and the Russian Parliament.[10] But, at this writing, the governments in Russia, Ukraine, and Romania are still wild cards, and the political future of their Orthodox peoples is unpredictable. The Orthodox Patriarchates in Moscow, Kyyiv, and Bucharest have not yet tasted complete, Western-style religious and political freedom.

Following a precedent in formerly Communist East Germany, the archives of the Soviet KGB (secret police) and Communist Party were opened for the first time toward the end of 1991.[11] Preliminary investigations have unearthed disturbing connections between active Russian Orthodox bishops and the deposed Communists, which the current patriarch of Moscow seems determined to keep under wraps.[12] These Churches remain very much prisoners of their own recent past. Thus their public moral witness in recent decades as chronicled in this study retains a more than historical interest. If the past is prologue, the immediate past in Russia, Ukraine, and Romania should indicate how the slow-to-change Orthodox Churches in these countries may perform in the immediate future.

To assess this performance fairly, however, we must first see how the Eastern Orthodox Churches historically have framed their moral doctrines pertaining to peace, freedom, and security. That is the task in chapter 1.

1

Peace, Freedom, and Security in Orthodox Moral Tradition

As a religious community of two thousand years' standing, the Eastern Orthodox Churches claim a rich doctrinal and moral heritage. This heritage is the yardstick against which the moral positions of contemporary Orthodox spokesmen must be measured.

Who are the Eastern Orthodox? They are, first, a **community of tradition**.

The Orthodox community is variously recognized in the West for its "mystical" sense, or rich liturgical practices, or "ethnic" identities, or fidelity to ancient Christian doctrines such as those proclaimed by the seven Ecumenical Councils held between A.D. 325 and 787. All these perceptions are correct, but even together they do not suffice to define a religious community that unabashedly proclaims itself "orthodox," much less "Orthodox."

Orthodox is a loan word from the ancient Greek language—a conflation of two words: *orthos,* meaning "correct," and either *dokein,* "to think," or *doxa,* "glory" (as in worship). Both meanings of the second word fit: Orthodox Christians everywhere and in every era share the same "correct thinking" about doctrinal and moral matters and the same "correct worship" of the God who has revealed himself as Father, Son, and Holy Spirit. Whether situated in the Eastern Mediterranean or Eastern Europe, or in more recent settlements in Western Europe, North and South America, and Australasia, the Orthodox Churches regard one another as equal heirs of the scriptural, patristic, canonical, hagiographical, liturgical, iconographic, and spiritual patrimony

11

derived directly from the ancient, undivided Christian Church of the first millennium after the life, death, and resurrection of Jesus Christ.

This emphasis on continuity with the ancient Christian past fosters among the Orthodox a fierce loyalty to **tradition**. They cherish that which has been "handed down"—as the Latin original of this loan word suggests—from generation to generation. This is not to say, however, that the tradition is monolithic or unadaptable to changing conditions. A cardinal principle of Eastern Orthodox theology rooted in the doctrine of the incarnation of the Son of God as the man Jesus is the necessity that tradition be "living."[1] Though *essentially* unchangeable, even as the divine nature of the Son of God is "unchangeable," tradition grows and matures organically, or "changes," as the Church appropriates it in different times. This intrinsically conservative—but not reactionary—approach theoretically prevents, on the one hand, rote repetition and stultifying rigidity and, on the other hand, radical, core changes in doctrine, piety, and ritual practices.

The Orthodox also stress their common experience of this living Tradition. The **community** called "Church" is thus the only proper locus of Orthodox doctrinal and moral reflection and the only authoritative source of public moral pronouncements. There is no room for unchecked, free-spirited "individualism" or the official proclamation of personal "opinion." Professor Christos Yannaras of Athens is one of many contemporary Orthodox moral theologians who insist that the ethic of the Orthodox Church is "a communal ethic, a social ethic." Sinful human beings cannot establish genuine communion even when they act "freely," because that freedom is constrained by sin. The Church transcends this problem by rejecting "every rationalistic criterion for participation in the life of communion." Anyone and everyone may become part of its community, which alone provides the necessary context for a genuinely free, personal response to God's transfigurative presence in the "holy mysteries," particularly what the Christian West calls the sacrament of holy communion, or the eucharist.

From Yannaras's seemingly radical but very Orthodox perspective, the "social ethic," or public morality of the Church is intended neither to "improve" nor to "reform" the condition of corporate life or the moral character of individual persons: "Its aim is to enable life to operate in the limitless scope of personal freedom, the freedom which can be existentially realized only as an event of communion." This "communal ethic" may, however, have a salutary impact on the wider societies in which Orthodox Christians live. "As people live the sacrificial ethos of the eucharist," he argues, "it suffuses economics, politics, professional life, the family, and the structures of public life in a mystical way. . . . And it transfigures them—it changes their existential presuppositions, and does not simply 'improve' them."[2]

Besides being a community of tradition, the Orthodox Churches are a **witnessing community**.

The emphasis on Orthodoxy as, above all, a community whose very presence is deemed to be uniquely efficacious in transfiguring the world leads to a preferred (though by no means exclusive) way of witnessing to the world that may be described as "centripedal" or "iconic." The Orthodox form of "centripedal" witness—a term borrowed from the Protestant theologian George W. Peters[3]—shares the life of Christ with non-Orthodox persons by attracting them to the "spritual beauty" that is presumed to exist in the Church community.[4] An invitation to others arises naturally from the virtue, holiness, and philanthropy that presumably characterize the personal lives and communities of Orthodox Christians. Thus the truth of Christ, whether theological or moral, is believed to be "caught" rather than "taught," modeled rather than explained, empowering rather than authoritarian.

"Mission is effective," wrote Fr. Dumitru Staniloae, a distinguished Romanian Orthodox theologian who died in 1993, "only when the power of the Holy Spirit radiates from the one who preaches Christ." When the Church fully actualizes "the power of the life of holiness" —by no means an unattainable ideal—then it is truly capable of winning souls to Christ.[5] The Eastern Orthodox faithful are called, therefore, to become a communal living "icon"[6]—a window to the Kingdom of God, a vehicle in which that Kingdom is present to the world-at-large, a means by which the world is transformed rather than merely reformed.

The other Orthodox way of witnessing to the world is probably more familiar to Western Christians. This dynamic approach, which Peters call "centrifugal," requires that believers both individually and in community make active efforts to gather people of the world into the Church. There is less a sense of "insiders" and "outsiders" than an awareness of the Church as the vanguard of the Kingdom to come, whose membership consists in both the "already" and the "not yet." This missionary impulse is expressed through personal and communal outreach, aggressive preaching, and pubic moral proclamations.

In the first millennium of Christianity, such proclamations appeared in the general statements and canons of discipline produced by assemblies of bishops, preeminently the seven Ecumenical Councils that convened in and around the imperial city of Constantinople. In the present century, however, the Orthodox Churches have also resorted to another forum. "Ecumenical" (meaning interdenominational) organizations have replaced the Ecumenical (from the Greek word *oikoumenē,* meaning "the inhabited world") Councils as the usual venue for the collective public moral witness of all the ancient patriarchates and national Orthodox Churches.

THE ORTHODOX WITNESS IN ECUMENICAL BODIES

The Orthodox Churches have become deeply involved in three controversial ecumenical organizations of Protestant provenance: the World Council of Churches, the Christian Peace Conference, and the National Council of Churches (U.S.).

World Council of Churches (WCC)

Among the founding member-churches of the World Council of Churches in 1948 were the ancient Orthodox Patriarchates of Constantinople, Alexandria, Antioch, and Jerusalem, the national Orthodox Church of Greece, and the émigré Romanian Orthodox Church in America. At first, the Moscow Patriarchate denounced the WCC as a tool of Vatican and Western capitalist interests. But by 1961, when the WCC Assembly was held in New Delhi, Soviet foreign policy had changed dramatically under Nikita Khrushchev, and the Russian Orthodox Church and all the national Orthodox Churches in the Soviet-bloc countries finally joined the WCC.

Based in Geneva, Switzerland, the WCC now boasts some 300 mostly Protestant member-churches that are said to represent non–Roman Catholic Christianity, or roughly a third of the world's 1.5 billion Christians. The WCC's predominantly Protestant power establishment continues to set the organization's agenda of theological, moral, and political concerns from a peculiarly liberal, and often radical, Protestant vantage that commonly is unrepresentative of the views of the growing evangelical and fundamentalist Protestant denominations as well as the Orthodox Churches.[7]

The role of the Orthodox Churches as moral leaders in this organization has been checkered at best. At the WCC Assembly in Canberra, Australia, in February 1991, Patriarch Parthenios of Alexandria was elected as one of the eight WCC presidents. Another distinguished Orthodox theologian, Metropolitan Chrysostomos of the Patriarchate of Constantinople, is one of the four officers of the Central Committee, the WCC's main policymaking arm between Assemblies (which are held every six to eight years). Priests and laymen such as Fr. Gennadios Limouris of Greece and Fr. Ion Bria of Romania serve as heads of various departments or sections in the Geneva bureaucracy.

Regrettably, before the demise of the Soviet Union in 1991, the Patriarchates of Moscow and Romania in particular exercised a distinctly leftist, pro-Soviet political leverage on the WCC Assemblies, especially those in Nairobi (1975) and in Vancouver (1983). The Orthodox Churches in the WCC that were not dominated by Communist governments had to endure, often in silence, all manner of politically motivated pronouncements and activities not only from the Protestant member-communions but also from their Orthodox brethren in former Soviet-bloc countries. In the aftermath of the 1991 Canberra Assembly, where a female Presbyterian minister from South Korea publicly invoked the "spirits" of the dead and those of trees and the earth, even some of the council's American Orthodox mainstays such as Fr. Leonid Kishkovsky, ecumenical officer of the Orthodox Church in America, have begun to question publicly the utility of continued Orthodox involvement in the WCC.[8]

Christian Peace Conference (CPC)

The ecumenical witness of the Orthodox participants in the Christian Peace Conference has been even more dubious. This organization began in June 1958 when some forty Protestants from West Germany and the Soviet bloc met in Prague, Czechoslovakia, to demand the elimination of all "weapons of mass destruction" and the establishment of "nuclear-free zones."[9] The movement mushroomed, and its declared goals soon encompassed a supposedly pacifist-inspired abolition of all weapons and armies.[10] By 1966 this aspiration had given way to explicit support for "revolution" as divinely sanctioned and rejection of "the so-called counter-revolution"—an attitude obviously derived from the "socialist" ideology to which the majority of delegates subscribed—as inherently unjust.[11] When representatives of the Orthodox Churches in the Soviet bloc joined the CPC in 1961 and participated actively in the first All-Christian Peace Assembly in Prague, they enhanced the organization's ecumenical flavor, if not its political diversity.

The CPC has been dismissed by many as either a Communist front or a congeries of ideologically one-sided, politically irrelevant activists —well-intentioned, perhaps, but dangerously naïve.[12] Among the CPC's defenders, however, is the Russian Orthodox priest-theologian Vitaly Borovoi, who vigorously denied the charge of ideological sub-servience to the Soviet regime and defended the participation of his Church in the CPC as follows: "[O]ur movement is not an artificial superstructure over political combinations of the 'Eastern bloc,' as some say, but a Christian movement which sprang from our deep sense that it is organic for our Churches and the whole of Christianity to minister to love and reconciliation."[13]

Eminent Russian and Romanian Orthodox have figured promi-nently in the deliberations of the CPC since 1968. In that memorable year, Metropolitan Nikodim Rotov of Leningrad assumed the presi-dency after the CPC's founding president, Czech Protestant theolo-gian Josef L. Hromádka, resigned to protest the Soviet invasion of his native land. Included on the present "presidential board" of the CPC are Metropolitan Nicolae Corneanu of Banat, Romania, as one of nine vice-presidents, and Metropolitan Filaret Denisenko of the Ukrainian Orthodox Church, Kyyivan Patriarchate (but "defrocked" by the Moscow Patriarchate in April 1992), as chairman of the "continuation committee." No Orthodox Christians from North America, however, have had any connections with this organization.

In the post-Communist era, the CPC may have a short life expec-tancy. In its three decades of existence prior to the collapse of Soviet Communism in 1991, its membership—churches, Christian peace groups, and individuals—was drawn primarily from the Orthodox

Churches and Protestant denominations in the Soviet bloc and from Protestant churches in Africa, Asia, and Latin America that felt a special kinship with Moscow and international socialism. In October 1991 —just two months after the failed Soviet coup—only ninety persons attended the CPC meeting in Celakovice, Czechoslavakia. And instead of meeting in the more familiar surroundings of first-class Prague hotels, the CPC this time gathered in a student dormitory on the campus of an American university.[14]

National Council of Churches (NCC)

The ecumenical organization in which the Orthodox Churches in the United States are most deeply involved is the National Council of Churches. First convened in 1950, this organization describes itself as "the primary national expression of the ecumenical movement in the United States." Its thirty-two "communions," or member-churches, which claim a total membership of some 40 million, subscribe to a constitution whose preamble commits them to "covenant with one another to manifest ever more fully the unity of the Church" in a "common mission."[15]

Six Eastern Orthodox jurisdictions and three Oriental Orthodox bodies (that is, those Eastern Churches that bolted in the fifth century from the Church centered in Constantinople, capital of the Byzantine Empire) have, on and off, maintained full voting membership in the otherwise "mainline" Protestant NCC. The Ukrainian Orthodox Church of America and what is now the Orthodox Church in America were founding member "communions" in 1950. The Greek Orthodox Archdiocese joined the NCC in 1952, the Serbian Orthodox Church in the U.S.A. and Canada in 1957, the Antiochian Orthodox Archdiocese in 1966, and what is now known as the Patriarchal Parishes of the Moscow-based Russian Orthodox Church also in 1966. The three Oriental Orthodox member-churches include American branches of the Armenian, Coptic, and Syrian Orthodox Churches in the Middle East.

A bittersweet milestone in the history of Orthodox participation in the NCC was the election of Fr. Leonid Kishkovsky of the Orthodox Church in America as president of the organization for the two-year period beginning in November 1989. Fr. Leonid was the first Orthodox, priest or layman, to serve in this capacity. The NCC had become the object of fierce criticism from otherwise ecumenically inclined Christians who oppose the pronounced liberal leaning of its resolutions on moral and social issues,[16] and at about the time when Fr. Leonid began his term, its Governing Board (renamed General Board in 1990) commenced a period of introspection and administrative reorganization.

But neither this move nor the Kishkovsky presidency seemed to move the NCC toward theological and moral concerns that harmonize better with traditional Orthodox interests. At least that was the preliminary conclusion of the widely esteemed Archbishop Iakovos Coucouzis, primate of the Greek Orthodox Archdiocese of New York and North and South America. Archbishop Iakovos announced in June 1991 that the Archdiocese had "suspended" its participation in the NCC. In a surprisingly terse letter to Fr. Leonid, Iakovos referred to "the extreme liberties" of the largely liberal Protestant organization, which "make our association and membership impossible."[17]

At a meeting of the Standing Conference of Canonical Orthodox Bishops in the Americas (SCOBA) on October 24, 1991, the other Eastern Orthodox member-communions of the NCC decided to follow Archbishop Iakovos's initiative by suspending their participation pending the report of a special six-person theological commission to the next meeting of SCOBA in March 1992. The commission was staffed by known supporters of the NCC. Not surprisingly, their report recommended lifting the suspension for two years and exacting from the NCC a pledge to publicize "minority" (read Orthodox) dissents from majority statements on controversial issues. SCOBA voted unanimously to follow this recommendation, to the grave disappointment of Orthodox critics of the NCC who hoped the American Orthodox had finally crossed an ecumenical Rubicon.

The NCC continues to send mixed signals to the Orthodox Churches in this country. At a meeting of the General Board in November 1992, the NCC announced an endowment fund of $10 million named after Archbishop Iakovos, thus wedding him—and, presumably, the Greek Orthodox Archdiocese—to this ecumenical organization for the rest of his life. Iakovos quickly demonstrated his renewed commitment to the NCC by helping to recruit former presidents Jimmy Carter and, astonishingly, Ronald Reagan as honorary co-chairmen.[18] The

NCC's well-known hostility to policies of the Reagan and Bush administrations was still in evidence in October 1993, when NCC General Secretary Joan Brown Campbell said about President Bill Clinton, "We now have a president who in many ways is putting forth legislation that is consonant with some of the things we have said."[19] With a more friendly liberal Democrat in the White House and the Orthodox more deeply involved than ever, it promises to be business as usual for the NCC and its distinctly liberal social and political agenda.

Perhaps the only consolation for Orthodox critics of the NCC is the occasional *mea culpa* that its leaders are now willing to offer, albeit belatedly. General Secretary Campbell finally admitted in October 1993, "We did not understand the depth of the suffering of Christians under communism. And we failed to really cry out against the communist oppression. I do give credit to people who called for that and did not get a response, at least from us."[20]

The "Ecumenical Agony"

What are the historic Orthodox interests in ecumenical forums such as the WCC, CPC, and NCC? The late Fr. Alexander Schmemann used the graphic phrase "ecumenical agony" to describe the gulf that separates the Orthodox ethos from those of the Western churches, despite their mutual hopes for unity within one visible Body of Christ called the Church.[21] The Orthodox themselves continue to be divided on the questions of why and how to bridge that gulf and to witness on behalf of the Orthodox tradition in ecumenical forums.[22]

The most conservative Orthodox ecumenical perspective would allow only for a *strict witness* **to** the truth of the living Tradition. Orthodoxy is equated with the fullness of divine revelation, and individual Orthodox Christians are expected to share their theological, spiritual, and moral riches with other Christians. They are to do this, however, without any compromise or ambiguity in proclaiming their message. At the WCC's Third World Conference on Faith and Order, held in 1952 in Lund, Sweden, the Orthodox delegates issued a separate statement that read in part: "We do not come to criticize other Churches but to help them, to illumine their mind in a brotherly manner by informing them about the teaching of the One, Holy, Catholic and Apostolic Church which is the Greek Orthodox Church, unchanged since the apostolic era."[23] Two decades later, in 1973, the bishops of the Orthodox Church in America (OCA) issued an encyclical entitled "Christian Unity and Ecumenism" in which they lamented what seemed to be the "singular task" of ecumenism — namely, "to manifest the minimum of unity which already exists among Christians rather than to recover the fullness of unity in God beyond all contradictions which, according to the Orthodox, has been lost."[24]

Other Orthodox ecumenists are seeking a *theological convergence* **in** the truth. This entails the recognition of an existing unity in certain doctrinal matters and at least a material agreement on various moral and social issues. These intersections are presumed to provide the impetus for continued progress toward the ultimate "reunion" of the churches on the basis of a common confession of faith to which none of the various communions may currently lay claim. Most of the Orthodox leaders — especially from the Russian and Romanian Orthodox Churches — who participate actively in the various international ecumenical organizations appear to subscribe to this innovative approach. "Convergence" ecumenism is most evident in their efforts to reach a common moral position on a myriad of issues concerning peace, freedom, and security.

ORTHODOX NORMS OF PEACE AND WAR

A fervent longing for peace has imbued the Eastern Orthodox community since the birth of the Church amidst the spiritual and political turmoil of first-century Jerusalem. More than the mere absence of war, "peace" (*eirēnē* in Greek) in Orthodox tradition means universal brotherhood, the well-being of the Christian community, spiritual serenity, and the tranquillity of order. The perennial moral problem confronting the Orthodox Churches, as well as other human communities, is how this peace can be achieved by individual members of the community, within the community itself, and in the world in general.[25]

Absolute Pacifism

Despite centuries of neglect and even hostility in mainstream Eastern Orthodoxy, **absolute pacifism**, a commitment to non-violence without exception, has endured in the quiet corners of monastic communities and individual souls. This is the prophetic norm governing the Orthodox approach to the moral problems of peace and war —the higher, revealed, "transfigurative" morality of the Gospel.

Old Testament revisionist scholars have argued persuasively that certain strands of Israelite religious tradition subscribed to the moral ideal of non-violence by Israel in deference to Yahweh, the *heavenly* "warrior." The New Testament contains specific injunctions by Jesus against violence, and apocalyptic elements—with their emphasis on God's, not man's, fight against evil powers—perpetuate the implicit pacifism of various prophets of ancient Israel, most notably Jeremiah. Explicit condemnations of human violence under any circumstances can be found in the patristic writings of St. Justin Martyr, St. Athenagoras of Athens, the mature Tertullian of Carthage, St. Hippolytus of Rome, Arnobius of Sicca, the early Lactantius, Pope St. Damasus of Rome, Prudentius, and St. Paulinus of Nola.

Further, the canonical corpus forbids clergy to participate in any form of violence or direct military activity; they stand apart in this way, not as a special moral caste, but rather as the vanguard of the peaceful, unbloodied, non-violent Church that will be a fitting "bride" of Christ when He returns to earth in glory. Numerous *vitae,* or lives, of soldier-saints such as St. Martin of Tours, and *acta,* or chronicles, of martyrs such as St. Maximilian document their refusal, in imitation of Christ, to engage in violent acts.

Implicit pacifism also characterizes the moral witness of medieval saints, most notably SS. Boris and Gleb (Hlib in Ukrainian), the "passion-bearers" of Kyyivan Rus. In Orthodox mystico-ascetic spirituality, virtues such as dispassion, stillness, and patience assist the Orthodox Christian in his "spiritual warfare" against demons and preclude any violent emotions or actual physical violence against mere mortals, however dangerous or ungodly. The modern Russian theological persective known as "kenoticism" (after the Greek verb *kenein,* "to empty," used by St. Paul in Philippians 2:6-7 to describe the voluntary humiliation of the Son of God) maintains this spirituality. It is most evident in the devotional writings of St. Tikhon of Zadonsk in the eighteenth century and in the novels of the great nineteenth-century writer Fyodor Dostoevsky.

More recently, the prolific American theologian Fr. Stanley S.

Harakas has argued in favor of a pacifist option for individuals along-side the ethic of justifiable war,[26] and the monks of the Finnish Orthodox Valamo Monastery have officially provided sanctuary to Finnish conscientious objectors to military service (much to the con-sternation of the five military chaplains from the Finnish Orthodox Church). The Orthodox absolute-pacifist ethic seems at last to be finding concrete expression today.

Justifiable War

As a concession to the omnipresence of human sin, the Orthodox Church has also developed a "civilizing" ethic of war that falls far short of the prophetic ideal. The ethic of **justifiable war** (unlike that of the "holy war" or "crusade," which is foreign to Orthodoxy) attempts to limit the use of military violence in the pursuit of necessary moral ends without automatically blessing war as a moral good.[27] It is clearly a lesser moral option than absolute pacifism, for those un-willing or unable to pay the full price of prophecy.

The justifiable-war ethic can claim an impressive array of advocates, including some Old Testament writers, various "warrior" saints such as St. Andrew Stratelates and St. Aleksandr Nevsky, and prominent Church Fathers like SS. Athanasios and Basil the Great in the East and SS. Ambrose and Augustine of Hippo in the West. Still, it has never been systematically elucidated in Orthodox moral theology.

I suggest that the justifiable-war ethic in its Orthodox form com-prises three key elements.[28] First, a *proper political ethos* is the Orthodox equivalent of "legitimate authority" in the *jus ad bellum* ("right to war") component of the Western just-war tradition.[29] A given government and society may be deemed worthy of defense by military means to the extent that they conform to the norms of the natural-law ethic and have positive relations with the Orthodox community.

The second condition establishes a sufficient cause for the resort to violence: *defense of the People of God.* As the divine-human Body of Christ, the Church may not suffer desecration. Each Orthodox Chris-tian, and the community as a whole, is morally obligated to defend the People of God wherever they are from any injustice, whether it be the violence that is endemic to foreign invasion, or domestic op-pression by those hostile to the free exercise of the Orthodox faith.

Such purely defensive violence may be considered by some, at worst, "a lesser evil" than that posed by the foreign or domestic enemy of the People of God. In the fuller political context, military defense — with its inherent risks to those who take up arms courageously and self-sacrificially — may be, at best, a virtuous enterprise.

Finally, a *spiritual intent* is necessary lest military action degenerate into mere revenge, self-righteousness, or conquest. Orthodox Christians may never regard national enemies as other than persons who were created, like themselves, in the image and likeness of God, and who therefore must never be reduced to the status of impersonal means to ends, however virtuous the ends. The ultimate goals of forgiveness and rehabilitation of the "enemy" must govern the decision to resort to force and the conduct of any military action.

If "mercy" is the virtue that the Orthodox absolute pacifist endeavors to maximize by refraining from all violence against human beings, the corresponding virtue that has priority for the Orthodox just warrior is "justice." Whereas the pacifist seeks to emulate Jesus as the Good Shepherd who allowed Himself to be slain unjustly by and for sinners, the just warrior perceives a higher duty: to defend the relatively innocent from unjust aggression. If the Orthodox pacifist can never do anything evil even for a reasonably just end, the Orthodox warrior cannot preserve his personal holiness by allowing evil to triumph through his own inaction.

Of course, this comparison puts a more positive face on the justifiable-war ethic than the historical record might warrant. As we shall see in chapters 5 and 6, even this relatively low-level morality has been honored more often in the breach.

ORTHODOX NORMS OF FREEDOM AND RIGHTS

Eastern Orthodoxy has not evolved a systematic, philosophical ethic of "human rights." As Fr. Stanley S. Harakas observes, "There is little in the sources of our Faith which highlight and emphasize claims for the fulfillment of rights."[30] In this century, however, several Greek Orthodox moral theologians, influenced by currents in Western philosophical thought, have appropriated modern concepts of "rights." For example, Panagiotes Demetropoulos of Athens and Chrestos Androutsos of Thessalonica emphasized the reciprocity of duties and rights. In contrast, Vasileios Antoniades of Constantinople grounded certain universal rights of human beings in the ontological fact of human existence and moral agency.[31]

Western formulations of certain human or "natural" rights since the eighteenth-century Enlightenment would seem to resonate well with several fundamental tenets of Orthodox moral theology. The American political philosopher J. Roland Pennock (emeritus, Swarthmore College) differentiates "natural" from "human" rights by suggesting that natural rights "are commonly said to be absolute, not subject to exception (once defined) or to be overridden," while human rights "may come into being" because of historical needs.[32] The Orthodox theological view of the inherent dignity of every human person created in the image and likeness of God provides solid ground for a concept of natural rights in Pennock's inalienable sense. Indeed, the doctrine of creation, by transferring the source of natural rights from the vicissitudes of human rationality to the absolute, revealed truth of God the Creator, may provide the only way of transcending more limited, secular appeals rooted in distorted, sinful human experience. The precepts of the "civilizing" natural-law ethic discussed in the Introduction, which imply a reciprocal right for each command ("do not murder," for example, implicitly acknowledges a "right" to life), assume in Orthodox moral theology a uniquely divine sanction.[33]

Another political philosopher, John W. Chapman (emeritus, University of Pittsburgh), contends that "moral equality implies that no one is to gain at the expense of another."[34] According to Orthodox moral theology, human or natural rights "reflect the triadic or communal pattern of the Trinity."[35] This fundamental dogma posits a "community," as it were, of three divine Persons, each distinct yet interrelated to the others, all equally possessing the one divine nature. Human beings, created in the image of this Holy Trinity, similarly share equally a common human nature and a dignity that demands mutual respect. St. Basil the Great taught in the fourth century that "we understand ourselves and realize that to every man belongs by nature equality of like honour with all men."[36] Particularly relevant in this context is the Orthodox emphasis on community, with its strong spiritual sense of organic corporate unity based on the biblical metaphor of the Church as the "Body" of Christ.

Certainly neither the Orthodox Churches nor individual Orthodox Christians may, in good conscience, benefit from the misfortune, much less political persecution, of others. The servants of the Suffering Servant who willingly died on a cross for the sins of humanity ought to appreciate, more than other persons perhaps, the right that men and women have not to be exploited, treated unfairly, or subjected to personal abuse against their wills by anyone for any reason.

A strong case can be made, therefore, that the Orthodox moral tradition contains an incipient teaching on natural or human rights without, however, couching this teaching in modern "rights" language. Chief among these rights is freedom of conscience and personal liberty. The Orthodox theological concept of the *autexousion* ("self-determining ability") posits that human beings are naturally endowed by God with free will and that their decisions and actions have moral meaning only when they are not coerced.[37] This implied right to freedom of thought requires of every human being the correlative duty to exercise what the post-Enlightenment Western world terms "tolerance."

In the ancient Orthodox Church, notwithstanding actual abuses in practice, the consensus of the Church Fathers was clearly in favor of religious tolerance, while adamantly opposed to coercion of any kind in the propagation of the faith or the exercise of moral conscience. The unknown author of the *Epistle to Diognetos* declared in the first half of the second century that God "out of kindness and gentleness" sent His Son into the world, because "He willed to save man by persuasion, not by compulsion, for compulsion is not God's way of working."[38] Lactantius, a contemporary of the Roman emperor St. Constantine the Great, compared Christian evangelism favorably to the pagan Roman practice of suppression: "There is no need of force and injury, because religion cannot be forced. It is a matter that must be managed by words rather than by blows, so that it may be voluntary."[39]

Even after the legitimation of Christianity in the empire, when the temptation to mimic the former imperial way of coercion obviously was great, several prominent Church Fathers taught forthrightly the proper Christian manner of conversion. St. Athanasios wrote in the fourth century that "it is of the nature of God not to coerce, but to convince."[40] St. Gregory of Nazianzos eschewed any attempts to "browbeat" in favor of trying to "persuade."[41] St. Gregory of Nyssa argued in his treatise *On the Making of Man* that "we are free from necessity, and not in bondage to any natural power"—a theme that echoes repeatedly in Orthodox theology. But he added a specific moral reference: "[V]irtue is a voluntary thing, subject to no dominion: that which is the result of compulsion and force cannot be virtue."[42] Early in the fifth century, St. John Chrysostom, referring to Judas, argued that Jesus "had the power to win the disciple over, but He did not wish to do good by constraint, nor to drag anyone to Himself by force."[43] Finally among the Fathers, St. Maximos the Confessor in the seventh century affirmed the need for human freedom: "Take from us the power of free choice, and we shall be neither images of God nor rational and intelligent souls, and our nature will be corrupted indeed, not being what it was meant to be."[44]

More recently, Greek Orthodox theologians such as Fr. Demetrios J. Constantelos, Archbishop Hieronymous Cotsonis of Athens, and Fr. John S. Romanides have unequivocally denounced evangelistic coercion and persecution in deference to the principle of religious liberty.[45] Another Greek, Archimandrite Vasileios of Mount Athos, summarizes this teaching dramatically: "Anything that exists outside freedom is hell and death."[46]

What the Church Fathers, in a spirit of tolerance and true charity, were so willing to extend to non-Christians they also vigorously claimed for the Christian community. St. Athenagoras of Athens, for example, appealed in A.D. 177 to the pagan Roman co-emperors Marcus Aurelius and Commodus: "What therefore is conceded as the common right of all, we claim for ourselves: that we shall not be hated and punished because we are called Christians. . . ."[47]

Though obviously lacking a modern conceptual framework for the enunciation of a systematic moral doctrine of natural or human rights, Eastern Orthodox moral tradition unequivocally upholds as a prophetic norm the right of individuals and communities to freedom of conscience and religion.

ORTHODOX NORMS OF SECURITY

The term "national security" is of recent vintage, having become widespread among policymakers only since the Second World War. It connotes, minimally, the protection of the people and territory of a nation from external or internal aggression. A more extensive meaning, as elaborated by two national-security experts, would allow for "protection, through a variety of means, of vital economic and political interests, the loss of which could threaten fundamental values and the vitality of the state."[48] The security of these "interests" constitutes the *telos,* or end, of national security, and the appropriate means to achieve this end range from the projection of political power and the unilateral use of military force to less direct, more collegial international measures such as alliances and coalitions, collective security organizations such as the United Nations, and appeals to international law.[49]

The moral problem of whether and how to guarantee the national security of modern states requires of the Eastern Orthodox Christians who live in them a response grounded in the normative Orthodox tradition of proper Church-state relations. That history yields an ideal prophetic norm for the political realm, with "political" referring to the institutional exercise of power by the governing authorities within a geographic entity. Lesser moral choices, however, predominate in the historical record.

Classic 'Symphonia'

Fr. Harakas has defined the Byzantine concept of *symphonia* as the principle "according to which Church and State cooperate as parts of an organic whole in the fulfillment of their purposes, each supporting and strengthening the other without this causing the subordination of one to the other."[50] This seems foreign to Americans accustomed to a "strict separation" of Church and state or, at best, a relatively distant, moderate degree of "accommodation" of religious practice by the state. To be sure, preserving the independence and sufficiency of the ecclesial and political hierarchies, while not separating the two into spiritual and secular authorities respectively, is no mean feat. There has, in fact, been no lasting implementation of it anywhere in Orthodox historical experience.

Scripture is nearly silent on this way of ordering a Christian commonwealth, owing undoubtedly to the peculiarly inhospitable political climate during the New Testament era. The only passage that may have served as a starting point for this political ethic is St. Paul's magnificent metaphor of the diversity within the Church as the

"Body" of Christ (I Cor. 12:12-31). As in the concept of *symphonia,* divine assignment of roles according to function is the underlying principle here. But the Apostle clearly has in mind only the Church.

The classic presentation in Byzantium of the symphonic ideal was the *Epanagogē* ("Introduction") of St. Photios, patriarch of Constantinople in the ninth century during the reigns of Emperors Basil I and Leo IV. Photios defined the Christian emperor as "a legal authority, a blessing common to all his subjects, who . . . behaves like an umpire making awards in a game." He must be Orthodox and pious and "is presumed to enforce and maintain" the scriptures, Church doctrine, and the civil laws. But he is bound to follow canon law as well. The patriarch of Constantinople (by this time the only Eastern patriarch free from Muslim domination) is described as "a living and animate image of Christ by deeds and words typifying the truth." His role is to protect and witness in behalf of the faith, care for the salvation of the faithful, interpret the Church canons, and supervise "all spiritual matters." In terms reminiscent of St. Paul's cited above, Photios declared that the emperor and the patriarch are "the greatest and most necessary" parts and "members" of the Christian polity.[51]

The theory is clear enough. Several problems arise, however, with respect to the implementing of this norm in Byzantium and its continued utility in the modern world. The role of the patriarch of Constantinople as St. Photios described it was perhaps too elevated for the traditional collegial preference in Orthodox Church polity; as Steven Runciman observes, it was "more suited to a Roman pontiff than to a Byzantine prelate."[52] Photios also presumed the existence of an emperor and assigned perhaps too much of a positive religious role to him. Although some contemporary Orthodox theologians such as Fr. Michael Azkoul still insist that monarchy is essential to the Orthodox political ethic, others, including Frs. Sergius Bulgakov and Stanley S. Harakas, have pronounced the idea of an Orthodox empire and monarchy dead and irrelevant to the divine plan of salvation.[53]

Nevertheless, the principle of *symphonia* is thoroughly grounded in the Orthodox teaching about Christ.[54] The Church *(sacerdotium)* and state *(imperium)* are presumably ideally united in the one Christian commonwealth, even as the divine and human natures of Christ are united in the one Person of the Incarnate Son of God. To abandon the symphonic ideal of Church-state relations is to divorce Christology from social ethics. Contemporary Eastern Orthodox moral theologians who take their own history seriously will, therefore, find themselves challenged to devise a political ethic that at once affirms the necessity of an organic relation between the Church and the state, respects the integrity and freedom of the Orthodox Christian community, and safeguards the religious liberties of non-Orthodox citizens in the given society.

A nation led by this kind of supportive government would rightly claim "a proper spiritual ethos" worthy of protection by the Orthodox community within it. The national security of such a state would seem to be a high priority for those Orthodox Christians in particular who embrace the justifiable-war ethic.

Contemporary Alternatives

Political realities in modern states are, however, hardly conducive to an implementation of the symphonic ideal. In Eastern Europe, Orthodox Christians, long accustomed to oppression in the Balkans by the Ottoman Turks, have in this century had to endure virulently hostile Communist regimes. With the overthrow of these regimes the situation of the Churches has improved greatly, but, as we shall see, problems remain. In Western Europe and the United States, the minority Orthodox communities are challenged by governments that are, at best, secular, pluralistic, and indifferent to religious values.

In these less than ideal circumstances, Orthodox leaders tend—prematurely, to be sure—to dismiss the symphonic ideal as unattainable. They generally settle for morally inferior patterns of Church-state relations.

The so-called strict separation of Church and state, an American hallmark, is certainly of recent lineage. In the history of the Orthodox Churches, the only possible precedent occurred during the first three centuries of their existence. During this formative period, the Church, having been born into generally hostile Jewish and Roman political environments, had to struggle under intermittent persecution by the established authorities. To survive, it seemed to many, the Church had to detach itself from the Roman political and social apparatus. In the modern era of mass persecution, many Orthodox leaders have sought refuge in a similar sectarian "separation" from the political and social ethos of their societies. Others have simply allowed the political or intellectual elites to circumscribe or marginalize their role in society.

Another deviation from the prophetic norm has been customarily though incorrectly called "theocracy." If that term is defined as a close harmony of Church and state with an underlying religious principle, the preferred term would be *symphonia*. But what critics perceive in Orthodox Church history as theocracy would be better described as "cosmocracy": the rule not of "God" *(theos)* but rather of the "world" *(kosmos)* in the form of political authorities.

The concept of the Roman emperor as the political image of God on earth, which Eusebios of Caesarea first formulated in his encomium for St. Constantine the Great,[55] reflected an iconic understanding of structure and order in the universe under God's monarchy. But, coupled with a simplistic interpretation of New Testament texts such as Romans 13:1-7 and I Peter 2:13-17 that urge the early Christians to obey the "governing authorities," this exalted view of emperors gave rise to unforeseen abuses of imperial power in relation to the Church (though never to the extent that the misleading term "caesaropapism" connotes[56]).

Conversely, this curious conceptual alloy has engendered all kinds of justifications for political conservatism in support of whoever happens to be in power at the time. Submission to the given political structure has become a historical commonplace for large segments of the various Orthodox Churches. Some Church leaders have hidden behind the belief that divine providence is somehow guiding the actions of even the most heinous anti-Christian rulers as a chastisement for the sins of the Orthodox. Other Orthodox hierarchs and theologians, particularly those in the formerly Communist-dominated states, have welcomed the rule of atheistic Communists as if they were Byzantine or Russian emperors in Marxist-Leninist garb.

The temptation to succumb to the "separation" or "cosmocracy" models of Church-state relations has proved overwhelming for those Orthodox Church leaders unwilling or unable to pay the price of prophecy. Unfortunately, as we shall see, in recent decades such leaders have more often than not governed the Orthodox communities in the former Soviet Union, Romania, and the United States.

2

The Moscow Patriarchate and Religious Freedom

The amazing collapse of the Soviet Union as a political and ideological force in 1991 promised the first real opportunity for religious freedom in the successor states in more than seventy years.

Prior to the ascendancy of the enigmatic Mikhail Gorbachev in 1985, religious freedom as a unique moral concern seemed to preoccupy the relatively few religious visionaries and human-rights activists in the world's first Communist state. But the virtual revolution that Gorbachev sparked in the Soviet Union—which Boris Yeltsin as his successor since December 1991 appears determined to perpetuate—has raised the hopes of every friend of liberty in Russia and Ukraine, including some of the Russian Orthodox bishops who dutifully served Gorbachev's more ruthless predecessors.

The endurance of this rebirth of religious freedom may depend upon Yeltsin and his fellow democrats' hold on the reins of political power. The failed coup by Soviet hard-liners in August 1991 revealed the persistence (though in this case not the competence) of the dangerous forces of Communist reaction. The sudden rise of Vladimir Zhirinovsky as a serious political force in the December 1993 parliamentary elections poses an unexpected threat from the extreme right. If the future is still painfully uncertain, memories of the past are too painfully clear.

Past Persecution, Present Promises

The Bolsheviks consolidated their power at the end of the Civil War in 1921, four years after the coup d'état known as the October Revolution. For almost seven decades after that, the Soviet government systematically pressured the Russian Orthodox Church to abandon its earthly mission, or at least to submit completely to the secular authority. Although successive Soviet constitutions guaranteed the freedom to practice religion and the separation of Church and state, actual Soviet practice was a very different matter.

The chronicle of restrictions on and persecution of the Orthodox Church and other religious groups in the Soviet Union reads as one continuous war on religion. That war waxed or waned according to the current needs of the government. Waves of persecution alternated with ebb tides, at best, of relative neglect. This sorry tale has been amply documented elsewhere and need not be recounted here.[1] Let it suffice to say that the ranks of Russian Orthodox martyrs swelled by the millions during the Soviet era, notwithstanding the active collaboration of most of the hierarchy with the Soviet regime from 1927 on. The hierarchy itself had almost disappeared by 1943 when Josef Stalin, confronted with Nazi German invaders, suddenly reversed course and allowed the four remaining bishops (out of a pre-Soviet total of seventy-eight) to replenish their numbers, the better to support the war effort.

At the behest of Mikhail Gorbachev, the behavior of the Soviet ruling elites toward their erstwhile enemy, the Church, softened considerably at the end of the 1980s. Holding the dual reins of power in the Soviet state—general secretary of the Communist Party and president of the state—the all-powerful Gorbachev launched a triple-pronged attack on the ills of Soviet society that promised not only "new thinking" throughout this intellectually moribund land, but also new paradigms for Church-state relations and for the ordering of social values such as liberty and justice. Gorbachev introduced an unprecedented tolerance of diverse opinion and the unhindered public expression of it (*glasnost'*, "openness," or literally, "giving voice to") as the necessary condition for the "restructuring" (*perestroika)* of a Soviet economy in its death throes. The professed goal was *demokratizatsiya,* enhancing the "democratic" quality of socialist life for the masses of Soviet citizens.

The first evidence of this sea change in the Soviet "initiative" toward the Moscow Patriarchate occurred in 1988, the year that marked a millennium of Christianity in what was then Soviet territory. The millennial events commenced auspiciously with a highly visible meeting on April 29 between Gorbachev and Patriarch Pimen Izvekov of Moscow together with the five other members of the Holy Synod of bishops of the Russian Orthodox Church—the first tête-à-tête between the leaders of Church and state in forty-five years. Amidst the usual pleasantries, platitudes, and bombast that accompany such diplomatic exchanges was a surprisingly candid confession by the Soviet leader: "Mistakes made with regard to the Church and believers in the 1930s and the years that followed are being rectified."[2]

To be sure, Gorbachev's earlier pledge to restore "the Leninist principles of attitude to religion, to Church and believers" was not very encouraging to Orthodox leaders, who remembered too well the murderous persecutions of the Church in the several years after Lenin seized control of the government in 1917.[3] But the pace of reform evidently outstripped Gorbachev's original intent. In the spring of 1990, the Institute of Marxism-Leninism admitted that the Communist Party had suppressed a classified letter from Lenin in 1922 urging the Politburo to use the terrible famine of that year as a pretext for "the expropriation of church valuables with the most furious and ruthless energy."[4] Equally amazing was the official confirmation in November 1990—after seventy-two years of denial by the Soviet government—that Lenin ordered the murder of the royal family of Tsar Nicholas II.[5]

After the failed coup in August 1991, the pace of the nation's disavowal of Leninism quickened. Statues of Lenin and his Bolshevik henchmen came tumbling down. The city of Leningrad reverted to its pre-Communist name, St. Petersburg. And on November 7, 1991, the anniversary of Lenin's coup in 1917, President Boris Yeltsin of the Russian Republic formally decreed the permanent abolition of all activities and organizations of the Communist Party on Russian territory and the seizure of all Party property.[6] This was followed a month later by the formation of the Commonwealth of Independent States (CIS), the resignation of Mikhail Gorbachev as national and Communist Party leader, and the end of the Soviet era.

Prior to his sudden exit from power, Gorbachev kept many of his promises to the leaders of the Russian Orthodox Church. His government returned to proper Church care a section of the venerable Kyyiv-Pechersky Monastery of the Caves, the Optina Pustyn Monastery in Kaluga region, the Tolgsky Convent in Yaroslavl region, one of the Solovetsky monasteries near Arkhangelsk, relics from the churches-turned-museums in the Kremlin, and, most spectacularly, on February 7, 1991, the relics of St. Serafim of Sarov († 1833), the beloved hermit canonized by the Church in 1903.[7]

Other signs of *glasnost'* in action included the reopening or reconstruction of at least 3,000 closed Orthodox churches, although two-thirds of these were in the contentious Ukraine, where anti-Russian nationalist sentiment was boiling; the reopening of at least sixteen seminaries; a more liberalized publication schedule of Bibles, liturgical books, and Church newspapers; public *mea culpas* by Communist officials and publications for past mistreatment of believers; stricter enforcement of the legal prohibitions against harassment of believers; the release from prison of hundred of political prisoners and notable religious dissidents, such as the prolific Orthodox confessor Fr. Gleb Yakunin; and the canonization in October 1989 of the first Soviet-era saint — Patriarch Tikhon Belavin of Moscow, who died in 1925 under mysterious circumstances. Perhaps the most visible event was the national celebration of the Orthodox Pascha (Easter) on April 7, 1991, in which St. Basil's Cathedral in Moscow, sacrilegiously misappropriated for so many years a symbol of Sovietism, was put to sacred use for the first time since the Revolution. The four-hour midnight liturgy at Epiphany Cathedral was broadcast on television, accompanied by explanations; conspicious among the worshipers was an official delegation led by Russian president Boris Yeltsin.[8]

Meanwhile, prominent leaders of the Moscow Patriarchate assumed unprecedented civic positions. In the dramatic open elections for the Congress of People's Deputies on March 26, 1989, Metropolitan Pitirim Nechaev of Volokalamsk was elected to represent the Soviet Cultural Fund and Metropolitan Aleksii Ridiger of Leningrad and Novgorod — who in June 1990 became Patriarch Aleksii II of Moscow — was chosen to represent the Soviet Charity Fund. Patriarch Pimen was elected to one of the five seats allotted to the Soviet Peace Committee; after his death in May 1990, his place was taken by Metropolitan Filaret Vakhromeyev of Minsk and Grodno.[9]

More importantly, several so-called dissidents also won elective offices. Fr. Gleb Yakunin, who as recently as 1987 was in prison, was elected to the parliament of the Russian Republic. An Orthodox layman, Valery Borshchov, became chairman of that parliament's Committee on Freedom of Conscience; and another devout layman, Victor Aksyuchits, chaired the Russian Republic's most prominent Christian Democratic political party—the Russian Christian Democratic Movement—until an internal power struggle led to his ouster.

The statutes of a new *ustav* (or Church "constitution") drafted for the millennial *sobor* (or clergy-laity "council") in June 1988 by the dynamic, young Metropolitan Kirill Gundaev of Smolensk reinstated the parish priest as president and head of the parish assembly in accordance with centuries-old Orthodox tradition.[10] Since the *sobor* could not, at that juncture, have so acted without the prior approval of the state's Council on Religious Affairs (CRA), these internal Church reforms presaged the momentous changes in the new "all-Union," or Soviet, Law on Freedom of Conscience and Religious Organizations passed on October 1, 1990, and the new Law on Freedom of Denominations approved by the Supreme Soviet of the Russian Soviet Federated Socialist Republic (RSFSR) on October 25, 1990. These laws, the latter even more democratic than the former, together supercede the repressive 1929 law that was revised in 1975.

This extraordinary turn of events has effectively restored many, albeit not all, of the particular freedoms pertaining to pastoral, educational, evangelistic, prophetic, and liturgical ministries that Western Christians take for granted as "rights." The 1929 law proscribed any religious activity construed by the government as "impairing the health, integrity, and rights of citizens" or contributing to "the systematic dissemination of slanderous allegations denigrating the political and social system."[11] The new RSFSR (and now simply "Russian") version: finally cedes to registered religious communities the much desired right of "juridical personality," which gives congregations official legal standing before civil authorities and in court proceedings; prohibits the control of religion by state organizations such as the infamous CRA; establishes effective equality between believers and atheists; allows for voluntary religious classes in state schools conducted by representatives of the religious communities; provides for the celebration of religious rites in the military; and removes strictures that prevented religious feasts from becoming national holidays.[12]

Prospects and Perils

Prior to his humiliating arrest during the short-lived coup in August 1991, Gorbachev tried in vain to maintain a balance between the radical reformist elements led by Boris Yeltsin—who, two months after his election as president of the RSFSR in May 1990, literally walked out of the Communist Party—and the hard-line reactionaries, particularly within the Soviet military, who in January 1991 apparently had persuaded him to crack down on the Lithuanian and Latvian independence movements, a violent and, fortunately, ill-fated step. Gorbachev seemed unable to grasp that his political fence-straddling could not last. In the born-again Russia that emerged in the waning months of 1991, Boris Yeltsin, the burly hero who had spoken to the people from atop a Soviet tank in August, finally eclipsed the enigmatic innovator of "new thinking."

During his rather dramatic tenure as president of the Russian Republic, Boris Yeltsin has accelerated the rapprochement between Church and state. Often appearing in photographs with Patriarch Aleksii II, Yeltsin returned to the Moscow Patriarchate for its permanent use six of the seven venerable churches within the walls of the Kremlin, as well as the spectacularly onion-domed St. Basil's Cathedral in Red Square. In a concordat signed on November 15, 1992, by Patriarch Aleksii and the Minister of Culture of the Russian Federation, the government also pledged "to fund, from the state budget, current maintenance, repair and restoration work" of these churches![13] Perhaps the moral high point of the post-Communist era occurred in June 1993 when Yeltsin publicly accepted full blame and apologized for the government's abuse of the Church during the Communist era.

Whether the fragile Commonwealth of Independent States (CIS) that supplanted the Soviet Empire in December 1991 eventually disintegrates into a congeries of warring ethnocentric nations and political factions or proceeds toward a peaceful dissolution into several sovereign but cooperative neighboring states, the new post-Communist era wrought by Gorbachev affords the Church a golden opportunity finally to come of age in the twentieth century.

This chapter will focus on the historical record of responses by both the hierarchy and dissidents of the Russian Orthodox Church to the violations of the principles of religious freedom by Soviet authorities. Although it may be a bitter medicine, this examination is a necessary condition for genuine healing and for the spiritual growth of the Russian Church. The public moral witness of the Moscow Patriarchate during the seven terrible decades since the October Revolution must be confronted in its entirety—failures as well as triumphs.

Many well-meaning leaders and friends of the Russian Church—both in Russia and in the United States—seem all too willing to whitewash a very checkered moral record. Western observers must, of course, appreciate the unique exigencies of the Church under Communist rule. Religious communities in the Soviet Union were forced into the unenviable position of merely responding to the strenuous initiatives of a government controlled by an ideologically motivated, inveterately hostile Communist Party. Ranging from derisive propaganda to the mass murder of believers, these governmental initiatives posed the gravest threat to the moral and religious integrity of the Church since the periodic mass persecutions of the ancient Church by the pagan Roman caesars. To many of the principal leaders, their survival—and, more importantly, that of the Church itself—was at stake.

OFFICIAL WITNESS OF THE PATRIARCHATE

The Moscow Patriarchate has at least 120 bishops currently active and an additional seven who have retired. Among the active bishops, five are permanently assigned to exarchates abroad and, unencumbered in the past by Soviet citizenship, have been able to speak more freely and to act with relative impunity.[14]

Three key questions help us to frame the prophetic quality of the hierarchy's public moral witness on issues of peace, freedom, and security during the Soviet era. First, in regard to any bishop, particularly if he enjoyed prominence as a spokesman for the Church: Was he an authentic religious leader, an agent of the KGB, or a misguided soul who tried in vain to be both? The question is not frivolous. In

1988 a former KGB officer using the pen name "Victor Orlov" cited his own experience as evidence that the Church hierarchy, at least since the mid-1950s, had been "penetrated by the KGB": as a young KGB intelligence officer, he was offered a "splendid career" as an undercover agent in the Church.[15]

More recently, two distinguished members of the Russian Parliament disclosed the preliminary findings of their unprecedented research in the files of the KGB and the archives of the Communist Party of the Soviet Union. The two are Fr. Gleb Yakunin, the celebrated dissident priest, and Lev Ponomarev, a non-Christian physicist, who is the chairman of a special investigatory commission appointed by the parliament. Their findings, first announced in the United States at a March 1992 press conference on Capitol Hill co-sponsored by the Ethics and Public Policy Center and the Jamestown Foundation, confirmed what many observers in the West had suspected for decades. No fewer than thirty bishops of the Moscow Patriarchate had official code-names as "agents in cassocks" of the KGB. In deference to his own hierarchy, Fr. Gleb declines to identify the living bishops who are implicated by the KGB files, but neither his fellow dissident Zoya Krakhmalnikova nor resourceful journalists in Russia and in the West—including Michael Dobbs of the *Washington Post*—have been so deterred.[16]

The second question is a corollary to the first: What were the relative ecclesial and political loyalties of Church spokesmen? This raises the delicate problem of personal motives—an elusive pursuit even in less byzantine circumstances than those in the Soviet Union. Specifically, why did the hierarchs of the Patriarchate speak and act as they did? And how sincere were their professions of loyalty to the Orthodox Church and to the ideology and policies of the state? The complexities of this question were underscored by an observer who might have been expected to pronounce a simple anathema. Archbishop John Maximovitch of the Russian Orthodox Church Outside Russia—émigré rival of the Moscow Patriarchate—wrote in 1972:

Even among the hierarchs outwardly subject to the Soviet regime, many are inwardly tormented by this and when the opportunity will come, they act according to the example of those at the Council of Chalcedon [A.D. 451] who declared with tears that they had given their signatures at the Robber Council [A.D. 449] under coercion.[17]

The third question is, How genuinely Orthodox were the public moral pronouncements of those who purported to be authentic spokesmen for the Russian Orthodox Church?

Furov's Categories

The now legendary "Furov Report" appeared originally in 1974 as a secret report to the Central Committee of the Communist Party of the Soviet Union. Its author, V. Furov, was deputy chairman of the Council for Religious Affairs (CRA), which was the government agency in charge of regulating religion. Furov classified the hierarchs of the Moscow Patriarchate in three camps according to their loyalty and usefulness to the Soviet regime. Somehow the document was "leaked" and was smuggled out of the Soviet Union. An English translation first appeared in 1980-81 issues of *Religion in Communist Dominated Areas*.[18]

Furov boasted to his superiors that the CRA "controls the Synod," that is, the group of eight senior bishops who govern the Church. Specifically, the CRA was directly responsible for selecting its members, choosing its topics for discussion, approving final decisions, and shaping the bishops' "patriotic views and attitudes." Although the CRA professed primary interest in the "political aspect" of the episcopate— that is, its posture toward the state and its role in Soviet foreign policy — Furov added, in clear violation of the 1918 Decree on Separation:

> There is no consecration of a bishop, no transfer without thorough investigation of the candidate by appropriate officials of the Council in close cooperation with the commissioner, local organs and corresponding interested organizations.

Furov may have exaggerated the effectiveness of his own organization to impress his superiors. Further, under Konstantin Kharchev, who became its chairman in 1984, the CRA began at last to loosen its iron grip on the Synod. But the "Furov Report" remains invaluable as an index of the way that the Communists assessed the collaboration of the Orthodox hierarchs.

1. *Unrestrained Loyalists.* The first of Furov's classifications was that group of bishops most devoted to the Soviet state, for whatever reasons. Furov described the hierarchs whom he had in mind as

the ruling bishops whose words and deeds attest not only to their loyalty but also to their patriotism to our socialist society, who strictly observe the laws on cults and who foster the same spirit in their parish clergy and believers, who realistically acknowledge that our government is not interested in expanding the role of religion and church in our society, and who, realizing this fact, are not personally involved in spreading the influence of the Orthodoxy among our population.

This amounted to damning praise of bishops who, at best, were not doing their job. A harsher judgment would depict these bishops as loyal sycophants or, worse, kindred ideological servants of the regime, who abandoned all but the pretense of devotion to the virtue of religious freedom.

In this camp Furov placed seventeen hierarchs, including six who will figure prominently in this study: (1) Pimen, the late patriarch of Moscow; (2) Metropolitan Aleksii of Tallinn and Estonia (the present patriarch), whose KGB code-name "Drozdov" was deduced and revealed by Russian dissidents and journalists in March 1992; (3) Metropolitan Yuvenaly Poyarkov of Tula (now Krutitsy and Kolomna), whose KGB code-name "Adamant" was revealed in February 1992; (4) Metropolitan Serafim of Krutitsy and Kolomna († 1979); (5) Metropolitan Sergii of Odessa († 1990); and (6) Archbishop (now Metropolitan) Pitirim of Volokolamsk, code-name "Abbot" in the KGB files.

Patriarch Pimen Izvekov conducted a notoriously mediocre reign from 1971 to 1990 as first-among-equals in the Russian Orthodox hierarchy. The Furov Report only confirmed the popular view advanced even by his eventual successor, then Archbishop Aleksii of Tallinn, that the patriarch, though respected for his apparent piety and liturgical skills, lacked an independent will and had no adminstrative ability or leadership qualities.[19] According to confidential CRA documents that surfaced only in 1988, a retired KGB colonel named A. S. Plekhanov reported in 1967 that Pimen, then Metropolitan of Krutitsy and Kolomna, had been "put on trial for desertion from the Soviet Army" and imprisoned in 1937, had deserted again in 1943 while holding the rank of major and "lived with forged papers," and was finally sentenced to ten years' imprisonment. Only the amnesty granted by the government after the victory over the Germans in 1945 curtailed this sentence.[20]

Even more damaging was the reputed claim by Archbishop Aleksii, which Plekhanov recorded at the CRA in 1967, that "it is known that Pimen has women" in Moscow. If true, this would have automatically disqualified him from further service as a priest, to say nothing of future election as patriarch.[21] These contentions lacked independent corroboration. But Pimen himself on various occasions provided conflicting details about his past, suggesting that he might have had something to hide. Dmitry Pospielovsky, a church historian and member of the Orthodox Church in America who lives in Canada, concludes that Pimen's proclivity toward concealment "made it possible for the . . . CRA to 'hook' him"—that is, to secure his eventual "election" as patriarch in 1971, while guaranteeing that he would be singularly subservient to the interests of the Soviet regime.[22]

Two of Pimen's predecessors as patriarch would surely have been placed in this same category, that of loyal sycophants, had Furov reporting during their tenures. **Metropolitan Sergii Stragorodsky** of Moscow became patriarchal *locum tenens* (temporary administrator) in 1926 and patriarch in 1943, when Stalin, reeling from the Nazi invasion and in desperate need of help from the Church, finally allowed the Church to reestablish the dormant Patriarchate. His immediate successor, **Patriarch Aleksii I** (Simansky), ruled the Russian Orthodox Church from 1945 until 1970. Their consistent advocacy of the Soviet agenda will be chronicled below.

Among the patriarchs of Moscow in this century, only **Patriarch Tikhon Belavin** would have escaped Furov's damning praise. Tikhon was elected patriarch by lot in November 1917 while the October Revolution raged outside the doors of the Moscow *sobor* (Church council). He immediately confronted the new Bolshevik government with a stern anathema for its anti-religious atrocities, excommunicated the offenders from the sacraments of the Church, and prophetically warned Lenin and his minions that they would perish by the sword. Tikhon was imprisoned in 1923, and he seems to have changed his outlook between then and his death two years later. Among the pressures he experienced during that time were his Church's direct confrontation with the regime over the confiscation of sacred liturgical vessels, the mass persecutions of his clergy and people, a new threat posed by a schismatic rival "Church" propped up by the government, and the steady propaganda by the regime denouncing him for alleged connivance with anti-Soviet émigré groups in Europe. Whether the apparent retractions published in the government newspaper *Izvestia* as Tikhon's "Confession" and "Testament" were forced out of him through torture or lesser forms of intimidation, Tikhon's "official" posture vis-à-vis the state at his death in 1925 may be characterized as one of non-resistance. Some scholars view this final position as a realistic and wise recognition of new realities. Others dismiss it as a coerced collaboration and therefore morally and spiritually meaningless.[23]

Besides his alleged role as Plekhanov's source of rumors, **Patriarch Aleksii II** (Ridiger) boasted impeccable credentials as an unflagging supporter of the Soviet regime, especially its positions on human rights and peace.[24] Born of German-speaking parents in the Estonian city of Tallinn in 1929, Aleksii received an advanced theological degree (Candidate of Theology) in 1953 and became bishop of his native Soviet republic in 1961. In 1986 he was transferred to the more prestigious Leningrad metropolitanate. Patriarch Aleksii's extensive activities in ecumenical circles reflected the trust that the Soviet regime had in him. He served on the Central Committee of the World Council of Churches from 1961 to 1968. For twenty-two years beginning in 1964 he was a president of the Conference of European Churches, the main ecumenical organization on the Continent. Equally zealous in the mission of peacemaking, Aleksii has been an active member and sometime officer of numerous Soviet-abetted "peace" organizations such as the Estonian Peace Committee, the Soviet Peace Fund, the Council of the *Rodina* (i.e., "Motherland") Society, the U.S.S.R.-India Friendship Society, and the Leningrad Region Peace Committee.

The Soviet government showed its gratitude for Aleksii's patriotism and peacemaking by awarding him the Order of Friendship Among Nations and the Order of the Red Banner of Labor, and he has also received medals from the World Peace Council, the Soviet Peace Committee, and the Soviet Peace Fund. In March 1989, while he was Metropolitan of Tallinn, his election to the Congress of People's Deputies as one of only three Orthodox hierarchs indicated the prominence he had achieved among his episcopal colleagues. That eventually led to his election to the patriarchal see in June 1990.

Despite his dubious record of collaboration and direct service to the KGB as a metropolitan, by the spring of 1994 Aleksii, as patriarch, had sent several signals that he and the Russian Church may at last be coming of age. These positive developments will be chronicled later in this chapter.

2. *Moderate Loyalists.* The second of Furov's categories described a more nuanced mode of collaboration. Furov regarded these ruling bishops, to be sure, as loyal to the state and observant of Soviet laws on religious activity. But he also viewed with suspicion this group,

> who in their daily administration and ideological work are trying to activate the clergy and the church body, who are trying to expand the role of the church in the private, family and social life with the aid of modernized or traditional concepts, views and actions, who are recruiting for priesthood young zealots of Orthodox piety.

These hierarchs apparently were determined to establish a mutually beneficial *modus vivendi* with the regime. Consistently fervent public support for domestic and foreign Soviet policies was conjoined to subtle endeavors to promote a circumscribed version of the traditional agenda of the Church.

Among the twenty-three bishops whom Furov identified in this camp are two whose influence has been especially significant: Metropolitan Nikodim Rotov of Leningrad († 1978) and Metropolitan Filaret Denisenko, the Moscow Patriarchate's erstwhile exarch in Kiev (the Russian version of Kyyiv) and Galicia.

Metropolitan Nikodim Rotov was an unusually enigmatic personage.[25] His meteoric rise to prominence in the Moscow Patriarchate before his sudden death in 1988 at the age of 49 was checked only by his inability to secure the Patriarchal throne in 1971, despite widespread expectations that he had been groomed by Soviet authorities expressly for that position. His experience as head of the Russian Orthodox Mission in Jerusalem, head of the Department of External Church Relations of the Patriarchate, chairman of the Synod's Commission on Christian Unity and Inter-Church Relations, president of the World Council of Churches, and president of the Prague-based Christian Peace Conference afforded him an international perspective —and a voice—that was unique in the history of the Church in the Soviet era. Perhaps Furov's classifying Nikodim in the second camp revealed an uncertainty by the regime as to the peripatetic hierarch's ultimate loyalties.

Nikodim's strong Roman Catholic leanings also may have sabotaged his career. Not only was he the force behind the ill-fated decision of the Patriarchate in 1969 to provide holy communion to Roman Catholics in clear violation of the historic Orthodox canonical proscriptions against "inter-communion," but he literally died in the arms of Pope John Paul I during a papal audience in Rome on September 5, 1978. This ironically symbolic event certainly fueled the mounting speculation—advanced, for example, by the priest-monk Mykaylo Havryliv—that Nikodim was, in fact, a "convinced Catholic and clandestine Catholic bishop."[26]

His controversial relations with the Roman Catholic community notwithstanding, Nikodim was generally respected by Christians in the West as a man of genuine Orthodox faith. To be sure, critics such as the Russian dissidents Boris Talantov and Anatoly Levitin railed against the metropolitan as a liar and schemer unfit to serve as a bishop.[27] Even Dmitry Pospielovsky, who remembers Nikodim somewhat fondly, admitted, "I was once struck by the *naïveté* of his apparent acceptance of Marxism as a social expression of Christian ethics."[28]

Metropolitan Filaret Denisenko finished third in the balloting for the Patriarchal throne eventually won by Metropolitan Aleksii Ridiger in June 1990. Filaret had forged a negative image among his fellow Ukrainians as a traitor to their national interests, and, as reported openly now by scholars known for their discretion such as Fr. Anthony Ugolnik and John Dunlop, his clandestine living arrangements with his housekeeper and alleged "wife" have scandalized Ukrainians for years.[29] Further, Filaret's hostility toward Rome in ecumenical contacts is notorious. His statements on the so-called Uniate problem in Ukraine reflect the hard-line position within the Moscow Patriarchate and the revived Ukrainian Autocephalous Orthodox Church.

Filaret's other wide-ranging contributions to the debates on peace, freedom, and security issues during the Soviet era would seem to place him clearly in the camp of ideological collaborators with the regime. Furov's classification, however, suggests that Filaret may be more of a pragmatic collaborator. Even on the verge of possible election to the

Patriarchal throne, Filaret studiously avoided a reformist image. "It's naïve to expect revolutionary changes in the church," he was quoted as saying in a newspaper interview, "in comparison to those which took place after the election of Gorbachev."[30]

By mid-1992 the unpopular Filaret seemed to be on the verge of forced retirement. His KGB code-name, "Antonov," had been revealed by Russian and Western journalists. Perhaps this latest controversy, together with whatever pressure may have been exerted by reformers behind the scenes, moved him to announce his resignation at last. In a strangely equivocal decision on April 2, 1992, the *sobor* (or "council") of the bishops of the Moscow Patriarchate acknowledged receipt of Filaret's resignation as "Metropolitan of Kiev" (Kyyiv in Ukrainian), without specifying that it had been accepted. The bishops appeared to be waiting for the Holy Synod of the "autonomous" Ukrainian Orthodox Church (that is, under the supervision of the Moscow Patriarchate) to ratify Filaret's decision before acting on it themselves. Nevertheless, the official document of the April *sobor,* signed by Patriarch Aleksii II himself, thanked Filaret for his many years of service and "blessed" him for yet another episcopal assignment in the Ukrainian Church.[31]

But then Filaret, upon his return to Kyyiv, betrayed the Patriarchate by revoking his resignation, claiming he had been unfairly pressured into it by the Russian bishops. The Patriarchate swiftly deposed him from "all grades of priesthood" on June 11 and appointed Metropolitan Vladimir Sabodan as the temporary head of the autonomous Ukrainian Orthodox Church, which maintains canonical ties to Moscow. It is a sad reflection of the Moscow Patriarchate's sense of moral and canonical propriety that only *after* Filaret had bolted from its jurisdiction did the Russian Church hierarchy finally defrock this miscreant on moral and canonical grounds.[32] Vladimir, who finished second in the June 1990 balloting for patriarch, was subsequently elected primate of this Ukrainian Church and arrived in Kyyiv on June 20, 1992, to lead his new flock. He has since de-Russified his name and is now known to his fellow Ukrainians more appropriately as Metropolitan Volodymyr.

Undaunted, Filaret scripted a new act in this ecclesial soap opera when he joined forces with Metropolitan Antony Masendych of Sichoslav and Pereyaslav, a bishop of the Ukrainian Autocephalous

Orthodox Church that was reestablished in October 1989 in opposition to the Moscow Patriarchate. Filaret apparently had the backing of President Leonid Kravchuk of Ukraine (this ex-Communist was a powerful political albeit not very religious figure). But Filaret's unsavory political and moral reputation was too much for the late Patriarch Mstyslav Skrypnyk, primate of the Autocephalous Ukrainians in Kyyiv: on October 31, 1992, Mstyslav publicly repudiated Filaret's role in his Church. Thus a schism ensued within the fledgling Ukrainian Autocephalous Orthodox Church. After Mstyslav's death in June 1993, the pro- and anti-Filaret factions elected rival "patriarchs," neither of whom is recognized as canonical by any autocephalous Orthodox Church! We shall attempt later in this chapter and in chapter 4 to unravel these confusing strands of Ukrainian Church life. Suffice it to say here that Filaret has left a trail of bitter controversy in both Moscow and Kyyiv that—as of June 1994—shows no signs of disappearing.

3. *Mavericks.* The last of Furov's categories belongs to seventeen bishops who apparently exceeded the tolerable limits of pro-Church activity. These bishops sought "to evade the law on cults." Some Furov deemed "religious conservatives"; others were so uncooperative as to conceal the true nature of their religious activities in their dioceses, or "to attempt to bribe and slander the commissioners [of the Council] and officials of the local government agencies."

In this category Furov focused his ire on **Bishop Khrizostom Martishkin** of Kursk and Belgorod. In 1975, at the age of 40, Khrizostom was exiled to Siberia for remarks about his fellow bishops such as the following: "Although all of us were anointed with the same chrism, we became obedient slaves, doing what was 'recommended' by the civil powers—bowing down, bending our backs."[33] Khrizostom has since become archbishop of Vilnius in Lithuania, and we shall hear more of this "maverick" later.

Advocacy of Sovietism

The first dimension of the official public moral witness of the Patriarchate on the issue of religious freedom is the explicit advocacy of the Soviet system in all of its manifold socialist richness. We shall look at two aspects of this advocacy, citing representative statements: (1) *pledges of loyalty* to the Soviet state and its Communist leadership; and (2) *ideological proclamations* reflecting old-fashioned Russian nationalism and/or a Communist/socialist worldview.

Pledges of Loyalty. The event that determined the subsequent course of the Patriarchate in its relations with the state was the "Declaration" made by Metropolitan Sergii on July 29, 1927.[34] This seminal document did more than attempt to reach a *modus vivendi* with a regime that had ruthlessly endeavored to eradicate all traces of religious belief and practice. It also committed the Russian Orthodox Church to a pro-Soviet position on all issues of Church-state relations, particularly that of religious freedom in a totalitarian state.

Sergii's ostensible reason for his "Declaration" gave his collaboration a "pragmatic" tint, but the exuberance of his language in support of the Communist regime suggests either a "conventional" or, worse, an "ideological" form. He wanted to "secure for the Church the possibility of a fully legal and peaceful existence." Thus he felt he had to prove to the government in both word and deed that the Church leadership was "at one with our nation and government," and that even "the most fervent adherents of Orthodoxy" could become "faithful citizens" of the new Communist state. Sergii perceived no conflict in identities or loyalties:

> We wish to remain Orthodox and at the same time to recognize the Soviet Union as our civil fatherland whose joys and successes are our joys and successes, and whose misfortunes are our misfortunes. Every blow directed against the Union, be it war, boycott, or any other common disaster, . . . we acknowledge as a blow directed against us.

This document abounds with problematical presumptions and specious arguments.[35] Misappropriating the controversial reference to "conscience" in Romans 13:5 ("Therefore one must be subject [to the governing authorities], not only to avoid God's wrath but also for the sake of the conscience"), Sergii appealed to conscience as the ground of "our duty to be citizens of the Union." He asserted that providence, not chance, had swept the Communists into power and was leading Russia, like all other nations, "toward its pre-destined goal." He berated those republicans and monarchists at home and abroad who, by their demonstrable opposition to the Soviet regime, refused to recognize what he called "the signs of the times"—a dangerous phrase that may lead to the justification of all contemporary change in the name of the *Zeitgeist*. He cited I Timothy 2:2 as biblical support for his claim that a godly existence in peace and quiet is possible only through submission to the lawful government.

Perhaps to guarantee his trustworthiness to the regime, Sergii demanded from the Russian Orthodox clergy who had emigrated after the October Revolution "a written promise of their complete loyalty to the Soviet government in all their public activities." Those who refused he threatened to expel from the ranks of the clergy subject to the Patriarchate. Thus did unquestioned political loyalty to a hostile state become a test of Church membership.

The most favorable interpretation of Sergii's motives is that he had sacrificed his own integrity and soiled his public image for the sake of a pragmatic accommodation with a regime that literally had the power of life and death over him and his Church. Even that view, however, cannot disguise the tragic consequences of his policy. The prophetic voice of the Orthodox Church in Soviet society had been muted, and the Church could no longer enjoy any semblance of an independent political existence.

Sergii's subsequent infamous encomia to Josef Stalin merely symbolize this spiritual suicide. On the twenty-fifth anniversary of the October Revolution (November 7, 1942, according to the Gregorian calendar), Sergii "cordially and prayerfully" greeted Stalin, whom he praised as "the God-chosen leader of our military forces" and on whom he invoked God's blessings for his "great exploits for the sake of the motherland."[36] At this time, of course, the Soviet Union had been plunged into an unanticipated war with its former ally, Nazi Germany, and Sergii's Russian pragmatism enabled him to overlook the countless atrocities and violations of human rights perpetrated by Stalin, especially during the preceding decade. The metropolitan, whom Stalin would soon allow to be elected patriarch, extended a New Year's greeting to Stalin in 1943: "In prayer I wish you health for the new year and success in all your undertakings, for the welfare of the country is entrusted to you."[37]

In the ensuing decades, platitudes of this kind became a veritable convention in the public utterances of patriarchs and other bishops.

Whoever happened to occupy the highest position of authority in the Soviet government was, irrespective of his personal turpitude and the brutality of his regime, routinely praised as a great leader, a champion of peace, liberty, and justice, and a noble human being. Patriarch Pimen, for example, eulogized Yuri Andropov, who rose to supreme power through the ranks of the murderous KGB, as "a preserver of the sacred gift of life" who was completely dedicated to "strengthening peace and justice among all nations on Earth."[38] The patriarch may have offended the memory of the many Orthodox martyrs at the hands of the Soviet Communists in an address delivered in the Patri- archal cathedral of the Epiphany in Moscow on February 12, 1984, before a memorial service for the deceased Soviet leader—a rite usu- ally reserved for faithful Orthodox Christians. Patriarch Pimen ex- tolled Andropov's "spirit of lofty humanism" and his "outstanding abilities and lofty spiritual qualities." At a time when thousands of Orthodox and other religious believers were languishing in the gulags and in psychiatric prisons, he also credited the Soviet dictator with promoting "the spiritual growth" of the nation.[39]

Ideological Proclamations. The public moral witness of the Patriar- chate's leaders during the Communist era served the state's ideology in two distinct but related ways.

First, *appeals to Russian nationalism or Soviet national interests* appeared frequently in print. Patriarch Pimen boasted to Mikhail Gorbachev during their historic meeting in April 1988 that the Russian Orthodox Church had always educated her children in "the Gospel principles" while "instilling in them civic virtues," especially "concern about the integrity of our Motherland."[40] Echoing his predecessor Sergii's as- surance to Stalin, Pimen reminded the graduates of the Moscow Theological Academy and Seminary in June 1985 that they had a dual vocation as priests and patriots: "A true clergyman of the Russian Church has always been a patriot. Love for his Motherland and defence of her national interests are inalienable features of his minis- try."[41]

In this statement Pimen actually surpassed his predecessor Sergii's profession of loyalty, for now it seemed that the clergy were called to enhance the national security of the land of their birth—a require- ment nowhere to be found in the classic texts of Orthodox canonical tradition. The canonical corpus, moreover, expressly forbids clergy from engaging in worldly or military pursuits, since these are deemed incompatible with the fundamentally liturgical and spiritual dimensions of the priestly vocation.[42] William Van Den Bercken of the University of Utrecht has aptly described this kind of abuse as, on the one hand, a "nationalistic exegesis" and hence misrepresentation of the biblical heritage, and, on the other, a "patriotic ecclesiology" that replaces a genuinely Christian sense of collective sinfulness with a tendency toward "national self-glorification."[43]

To be sure, the leaders of the Moscow Patriarchate were not alone in their excessive patriotic fervor. The Russian émigré community, who were unreservedly opposed to the Communist regime in their native land, have tended to be at least as Russian as they are Orthodox. Their Russian nationalism, when combined with a fervent anti-Communism, has, on occasion, pushed some émigrés to the other political extreme. In 1939, for example, Metropolitan Anastasy Gribanovsky, primate of the Russian Orthodox Church Outside Russia, thanked Adolf Hitler profusely for permitting and financing the construction of a Russian Orthodox church in Berlin. "National values," Anastasy wrote to the Führer, "are the honour and glory of every nation, and, for this reason they find a place also in the everlasting kingdom of God." That was, to be sure, a debatable proposition. But the metropolitan went further:

> Your great achievements on behalf of the German people and towards the greatness of the German Empire have made you an example worthy of imitation, a model of devotion to one's own people and one's Fatherland, and of how one must stand up for one's national and spiritual values.[44]

The second way in which the public moral witness of the Patriarchate served ideology was by reflecting *a Communist/socialist worldview.* On one level, until 1991 or so the pages of the *Journal of the Moscow Patriarchate* were filled with paeans to socialism, echoing the rhetoric of the secular political authorities. In 1977, on the sixtieth anniversary of the 1917 Communist putsch, Patriarch Pimen extolled that event as "a guiding light for millions of people on earth who were oppressed, without rights, hungry, and poverty stricken." The "Great October Socialist Revolution" also signaled "the rout of colonialism and oppression" and "gave the peoples of the world an example they could follow, leading them to popular power and progress."[45] A decade later, in 1987, the patriarch praised the 1918 Decree on Separation of Church from State, which virtually eliminated all public activities of the Church, as a "democratic act" that "legalized the principles of freedom of conscience and the independence of the Church from state institutions."[46]

By the end of 1991, when the Patriarchate found itself left on the dock as the ship of state sailed toward greater democracy, Aleksii II and other Church leaders were scrambling to craft the exact phrasing that would demonstrate their continued support for the national political leadership while acknowledging the need for the "new thinking." But how can the Patriarchate's leaders advocate essential social change as glibly as they supported the status quo before Gorbachev? How can a society that supposedly was a beacon of light for the earth's oppressed require such a thorough rehabilitation as Gorbachev and Yeltsin have enacted?

A key to understanding this Orwellian posture was provided in 1987 by Archbishop Aleksandr, rector of the Moscow Theological Academy, in a speech commemorating the seventieth anniversary of the October Revolution. He affirmed the "necessity for Church conscience to try and correlate its traditional values with those of socialism within a positive dialogue." The Church in the present "period of new construction" must defer to "the values chosen by the historically creative and active part of the Russian nation, . . . the values of the victorious revolution."[47] Whether nationalism or socialism is the dominant partner in this new *modus vivendi,* the Church is clearly the subordinate participant. The archbishop could not have voiced a more succinct form of the "cosmocracy" type of church-state relations.

On another level, "ideological" collaboration best describes the way that bishops and theologians of the Moscow Patriarchate conceptualized human rights, particularly religious and political freedom, in the *ancien régime.* In his first speech at a regional meeting of the Prague-based Christian Peace Conference in 1963, Metropolitan Nikodim (then archbishop of Yaroslavl) made a veritable profession of faith in the "socialist" version of freedom, private property, and peace.[48] Displaying a penchant for hyperbole, he lambasted "the apologists for the unchangeability of unjust social orders," "the irascible voices of some 'Christian' statesmen of the West accusing socialist countries of violating civil right[s]," "these impatient accusers" who "often become zealous, but blind, defenders of tendentious anti-communist propaganda which has nothing in common with fundamental Christianity."

Nikodim's positive affirmations are no less shocking than his negative attacks to those whose point of socio-political reference is the liberal democracy characteristic of Western societies. The archbishop posited that "genuine freedom is a reasonable and voluntary service of truth and peace" but concluded in typical collectivist fashion: "Every civil right . . . is of genuine value only if it is used for the good of society, of one's country, of all mankind" instead of "to protect the interests of a selfish individual or of a privileged class." He specifically challenged, as an example of a false civil right, "private ownership of important national properties." This implicit Marxist premise surfaced more clearly in the following rhetorical question: "Is it possible, from a Christian standpoint, to consider true liberty the legal protection of a right for individuals to hold undisputed ownership over means of production which should belong to society as a whole?"

Then, as if to remove any doubt about his ideological outlook, Nikodim made the astonishing claim that socialism transcends ideology and immorality. Specifically, he declared as "fact" his personal belief that "in socialist states there is no 'freedom' to exploit the labour of another, no 'freedom' for a pernicious ideology to affect the surrounding world." Describing citizens of the socialist utopia he said:

> It is also impossible, for them to fall prey with impunity to the temptation of an idle life, a life of unbridled wantonness, of moral depravity and corruption. Christians cannot do other than regard these people who are freed from the temptation of living an un-Christian way of life as a great gift of God's grace.

A more recent argument by Professor Aleksii Osipov of the Moscow Theological Academy demonstrates the staying power of this skewed view of human freedom.[49] In a 1984 article Osipov defined "human rights" as "nothing more than 'material freedom,' i.e., the freedom of a person to perform a certain range of actions in the family, society and the state." As examples he listed "such vitally important human rights as the right to work, education, rest, free medical care, social security, etc." This amounts, of course, to the short list of what some political theorists call "social welfare rights," that is, "positive" rights *to* something; these are distinguished from "negative rights," the procedural rights deriving from principles of liberty—that is, the rights to be *free from* certain constraints or impositions of the government or social groups.

For Osipov, freedom was effectively teleological, based on ultimate ends: since "a genuine right" is intrinsically one that points toward "the ideal of the *new* man," true freedom must, as a conditional and not absolute right, enhance the development of what is good and uproot what is evil in man and human society. Unlimited freedom, therefore, is not a virtue, but rather the ground of the original sin of selfish pride. Freedom of speech, to cite one aspect of the right to liberty, remains a human right, Osipov argued, "only as long as it does not overstep its positive bounds" by allowing the advocacy of lies, slander, violence, and other evils. When this freedom exceeds these bounds, it "can no longer be called a human right and be allowed to exist in society." Freedom is, in this view, a strictly material right depending on its results (as judged, presumably, by some central political authority), and not the formal right to personal expression, irrespective of content, that is central to classic Western liberalism.

In light of these carefully crafted arguments for a socialist view of human rights, the following assertion by the Soviet authors of a 1988 popular history of Orthodoxy in Russia and the Soviet Union does not seem so radical: "The Moscow Patriarchate is developing, in fact, a concept of 'Christian socialism.' "[50]

Deceptions and Denunciations

The second dimension of the official witness of the Patriarchate on the issue of religious freedom is the duplicity that characterized many of the statements and activities of the hierarchy. Two particular forms of active collaboration in this regard will engage our attention here: (1) the proclamation of deliberate falsehoods concerning the religious freedom of the Orthodox Church, and (2) active measures in the suppression of Orthodox dissidents.

Deliberate Deceptions. Metropolitan Sergii established a scandalous precedent in a press conference with foreign journalists in February 1930. He denied the charges of the persecution of religion in the

Soviet Union and maintained that Orthodox clergy and laity were repressed only for their political activities against the government and "by no means for their religious convictions."[51]

This became a predictable refrain whenever Westerners broached the subject of religious freedom. Metropolitan Aleksii of Tallinn, for example, whitewashed the Brezhnev regime in 1980, as Sergii had exonerated Stalin: "In the Soviet Union citizens are never arrested for their religious or ideological convictions."[52] Even in the early years of *glasnost'*, the Big Lie continued unabated. Patriarch Pimen commented in 1987:

> [T]here is no truth in the assertions that the Church is oppressed in our country. Needless to say, there are instances of violation of believers' rights. But this does not reflect the state's attitude to the Church. Commonly, this is a consequence of deviation from law on the part of certain individuals or local bodies of authority. There are instances of law-breaking on the part of religious organizations too.[53]

Thus denial of persecution degenerated further into blaming the victims for their own oppression.

Another tactic for deflecting criticism was the counteroffensive, which Metropolitan Yuvenaly perfected. In an interview with the BBC recorded in January 1975, the metropolitan, then head of the Patriarchate's Department of External Church Relations, railed against "the tendency among certain circles in England, supported even by some officials of the Anglican Church, to present a biased and one-sided picture of Russian Orthodox Church life." This supposed preoccupation with "only the dark side" of Church life — an implicit admission in itself — was fostered, he contended, by dissident sources in the Soviet Union who had their own axes to grind.[54]

In international ecumenical circles, particularly the World Council of Churches, representatives of the Moscow Patriarchate used heavy-handed tactics to deter or deflect criticism of the human-rights record in their homeland. Perhaps the most controversial incidents of this sort occurred at the World Council of Churches' 1975 Nairobi Assembly and 1983 Vancouver Assembly. In each case the WCC received an appeal from Russian Orthodox dissidents imploring it to rally to the cause of persecuted believers in the Soviet Union. These cases have been reviewed thoroughly elsewhere.[55] Let it suffice to say here that the response of the Patriarchate scandalized even many of the usually left-leaning Protestant representatives. The concerted opposition—led by Metropolitans Yuvenaly and Nikodim—to any action by the Nairobi Assembly on the letter of appeal from Fr. Gleb Yakunin and Lev Regelson resulted in a toothless "compromise" resolution on religious liberty in Europe that virtually whitewashed the Soviet record. The Russian Orthodox delegation, in tandem with the Soviet Baptist, Armenian Orthodox, and Georgian Orthodox delegations from the Soviet Union, also managed to intimidate the WCC administration so much that at the Vancouver Assembly eight years later a similar letter of appeal from Deacon Vladimir Rusak was not allowed to reach the full assembly.

The case of Metropolitan Nikodim is particularly instructive. He reportedly revealed his approach to prevarication in public to a priest of the Orthodox Church in America: "Let us come to an accord on this question. You publicize these materials in the West, and we shall issue denials."[56] Nikodim rationalized his deliberate deceptions as a necessary compromise for the sake of the survival of the Church— an example of what we have called "pragmatic collaboration." In a private conversation with Professor Dmitry Pospielovsky, the well-traveled metropolitan dismissed the possibly adverse impact on believers of a bishop engaged in lies and distortions: "It is you people in the West that react this way. We're used to this sort of thing in the Soviet Union, and we don't react." Whether this practice was good or bad, Nikodim implied, it was the given reality there. He implied further that the criticism of Soviet abuses that comes from "such respected persons as, for instance, the Anglican Archbishop of Canterbury, can be of great use to us."[57] Apparently, these external voices of prophecy afforded Nikodim the "moderate loyalist" some leverage with the Communist authorities in his efforts to improve Soviet relations with the West and Soviet policies toward his fellow churchmen back home. If Patriarch Pimen had been cowed into an instrumental collaboration through KGB extortion, then Metropolitan Nikodim pragmatically allowed himself to become a voice of propaganda in the hope of achieving at least a modicum of prophecy.

Patriarch Aleksii II put a new spin on this perverse "spirituality of deception" in an interview in December 1990 with the Moscow journal *Literaturnaya Gazeta*. Aleksii repeated the now classic justifications of Metropolitan Sergii's 1927 Declaration, saying it did not harm the Church and, on the contrary, was commensurate with the political precedents established by the great Orthodox princes SS. Boris and Gleb (Hlib) and St. Aleksandr Nevsky. But he also applied the word "sin" to Metropolitan Sergii's efforts to preserve the Church: "The course was to burden one's conscience with a lesser sin in order to avoid a greater sin." Sometimes hierarchs must, Aleksii insisted, sacrifice their own "personal perfection" for the sake of their flocks. That may mean "shielding" the Church "by means of a compromise" such as "a declaration of loyalty." Readily acknowledging "that members of the hierarchy burdened their souls with a sin, a sin of silence, a sin of untruth," Aleksii mitigated the value of this public confession by insisting, "We have always atoned to God for this sin" and "we are not guilty before the people."[58]

Even after the failed coup in August 1991, Patriarch Aleksii II and the Holy Synod of the Moscow Patriarchate refused to make a clean break with their dubious past. On the one hand, the patriarch expressed what appears to be an unqualified repentance in an interview with the Italian weekly *Sabato* reprinted in the August 26/September 1, 1991, issue of the Moscow weekly *Golos:*

> From those who have suffered because of these concessions [by the Patriarchate], this silence, this forced passivity, or the appearance of loyalty on the part of church officials of this [Soviet] period — I ask forgiveness, understanding, and prayer from all these people and not just from God. I say to them: "Forgive me, beloved, forgive me, my children."[59]

But in the same week, on August 30, Aleksii and the Holy Synod issued an "Appeal" to the faithful in which they insisted that the Russian Orthodox Church "kept the faith pure" in the Communist era. They broached the question of collaboration gingerly:

> At the same time we recognize with humility that not all the servants of the Church were equal to the task of their vocation in the years of trials. Our Lord and Righteous Judge will reward everyone according to his deserts. We get down to the cleansing and reviving of our Church, and in doing this we should be guided

by a conciliar mind, canonical order and personal responsibility of everyone before God, one's own conscience and the people of God. . . .[60]

Patriarch Aleksii made another attempt at self-justification when he spoke at Georgetown University in November 1991, during his first trip to the United States. He had chosen not to "act resolutely" during the era of persecution, he said, in order to avoid the "deadly sin" of preserving "my own moral image" by abdicating his "diocesan responsibilities." And so he remained with his flock, however politically and spiritually fleeced they were by the "Theomachists" (that is, fighters against God), and was "happy" to report that "in those difficult years I was useful to my church."[61] The patriarch seemed determined to have it both ways: to issue *mea culpas,* while effectively congratulating himself for saving the Church by those same sins of commission and omission.

A long-awaited breakthrough finally occurred in Patriarch Aleksii's Lenten Message on February 28, 1993 (according to the Gregorian calendar). In the unequivocal language of repentance, he spoke from the heart:

> We repent for those of us who did not stand firm enough for the faith in the years of persecution, who [were] faint-hearted and even, God forbid, pandered to the persecutors who trampled on the Church of God, bringing to Christians suffering and death.
>
> Today when a sea of suffering has flooded us, we are guilty before every one who suffers, guilty of not always warming him with the warmth of our hearts, not always sacrificing ourselves for his good. . . .
>
> Every one has sinned against God. But, my fellow-brothers, the greatest blame lies with us, archpastors and pastors. We will have to answer for our flock at the Last Judgement. We carry the burden of both their sins and our failure to be always a good example and good teachers for them. . . .
>
> On this day of Cheesefast, the Sunday of Forgiveness, I make to every one of you, beloved in the Lord bishops, fathers, brothers and sisters, a humble appeal to forgive me for all my many sins before you.[62]

This public atonement of the patriarch of Moscow compares favorably with an earlier action by six of the metropolitans of the

Bulgarian Orthodox Church based in Sofia. In December 1990, Metropolitans Pimen of Novrokop, Stefan of Veliki Trnovo, Pankraty of Stara Zagora, Kalinik of Vratsa, Dometian of Vidin, and Kirill of Varna expressed contrition for their "personal transgressions both direct and indirect" during the Communist era. Even more remarkable was their admission that they acted unjustly in their March 1988 condemnation of Fr. Khristofor Sabev.[63] Fr. Khristofor, a controversial human-rights activist, founded the Committee for the Defense of the Rights of Believers in Bulgaria. The only prominent hierarch whose signature was conspicuously absent from this text was Patriarch Maksim himself.[64]

Denouncing Dissidents. Whether to prove their loyalty to the regime or to consolidate their own limited power base, prominent hierarchs of the Moscow Patriarchate turned on their less cooperative brethren with a viciousness surprising even for strict collaborationists. No one who, prior to the ascendancy of Gorbachev, dared to buck the Patriarchate's party line escaped the wrath of the leadership, not even esteemed bishops. Archbishop Yermogen of Kaluga was perhaps the best known episcopal casualty of these "active measures" of collaboration. In 1965 he submitted to the patriarch a petition, co-signed by seven other bishops, that protested the canonical irregularities of the revised Church regulations of 1961, particularly the requirement that a committee of twenty laymen—from which the parish priest was officially excluded—establish and govern a parish. As a result, Archbishop Yermogen was forcibly "retired" by the Holy Synod in 1967 and subsequently subjected to trumped-up charges of incompetence.[65]

Specific cases of punitive actions by the Patriarchate against its prophetic sons are legion. Patriarch Pimen intimated in 1975 that conscientious objectors during World War II were not tolerated by Church leaders; he commended his predecessor Sergii for "exposing and exhorting them, as we still do today."[66] At the 1975 Nairobi Assembly of the World Council of Churches, Metropolitan Yuvenaly, who chaired the Russian Orthodox delegation, not only categorically denied the charges of religious persecution presented to the WCC in the letter from Fr. Gleb Yakunin and Lev Regelson; he also questioned the credibility of the two Orthodox dissidents in *ad hominem* attacks against their standing in the Church and their views on ecumenism.[67] The "assistance" of Metropolitan Serafim of Krutitsy and Kolomna was, according to the Furov Report, crucial in the virtual silencing of the respected dissident priest Dmitry Dudko in 1974. Serafim removed the outspoken priest from his Moscow parish, banishing him, in effect, to a suburban district. Furov also credited the compliant metropolitan with persuading Fr. Dmitry to issue his notorious recantation.[68]

The most controversial—and infamous—public denunciation of a Russian Orthodox dissident by a spokesman of the Patriarchate was the Solzhenitsyn affair in March 1974. In a shocking letter to the London *Times,* Metropolitan Serafim denounced Aleksandr Solzhenitsyn, the great Russian writer, as "unchristian," "a prodigal son," and a traitor to his country.[69] The response was, predictably, swift and furious, all of it in defense of Solzhenitsyn's religious virtue and Russian patriotism.

More surprising, however, was the contrary witness of two of Serafim's colleagues in the hierarchy of the Moscow Patriarchate.[70] Metropolitan Anthony Bloom of Sourozh, esteemed author of several contemporary spiritual classics and London-based exarch of the Patriarchate in Western Europe, wrote to the London *Times* one week later, "I want, in my own name and in that of both my clergy and the believers, to disown the statements about Solzhenitsyn in the letter of Metropolitan Serafim. . . . [He] speaks for himself and those in the USSR who misguidedly choose to side with him." Similarly, the late Archbishop Vassily Krivocheine of the Russian Orthodox Church in Belgium (which is under the jurisdiction of the Patriarchate) wrote a letter to a Brussels newspaper in which he clearly broke ranks with his senior colleague from Moscow:

> I therefore declare that I find myself in complete disagreement with Metropolitan Serafim's declarations as a whole and with his justifying repressive measures against Solzhenitsyn in particular.
>
> Such declarations gravely wrong the good name of the Patriarchate of Moscow. It is dismaying to see a high dignitary of the Church approve measures of violence against a man whose only fault is to have told the truth.

These two bishops, to be sure, lived in Western Europe at the time, far away from the iron grip of the patriarch and his Holy Synod. But the authentic prophetic roles of the two exarchs cannot be gainsaid: at least some of the ruling hierarchs of the Moscow Patriarchate in the pre-Gorbachev era were willing to witness courageously on behalf of the truth—in public as well as in private.

Even in the post-Communist era some of these heavy-handed abuses of power seem to die hard. In the aftermath of Patriarch Aleksii II's 1993 Lenten Message, the only lingering doubt as to his full *metanoia* ("repentance" in Greek) concerns his unwillingness to acknowledge his KGB code-name and apparent refusal to ask forgiveness personally of Orthodox dissidents such as Fr. Gleb Yakunin, whose role in Russia parallels that of Fr. Khristophor Sabev in Bulgaria. In November 1991, during Aleksii's first visit to the United States, the Russian patriarch indicated ominously to Lawrence Uzzell, vice-president of the Jamestown Foundation, that he regarded Fr. Gleb's behavior through the years as questionable. Two years later, on November 2, 1993, the Holy Synod of the Moscow Patriarchate officially deposed Fr. Gleb from the priesthood, a decision that rocked much of the Orthodox world and the ecumenical community and that promises to have long-reaching effects. The ostensible reason for this dramatic initiative was that Fr. Gleb—unlike another politically involved priest, the monk Innokentiy Pavlov—refused to remove his name from the list of candidates in the December 1993 election of deputies to the lower house, or Duma, of the Russian parliament. Patriarch Aleksii and his fellow bishops clearly stood on firm canonical ground: priests are expressly prohibited by ancient Church canons still in force to hold political office.

But Fr. Gleb is determined to defy the Holy Synod and to fight this "illegitimate" and "unjust" decision by appealing to the next All-Russian *Sobor* ("Council") of the Patriarchate. He may have a case. The current patriarch himself and a number of other hierarchs and priests held political office in the Supreme Soviet of the Communist regime and in the Congress of People's Deputies of the RSFSR and its successor state. More to the point, however, is the flagrant hypocrisy of Metropolitan Filaret Vakhromeyev of Minsk and Grodno (KGB code-name "Ostrovskii"), one of the signatories to the decree of defrocking, who continues to hold political office as a deputy in the Supreme Soviet of the new Republic of Belarus. Further, Fr. Gleb believes that the canonical conundrum is a smokescreen to shield a personal vendetta against him waged by Patriarch Aleksii for the dissident priest's role in exposing the KGB connections of the hierarchy and for resisting the Patriarchate's attempt in 1993 to restrict the activities of foreign missionaries in Russia.[71]

Reaping the Rewards

The third dimension of the official witness of the Moscow Patriarchate on the issue of religious freedom is the opportunistic quality of its collaboration with the Communist state.

The unmitigated loyalty of the patriarchs was amply "rewarded" when it suited the regime to bestow its good graces. In 1943 the Russian Orthodox Church lay virtually prostrate before Stalin, having suffered a massive persecution at the end of which only four bishops remained in active service. The Soviet dictator, beleaguered by the invading Germans, granted a reprieve to the remaining shell-shocked Church leaders on condition that the Church support the Soviet war effort. Metropolitan Sergii was allowed to be elected patriarch, and the Patriarchal leadership roused the masses to a spiritual crusade that was tantamount to a very un-Orthodox, nationalistic "holy war" (see chapter 5). This was hardly an alliance made in heaven, to be sure, but the Church—and nation—were spared extinction by their respective enemies.

As a result of Gorbachev's sweeping reforms, the Patriarchate was again able to reap the rewards of its loyalty to the regime, including the return of confiscated Church properties and increased access to the mass media. The Soviet leader, beset by political opponents on both the reactionary "right" and the reform-minded "left," needed to curry the favor of the Church.

These material gains notwithstanding, the longtime pragmatic collaboration of the Moscow Patriarchate heavily taxed the moral capital of the Church. That the Patriarchate accepted "windfalls" resulting from the regime's persecution of other religious communities is historically indisputable. Even in mid-1992 most of the hierarchy still seemed unable or unwilling to right these wrongs.

The Ukrainian Catholic Church. The official liquidation of the Ukrainian Catholic Church of the Byzantine Rite in March 1946 was, from a broad historical perspective, one stage in a centuries-old struggle between Rome and Moscow for the spiritual allegiance of the Ukrainian nation. Violations of religious freedom and integrity have occurred from both directions, beginning with the Vatican's aggressive proselytism of this historically Orthodox region in the sixteenth century. But our subject here is the continued abuse of the Ukrainian Catholics by the Moscow Patriarchate in the post–World War II era.

The facts in this case, though disputed by both sides, seem to be as follows. A so-called People's *Sobor* ("Council") met in Lvov (Lviv in Ukrainian) March 8-10, 1946, ostensibly to revoke the decision of a controversial assembly 350 years earlier—the Union of Brest. At the 1596 assembly, a majority of the Orthodox hierarchy, but only a minority of the representatives of the Orthodox population in the Galicia region of the Polish-Lithuanian Commonwealth, opted for union with Rome as a national Church. This community was supposed to retain its Orthodox liturgical and doctrinal traditions, while acknowledging papal authority over the universal Church. The "Uniates," as the Orthodox came to refer to them derisively, seem to have been enticed into the Roman orbit by offers of political privileges and cultural benefits in the Catholic Polish state. Dissenters faithful to Orthodoxy were forcibly suppressed by the Polish authorities.

The 1946 Council of Lvov was organized by three Ukrainian Catholic priests, two of whom were swiftly consecrated to the episcopate by Russian Orthodox hierarchs. The assembly of 216 clergy and only 19 laymen declared the entire Ukrainian Catholic community "reunited" with the mother Church—that is, the Russian Orthodox Church—and all vestiges of the unique Catholic identity of this people, forged through three and a half centuries, were systematically purged.[72]

Despite the instigation and enforcement of this "decision" by the Communist regime, a substantial Ukrainian Catholic Church persisted, albeit underground and hence "illegally" prior to the historic agreement in December 1989 between Gorbachev's Soviet government and the Vatican. Precise statistics are unavailable, but a recent statement on Eastern Europe by U.S. Catholic bishops estimates a Ukrainian Catholic population of three to six million, concentrated in Western Ukraine and led by approximately 18 bishops and 1,000 priests.[73] Pope John Paul II enunciated the Roman Catholic position on this question as follows: "Membership in the Catholic Church should not be considered by some as incompatible with the good of one's own earthly country and with the inheritance of St. Vladimir."[74] St. Vladimir (for Ukrainians, Volodymyr) was the tenth-century prince of Kyyiv who founded the Church on what is now Ukrainian territory.

The present generation of Russian Orthodox leaders have, for the most part, viewed the action of the 1946 Council of Lvov as a matter of justice long overdue. Less convincingly, they also deem it a popular, democratic move in conformity with religious truth, having far-reaching, salutary consequences. In 1986, on the fortieth anniversary of the Lvov council, several hierarchs of the Patriarchate issued messages and reports extolling the 1946 action. First, they acknowledged their debt to the government insofar as the "joyful event was possible only after the reunification of the Western Ukrainian population with the people of the Soviet Ukraine and the Soviet victory in the Great Patriotic War" (that is, World War II).[75] Metropolitan Filaret Denisenko, then Moscow's exarch in Kiev and Galich, was, at best, disingenuous when he contrasted "the conditions of political freedom and national unity" under the Soviets to the "power of Rome" and the Polish Jesuits by which the Union of Brest had been "forced on our ancestors."[76] This posture betrayed an untoward reliance on the political authority—one that is antithetical to the Orthodox ethos in contravention of a traditional Orthodox teaching (the virtue of religious tolerance). This unfortunate politicization of an internal Church conflict also tended to undermine the rest of the Patriarchate's political and nationalistic appeal, specifically the bishops' contentions that during World War II the Ukrainian Catholic hierarchy "sided with the enemies of our Motherland the Nazi invaders" and that the original union in 1596 was "politically motivated" and an egregious act of aggrandizement by Polish Jesuits and a minority faction impressed by the material advantages extended by Rome.[77]

The Orthodox bishops also used a myth of unity clearly belied by the facts to justify the overt Russification of what had evolved during several centuries as a Church with a distinctive Ukrainian national identity. "For forty years," Patriarch Pimen declared, "we have all been one common Orthodox family."[78] Other hierarchs claimed, amazingly, that the undoing of the Union of Brest "put an end to enmity and hatred between brothers by blood."[79] And yet not only did millions of Ukrainians chafe in official silence under their forced reunion with Moscow: until quite recently many continued to suffer overt persecution by the Communist regime.

The notion of unity within the Patriarchate itself on this question is also a fiction. Orthodox "dissidents" such as Anatoly Levitin-Krasnov, Yelena Sannikova, Vladimir Poresh, Aleksandr Ogorodnikov, Fr. Georgi Edelshtein, and Fr. Gleb Yakunin have sided publicly with the Ukrainian Catholic community against their own Orthodox hierarchy. Even one of the Patriarchate's hierarchs broke ranks early with his brothers on this point, as Metropolitans Anthony and Vassily had done a decade earlier in the Solzhenitsyn controversy. Myroslaw Tataryn reported in the Winter 1989 issue of *Religion in Communist Lands* that Metropolitan Irenei of Vienna had written to him, denouncing the pretense that the Ukrainian Catholics did not exist underground in the Soviet Union and calling for the re-legalization of their church.[80]

In the wake of Mikhail Gorbachev's political pilgrimage to the Vatican in December 1989, the position of the Moscow Patriarchate appeared to soften. Metropolitan Kirill of Smolensk was the first Orthodox hierarch to signal publicly that the Russian Orthodox Church was willing to resolve the Ukrainian problem through direct negotiations with the Vatican. As early as July 1989, Kirill had stated his approval of "personal contacts" between Ukrainian Catholic and Orthodox clergy in Ukraine. "We need encounters," he said. "We need informal and formal meetings; we need to talk with each other as Christians."[81]

The Vatican and the Moscow Patriarchate took a dramatic step in this direction in January 1990, when representatives from each Church finally met in Moscow to seek an equitable settlement. This discussion ended abruptly two months later when Metropolitan Volodymyr Sterniuk, representing the Ukrainian Catholic Archbishop of Lviv, Cardinal Miroslav Lyubachevskij (then in "exile" in Rome), withdrew his delegation to protest what he claimed was foot-dragging by the Russian Orthodox representatives. In a stern statement issued on March 17, Sterniuk and the six other bishops in Ukraine insisted that the Patriarchate accede to three demands: (1) recognition of the Ukrainian Catholic Church as a juridical body and a "Particular

Church" instead of a mere "rite" in accordance with the teachings of the Second Vatican Council; (2) return of all properties confiscated from the Ukrainian Catholic Church since September 17, 1939; and (3) formal declaration of the 1946 "pseudo-synod of Lviv" as "uncanonical."[82]

These demands may be deemed respectable as an opening bid in what was sure to be a difficult negotiation. But Sterniuk showed signs of being as unreasonable in the present as the Patriarchate had been in the past. He seemed too willing to resort to the civil authorities to put pressure on the Patriarchate to relinquish the disputed church properties. Referring to the Ukrainian nationalist movement known as *Rukh* ("movement" in Ukrainian), which had achieved local electoral victories in western Ukraine, Sterniuk told an American Catholic reporter, "We don't want politics to interfere with our Church's spiritual life. But Rukh members *have* to support us, because they themselves are Eastern-rite Catholics."[83]

Nor does the return of Cardinal Lyubachevskij to his homeland promise much of an improvement in relations between the two Churches. Fr. Anthony Ugolnik, a priest of the Ukrainian Orthodox Church of America, reported that in an interview the cardinal "expressed a pre–Vatican II theology":

> He alluded to Orthodox as "schismatics" who "lied" about the Ukrainian Catholics; he maintained that the Orthodox had surrendered all claim to continuity with the Apostolic Church of St. Vladimir (again, not a position in line with conciliatory gestures Rome has made toward the Orthodox). His rhetoric was very different from that which the papacy has used toward Orthodox since the time of Pope John XXIII.

Cardinal Lyubachevskij suggested to Fr. Anthony that the civil authorities in Ukraine may be afraid of the Ukrainian Catholics. Speaking about the movement for an autocephalous Ukrainian Orthodox Church, he said it could "never survive" and was "based upon a politics, not upon Jesus Christ." And, in a remark certain to win him no friends among the Orthodox, he asserted that "the Orthodox never suffered under the Communists."[84]

These reactionary attitudes by the principal Ukrainian Catholic leaders in Ukraine pose a seemingly insurmountable obstacle to the religious ambassadors of good will on both sides of this Eastern divide. There are other obstacles. In western Ukraine, where the Ukrainian Catholics are most numerous, bitter, deep-seated memories of the Union of Brest on one side and the Council of Lvov on the other may die hard. Some Ukrainian Catholics manifested a militancy in late 1989 and early 1990 when, in the first flush of their political ascendancy, they "seized" Orthodox church buildings by force, even resorting to physical violence against their Russian Orthodox adversaries.[85] And yet Cardinal Lyubachevskij and those sympathetic to the Ukrainian Catholic cause in the West have never acknowledged such violence.[86] Ironically, shrill anti-Russian rhetoric was on the rise, even as the Moscow Patriarchate struggled at last to become more irenic toward the Ukrainian Catholics.

Still another setback occurred in spring 1991 when the Vatican announced the appointment of Roman Catholic bishops for sees in Russia. Although the Vatican's chief ecumenical officer, Cardinal Edward Cassidy, later admitted that this designation of "apostolic administrators"—instead of ordinary bishops to rival the Orthodox in four cities—was not handled "in the best way," the perception of renewed proselytism by Rome against the Russian Orthodox faithful led to an indignant public refusal by Patriarch Aleksii II—backed by all the other autocephalous Orthodox Churches save Constantinople—to send observers to the Vatican's special synod on the evangelization of Europe, held in November 1991.[87]

The Ukrainian issue managed to galvanize the Orthodox world. On March 15, 1992, an unprecedented assembly in Constantinople of the patriarchs or primates of every universally recognized autocephalous Orthodox Church except Alexandria and Georgia issued a concise eight-part "Message." The fourth and longest section complained bitterly about the renewed proselytism of "traditionally Orthodox countries" by the Roman Catholic Church and "certain fundamentalists and Protestants." The document specifically condemned the activities "against our Churches in The Ukraine, Romania, Eastern Slovakia, the Middle East and elsewhere by Uniates, who belong to the Church of Rome."[88]

Other Ukrainian Churches. To complicate matters further, how does the self-professed but still officially unrecognized and "uncanonical"

Ukrainian Autocephalous Orthodox community factor into this dialogue, especially since it elected American-based Metropolitan Mstyslav Skrypnyk as its first patriarch in June 1990? Mstyslav was reportedly greeted by tens of thousands of jubilant Ukrainians during a whirlwind visit to his native land in October-November 1990. Present at Patriarch Mstyslav's enthronement in Kyyiv's eleventh-century St. Sophia Cathedral on November 18 was an official government delegation that included Mykola Kolesnyk, chairman of the CRA of what was then the Ukrainian SSR.

In stark contrast, the visit to St. Sophia Cathedral by Patriarch Aleksii II three weeks earlier had led to mass protests and some violence by warring factions of Ukrainians for and against the Moscow Patriarchate.[89] Ironically, Aleksii had traveled to Kyyiv to announce the October 27 decision of the Patriarchate's Holy Synod to grant local autonomy to the Ukrainian Exarchate of the Moscow Patriarchate under Metropolitan Filaret Denisenko. Filaret took the title Metropolitan of Kiev and All Ukraine, and the Church there was renamed, perhaps disingenuously, the "Ukrainian Orthodox Church."

Dramatic developments in 1992 and 1993 further muddied the ecclesiastical waters. First, in rapid succession in April 1992, as noted above, Metropolitan Filaret offered to resign, was commended for his years in the episcopacy by the hierarchy of the Moscow Patriarchate, revoked his offer and denounced the Patriarchate, was deposed by the Russian bishops, announced the formation of yet another "autocephalous" Ukrainian Orthodox Church under his personal primacy, and forged a tenuous alliance with one of the bishops of Mstyslav's jurisdiction. In late May, Bishop Vsevolod Majdanski, head of the Ukrainian Orthodox Church of America—an autonomous émigré diocese under the jurisdiction of the Ecumenical Patriarchate in Constantinople—participated as a "private observer" in a meeting of the Synod of Bishops of the Ukrainian Catholic Church in Lviv. His praise for the Uniate synod was effusive, perhaps even excessive from an Orthodox ecclesiological perspective: "You guard an ecclesiastical treasure which belongs to us all. Your synod is heir to the Metropolitans of Kyyiv."[90] Then, in August, a delegation from the Ecumenical Patriarchate met in Oxford, England, with representatives of the Ukrainian Catholic Church, their first official contact since 1596.[91] The precise significance of these irenic actions emanating from Constantinople is unclear, but they did introduce yet another Orthodox player into the complex drama unfolding in this troubled region.

By autumn 1993, however, the death of the widely respected nonagenarian Mstyslav had accelerated the unraveling of the fragile Ukrainian Orthodox unity.[92] There are currently no fewer than three rival Ukrainian Orthodox bodies—which neither recognize nor respect one another—competing for souls with the Ukrainian Catholics: (1) the Moscow Patriarchate's satellite "autonomous" Ukrainian Orthodox Church (UOC-MP) under Metropolitan Volodymyr Sabodan, who claims 6,000 parishes, 30 bishops, and 5,000 clergy in 28 dioceses; (2) the Ukrainian Orthodox Church—Kyyivan Patriarchate (UOC-KP), led by Patriarch Volodymyr Romaniuk, a distinguished former political prisoner of the Communist regime, who claims some 3,000 parishes, 2,500 priests, and 15 million out of the 35 million Ukrainian Orthodox faithful (with, however, the Ukrainian *bête noire* Metropolitan Filaret Denisenko lurking in the immediate background); and (3) the Ukrainian Autocephalous Orthodox Church (UAOC), the surviving remnant of the original group loyal to the wishes of the late Patriarch Mstyslav, currently led by Patriarch Dmytrii Yarema, who claims 1,500 parishes and 5 bishops in 8 dioceses.[93]

The Outlook in Ukraine. The only serious hope for an amicable settlement of historic differences in Ukraine in accordance with universal principles of religious freedom and justice rests with the religious hierarchies in Rome, Moscow, Constantinople, and now Kyyiv itself. A particularly hopeful sign is Pope John Paul's II apparent impatience with his own Ukrainian Catholic contingent in the ecumenical negotiations in Ukraine. At a historic meeting of twenty-nine Ukrainian Catholic bishops in Rome in June 1990, the pope asked them to "forgive" their Russian Orthodox counterparts in the interests of ecumenical dialogue. He also issued a firm command: "Be a bridge, then, and in no way an obstacle!"[94]

Cardinal Lyubachevskij may at least be listening to his own Holy Father. At the May 1992 synod in Lviv, the Ukrainian Cardinal declared his "lively hope that the Ukrainian Greek Catholic Church can attain full communion with the Churches of Ancient and New Rome" —that is, Constantinople and the Vatican.[95] On the Orthodox side, if reasonable ecumenists like Metropolitan Kirill of Smolensk and

Patriarch Bartholomaios of Constantinople can wield influence on the Moscow Patriarchate's negotiating posture, Moscow may prove willing, at last, to meet the Vatican at least half-way on the issue of religious freedom. With the Communist Party now defunct, Russia and Ukraine drifting further apart, and the democratic governments of these countries virtually out of the anti-religion business, the Churches themselves no longer have any political excuses for failing to reach a just, amicable accord.

More Than a Whisper

By far the most hopeful indications that Patriarch Aleksii II may have finally assumed the mantle of prophet as well as priest occurred during the two most wrenching political events in Russia since August 1991.

As recently as December 22, 1990, Patriarch Aleksii had joined more than fifty political, academic, and literary luminaries in a written appeal to Gorbachev "not to permit the break-up of the state" by a "destructive dictatorship of people who are shameless in their striving to take ownership of territory, resources, the intellectual wealth and labour forces of the country whose name is the USSR."[96] But this step backward appears to have been a temporary aberration. Aleksii's speech to the Congress of People's Deputies on June 1, 1989, had already included the following remarkable admission: "As is known, our history has corroborated the old truth that it is impossible to implement the finest social ideas by forced methods, without appealing to man's morality, his conscience, reason, disregarding moral choice and inner freedom."[97] On June 12, 1990, in a speech delivered to Mikhail Gorbachev, the newly elected patriarch waxed hopeful: "The favorable changes which are taking place in our country are opening up vistas enabling the Church to effect her ministry in full measure."[98]

In his first news conference as patriarch, Aleksii specifically vowed to engage in enhanced educational activities such as the inculcation of the spirit of mercy and charity, heretofore reserved to the state. He also urged, according to a broadcast in June 1990, that the new Soviet law on religious freedom "grant the right of juridical person to the whole church and not its separate structures."[99] Indeed, his name appeared on a candid critique of a draft of that law one month later. This document, expressing the views of the Patriarchate's *sobor*, criticized the proposed law for failing to guarantee to the entire Church such rights as "juridical personality," access to mass media, ownership of real estate for religious purposes, and the performance of religious rites and ceremonies at public events.[100]

When the hard-line Communists seized power on August 19, 1991 —the Orthodox feast day of the Transfiguration, according to the Julian calendar—all this progress seemed to come to a screeching halt. The Patriarchate was confronted with yet another challenge to exercise its prophetic conscience.

The opportunity came from an unexpected quarter. Boris Yeltsin, president of the Russian Federation and political hero of the hour, had issued an extraordinary personal appeal to Patriarch Aleksii that was broadcast over domestic Soviet radio on August 20, the second day of the attempted coup. "We call upon you to use your authority among all religions and believers," he exhorted Aleksii, "as well as the influence of the Church, to not be bystanders to what is happening. . . . Believers, all Russian people, the whole of Russia awaits your words."[101]

The day before, Aleksii had omitted the usual reference to the governing authorities in the liturgy for the Feast of the Transfiguration, a signal to the most attentive that something was awry. Yet the patriarch's initial public statement was, contrary to widespread news accounts in the West, rather muted. The purported "withdrawal" of Soviet leader Mikhail Gorbachev, the patriarch observed in carefully crafted language, "disturbs the conscience of millions of our compatriots, who call in question the legality of a newly formed State Committee for the State of Emergency." Expressing his hope that the Supreme Soviet "would take strong measures for the stabilization of the situation in the country," Aleksii said that "it is necessary at the moment to hear the voice of President Gorbachev and to find out what is his attitude to the current events."[102]

This apparently tepid opposition to a coup-in-the-making must have disappointed the millions of Russian Orthodox faithful who desperately wished that their spiritual leader would indeed take the initiative for a change. These faithful may still wonder wistfully what kind of video icon might have been fixed in minds around the world if the patriarch, or *any* Russian Orthodox bishop or priest, had joined the defiant Yeltsin atop a tank while the coup was in full sway.

But Aleksii quickly gathered his courage. On the third day of the coup, half an hour before the time when coup resisters expected an armored assault, a second statement by the patriarch was read over the public-address system at the barricades surrounding the RSFSR parliament building. Speaking directly to the "soldiers and commanders" about to commit "the horrible sin of fratricide," Aleksii declared that it was his duty as patriarch "to warn . . . that those who take up arms against their neighbor, against unarmed people, take the gravest sin upon their souls, the sin which excommunicates them from the Church and from God." (This action contrasted markedly with Metropolitan Filaret of Kiev's sermon on the first day of the attempted coup, welcoming it as a return to order.[103]) If the customary prophetic witness by Orthodox patriarchs to Byzantine emperors or Russian tsars entailed "whispering" in their ears, Patriarch Aleksii II broke that mold on August 21, 1991. His bold exhortation to the army of the commissars was a veritable shout.

A second opportunity for Patriarch Aleksii to exercise strong moral leadership came during the dangerous—and ultimately violent—political showdown throughout 1993 between Russian president Boris Yeltsin and the radicals and reactionaries (the so-called Red-Brown) forces in the Russian parliament. On March 25, during an earlier phase of the brewing political battle, Aleksii delivered an address on national television that urged the Russian people and their government to work for "a state which would not allow a return to the past, to dictatorship, to suppression of personal freedom and freedom of the people." He exhorted the army neither to participate in "political confrontation" nor "to come under the extremists' influence," and he advised the government authorities "to reach a compromise" to avert bloodshed and civil war. Aleksii specifically commended President Yeltsin for proposing a referendum as "the only way to elect a new parliament and a president."[104]

Later, in autumn, as the political struggle reached critical mass, Patriarch Aleksii's proven fairness and moderation earned him an unusual role in the last-ditch efforts to stave off violence. Cutting short his second visit in as many years to the United States, Aleksii returned to Moscow on September 27 to attempt to mediate the conflict. For two days he presided over marathon roundtable talks between the two factions in his official residence in the Danilovsky Monastery. When the talks failed, Aleksii requested that food, water, and medicine be allowed through the blockade of the parliament building, where the anti-reform faction was under siege by the pro-Yeltsin military. On Sunday, October 2, in his main cathedral, the patriarch himself carried the icon of the Vladimir Mother of God in a procession customary only in times of extreme crisis and prayed for the reconciliation of the opposing sides. On October 3, the eve of the eventual military assault on the parliament building, representatives of the Patriarchate tried desperately to forestall any violence by meeting individually with various political officials in both factions, all to no avail.

Patriarch Aleksii collapsed at the end of the Divine Liturgy on October 3, succumbing to a "viral infection" and, doubtless, the stress of the moment. Although he had "failed" to maintain the precarious peace, Aleksii rose in moral stature as a result of his untiring efforts to mediate the conflict. In classic prophetic form, he pronounced judgment on the nation after the outbreak of violence on October 4: "[The] wrath of God has fallen on Russia; . . . as a result of our sins, the Lord has allowed this tragedy to take place."[105]

VOICES FROM THE DISSIDENT WILDERNESS

Ever since the Khrushchev era in the early 1960s, while the official leadership of the Moscow Patriarchate was engaging in various sorts of collaboration with the Communist regime, undercurrents of dissent have rippled through the Russian Orthodox Church.[106] The expression of dissent has varied in accordance with the state's anti-religious strategies. During the Leninist and Stalinist periods, brutal persecution compelled many Orthodox Christians to assume the crown of martyrdom. In the most recent pre-Gorbachev regime, that of Leonid Brezhnev, the state relied more on sophisticated legalistic ploys, though persecution continued to oppress the Church.

A growing number of Orthodox citizens were outraged by their government's flagrant violations of universal human rights and even Soviet law, and by the complicity of their own Patriarchal leaders in the oppression of their Church. But unlike the earlier, unyielding anti-Soviet martyrs and confessors who resisted the establishment of an inherently anti-religious Communist state, the latest generation of Orthodox "dissidents" had, for the most part, accepted the reality of the Soviet state in which they lived. They continued to hope, however, that the political and religious establishments could be persuaded to recognize in practice the rudimentary religious freedom "guaranteed" by Soviet law.

The number and variety of Russian Orthodox dissidents grew steadily after the Khrushchev era. We shall consider the witness of five of them.

Aleksandr Solzhenitsyn. Nobel laureate Aleksandr Solzhenitsyn is only the most famous among a chorus of prophetic voices whose devotion to the principles of religious freedom and public tolerance of religious diversity is grounded in their Orthodox faith. The author of the multi-volume chronicle of Stalinist atrocities, *The Gulag Archipelago,* Solzhenitsyn also reflected the common piety and experience of ordinary Orthodox believers in his deeply moving "Lenten Letter" to Patriarch Pimen in 1971. In this plaintive appeal to the head of his Church, Solzhenitsyn humbly complained about the persecution of the Orthodox Church by the state and the compliant role of the hierarchy, without, however, directly accusing Pimen of anything or suggesting irreparable spiritual damage.[107]

The course of action that Solzhenitsyn encouraged Pimen to take — the way of suffering and martyrdom — is descriptive of his own life as a political prisoner and later, from 1974 until his long-awaited return in May 1994, expatriate in the West. The price of prophecy for Solzhenitsyn included a fate that for him was second only to death — forced exile from his beloved native land. He may have only narrowly escaped death itself: in April 1992 a writer in a Russian tabloid claimed that the KGB had almost succeeded in poisoning Solzhenitsyn as long ago as 1971.[108]

Solzhenitsyn has not lacked for critics in the West, especially among non-religious Russian émigrés such as Valery Chalidze and Mihajlo Mihajlov, who try to portray him as a potentially dangerous authoritarian reactionary.[109] To be sure, his opposition to Communist tyranny and his appeal to religious freedom are hardly based on the classic political theories operative in Western liberal democracies. Although he was born after the demise of Holy Russia in 1917, Solzhenitsyn is thoroughly grounded in the political ethos of the thousand-year-old Russian-Kyyivan Orthodox tradition and its Byzantine precursor. His vision of Church and state is the *symphonia* model of a harmonious, homogeneous society that strives to image the collegiality within the Holy Trinity as the Kingdom of God on earth without resort to political or religious coercion.

Whether this vision is at all realistic for a Russia that has experienced nearly a century of militant atheistic Communism is certainly an open question. Similarly quixotic may be his widely publicized plea in September 1990 for a much reduced, separate Slavic state comprising only the historic Russian, Belarussian, and perhaps Ukrainian lands, together with the Russified areas of Kazakhstan.[110] What is not, or ought not to be, subject to serious doubt is Solzhenitsyn's commitment to the ancient Orthodox Christian version of the virtue of religious freedom.

Deacon Vladimir Rusak. Another Orthodox dissident who suffered expulsion from his country is the former deacon Vladimir Rusak. He became known in the West when, in July 1983, an "open letter" that he had addressed to the Vancouver Assembly of the World Council of Churches generated an international controversy in that ecumenical body. Urging the assembled delegates to refrain from regarding the official Soviet delegations at such events as the sole voice of the Russian Orthodox Church, Rusak implored the WCC to examine the problem of religious freedom in the Soviet Union without political constraints.[111] Having been brought into line, apparently by the Russian Orthodox delegates after the Yakunin/Regelson affair at the 1975 Nairobi Assembly, the WCC leadership refused to allow discussion or official publication of the Rusak letter. But the witness was not entirely muted. The letter to the WCC was printed elsewhere, and Rusak was personally vindicated by the Anglican Archbishop of Canterbury at a press conference and in a BBC radio broadcast.

In a poignant conclusion to his letter, Rusak expressed his motivation in tackling the leadership of his own Church:

> I believe in God. I love my Church, I grieve for Her fate, and I want to serve Her, but, of course, not at the price of subservience, that terrible price which our Church leadership is paying and which it proposes that I also should pay.[112]

The Patriarchate's leaders exacted a different price from Deacon Rusak. When the KGB confiscated the original manuscript of his three-volume history of the travails of the Russian Orthodox Church under the Soviet regime beginning with Lenin (*Svidetel'stvo Obvineniya*, "Witness for the Prosecution"), Rusak managed to have a copy smuggled abroad. The Holy Trinity Press of the Russian Orthodox Church Outside Russia published the manuscript in 1987. Not long afterward, Rusak was removed as a deacon in his Moscow parish and fired from his job on the editorial staff of the *Journal of the Moscow Patriarchate*. His wife, who had tried in vain to convince him to destroy the manuscript, left him. Rusak was convicted on a charge of violating Article 70 of the Criminal Code of the RSFSR—which prohibits "anti-Soviet agitation and propaganda"—and sentenced to seven years in a labor camp beginning in April 1986.

Although he refused to recant or sign a confession, Rusak, obviously suffering the effects of malnutrition, was released early from prison. With no means of livelihood in his native land, he and his second wife emigrated to the United States in April 1989. He settled in Jordanville, New York, where he teaches Church history at the Holy Trinity Seminary of the Russian Orthodox Church Outside Russia, edits the Russian-language journal *Orthodox Russia*, and continues to work on his multi-volume history of the Russian Orthodox Church under Communism.

Zoya Krakhmalnikova and Felix Svetov. The Orthodox married couple Zoya Krakhmalnikova and Felix Svetov may be likened to SS. Prisca and Aquila, fellow laborers for the Gospel with St. Paul (I Corinthians 16:19). If the ancient Jewish Christian couple found the pagan culture of Rome inhospitable, the Russian pair has certainly found modern Soviet society an equally difficult mission field.

Krakhmalnikova and Svetov are not properly classed as "dissidents," for they never overtly opposed the Soviet government, preferring to let their positive personal witness on behalf of the truth of Orthodoxy speak for itself. And yet each suffered the penalty visited upon the most outspoken dissidents—imprisonment.

Zoya Krakhmalnikova is a former member of the Communist Party, an adult convert to Russian Orthodox Christianity, and an academically trained literary critic with a Ph.D. in philology. The author of three books on literary criticism and numerous scholarly articles, she became nationally renowned for her anthologies of classic Orthodox spiritual writings, personal testimonies and stories of conversion to Orthodoxy, and pious essays. These collections were self-published *(samizdat')* between 1976 and 1982 under the title *Nadezhda* ("Hope"). Archbishop Anthony of Geneva and Western Europe (Russian Orthodox Church Outside Russia) provided an external imprimatur for her work:

> In 1978 we blessed the publishing of this collection, which was so needed by the faithful. . . . We would like to draw everyone's attention to the fact that the *Nadezhda* collections do not contain any other materials besides those that are strictly religious.[113]

Krakhmalnikova was suddenly arrested at her summer cottage near Moscow in August 1982 on the same charge leveled against Deacon Vladimir Rusak—"anti-Soviet agitation and propaganda." She was taken to Lefortovo prison and in April 1983 was sentenced to one year in prison and five years of internal exile.

Her husband, Felix Svetov, a Jewish adult convert to Russian Orthodoxy, appealed for help in open letters to Russian writers and to the primates of the autocephalous Orthodox Churches throughout the world. To the latter, he eloquently professed his belief in the virtues of religious and intellectual freedom:

> The tragic fate of *Hope* is very characteristic of our life when a contemporary religious book is suppressed in general. Suppression of a book, destruction of a book, and the persecution of people because of a book is truly frightening. It is especially frightening in Russia, whose history began with a Book [i.e., the Bible]. The Book became the destiny of Russia, it was copied and preserved, it was a Russian's salvation during the most arduous twists of his fate.[114]

Felix Svetov himself was arrested in January 1985 after the authorities searched his home and found religious literature. Two years later in an early demonstration of Mikhail Gorbachev's new policy of *glasnost'*, both Krakhmalnikova and Svetov were granted reprieves. They chose to remain in their native land rather than emigrate, refusing to "abandon" their co-sufferers for the faith.[115]

Although these modern confessors maintain a positive, "centripedal," iconic witness to the truth they have found in Orthodoxy, that witness took a decidedly critical turn in the Gorbachev era. Their faith in religious and intellectual freedom led Krakhmalnikova, for example, to denounce their local bishop, Sevastian Pilipchuk of Kirovograd, in an open letter to Patriarch Pimen published in early 1990 in the journal *Glasnost*.[116] "All believers," she wrote, "are agitated by the cold-blooded attitude exhibited by the spiritual leadership in Moscow toward matters holy." The bishops "do not value our priests and churches" but prefer instead to "pursue earthly glory, earthly awards and, of course, large salaries." Her own bishop, she said, had closed a church in Yelizavetgrad in June 1986 and allowed Soviet bulldozers to demolish it, yet had been awarded the Order of St. Sergius by Patriarch Pimen. She herself had something else in mind for the errant bishop: "We hope that God's Archangel Michael, in whose honor our church was named, will smite with his fiery sword the head of Bishop Sevastian."

Another jeremiad by Krakhmalnikova followed the the disclosures of the KGB files early in 1992. She denounced the collaboration of the hierarchy of the Moscow Patriarchate with the Communist regime without mincing words:

> It is a catastrophe. A national moral catastrophe. . . . This is a spiritual Chernobyl', an infection with the sin of Judas. The Lord said concerning Christians that they are the salt of the earth, the light of the world. And if we Christians behave ourselves so shamefully, so immorally that our clergymen collaborate with the secret police, that our hierarchs turn out to be agents of the KGB, then what can we expect from our people, of whom we are a part? . . . [A] patriarch who has turned out to be a KGB agent cannot repent only before God. He must repent [publicly] before the church people.[117]

A year later, as we have already seen, Patriarch Aleksii, like a modern-day David to Krakhmalnikova's Nathan, did precisely as she prophesied (though without, however, confessing that he was indeed KGB agent "Drozdov," as Krakhmalnikova herself had deduced).

Fr. Gleb Yakunin. Among the better-known Orthodox dissidents are the laymen Boris Talantov, Anatoly Levitin-Krasnov, Vladimir

Osipov, Aleksandr Ogorodnikov, Vladimir Poresh, and Lev Regelson (who also, in 1980, recanted his "anti-Soviet" activities), and the priests Georgi Edelshtein, Dmitry Dudko (who, in 1980, also recanted, unexpectedly and under mysterious circumstances), and the saintly Aleksandr Men (who was brutally murdered in October 1990). But the most persistent and consistent advocate of religious freedom for the last quarter-century has been Fr. Gleb Yakunin.[118]

Fr. Gleb's career as a nonconformist priest began in earnest in November 1965 when he and another Moscow priest, Fr. Nikolai Eshliman, issued an "open letter" to Patriarch Aleksii I critical of the complicity of the Patriarchate's leaders in the weakening of the Church by the regime. A "declaration" the following month to Chairman Podgorny of the Presidium of the Supreme Soviet protested the illegality of restrictions on Church life enacted in 1961. This action vaulted the two priests into public visibility and effectively launched the religious movement for human rights in the Soviet Union. Five months later, in May 1966, Patriarch Aleksii I relieved them of their priestly duties and prohibited them from serving as clerics until they were willing to repent and change their ways.

Fr. Gleb's prophetic actions, however, did not come to an end. In 1974 he wrote critical letters to individual bishops of the Patriarchate. In April 1975, together with two Orthodox laymen, he protested directly to the Politburo the regime's decision that Soviet citizens must work on Pascha (Easter). Later that same year, Fr. Gleb and Lev Regelson dropped their ecumenical bombshell at the Nairobi Assembly of the World Council of Churches.[119] Their "message," firmly rooted in the "convergence" tradition of Orthodox ecumenism mentioned in chapter 1, sorely tested the commitment to universal human rights of that assembly.

In December 1976, Fr. Gleb led a small group of Russian Orthodox Christians in founding the Christian Committee for the Defense of Believers' Rights (CCDBR). This confessional organization was closely allied to the Moscow Helsinki Watch group set up to report on violations of the 1975 "Helsinki Agreement" on human rights, and to the more liberal, secular Democratic Movement for human rights in the Soviet Union. The example spurred other faith groups, especially Lithuanian Catholics, to form their own human-rights committees. The ecumenical concerns of the CCDBR also earned for this

Orthodox body the respect of activists from the Roman Catholic, Baptist, Pentecostal, and Adventist communities.[120]

Fr. Gleb's "report" to the CCDBR in August 1979—a detailed document lamenting the various facets of Russian Orthodox life under the Communists—led to his arrest by the KGB in November during a massive purge of dissidents that began, curiously, on the eve of the Soviet invasion of Afghanistan. Tried the following August on the familiar charge of "anti-Soviet" activities, Fr. Gleb was sentenced to five years in a labor camp and another five years of internal exile. This drew protests worldwide; among the protestors were a group of Soviet human-rights activists led by the late Andrei Sakharov and the British Council of Churches.

Having signed a pro forma document promising not to resume his "illegal" activities—he, of course, considered his activities legal—Fr. Gleb was released "early" from internment at Mikhail Gorbachev's behest in February 1987, along with 139 other prisoners of conscience. He also was reinstated as a priest by the Holy Synod of the Moscow Patriarchate and assigned to a parish near Moscow.

Fr. Gleb resumed his prophetic ministry almost immediately. He sent public letters to Gorbachev and the Supreme Soviet arguing on behalf of the necessary unity of legal and moral principles in social practice. During the millennial celebrations in the summer of 1988, he audaciously proposed that Patriarch Pimen resign his office since poor health, together with his demonstrable lack of will to lead, had rendered him incapable of functioning effectively. In 1989, the activist priest was the first signatory to a press release summoning the entire Russian Orthodox Church to support the creation of a new movement called "Church and Perestroika." This latest venture into the always dangerous waters of human rights would apply the goals of *perestroika* ("restructuring") to a Russian Orthodox Church desperately in need of restructuring from the top down.

As the political process grew increasingly democratic under Gorbachev, Fr. Gleb turned to public oratory and political involvement. In April 1990 he addressed a huge crowd assembled in Manege Square near the Kremlin, declaring that the time had come for God to lead the Russian people out of totalitarian Marxist-Leninist captivity, as Moses had liberated the Hebrews from totalitarian Egypt.[121] The following month, as a founding member of the Russian Christian

Democratic Party—but without the blessing of his diocesan bishop —he ran for parliament. He was elected by a wide majority as a "people's deputy" to the parliament of the RSFSR and subsequently to the Supreme Soviet of the RSFSR. He also became deputy chairman of the republic's Standing Committee on Freedom of Conscience, Religion, Philanthropy, and Charity. Thus in three years, this remarkable priest's odyssey took him from internal exile as a prisoner of conscience to the halls of political power.

In all his myriad public activities, Fr. Gleb Yakunin has consistently proclaimed the political and ecclesiastical necessity of religious freedom for every Soviet citizen. In his open letter to Patriarch Aleksii II in 1965, he rebuked an "active and growing group of 'evil pastors'" —a contingent of bishops and priests who "would like to turn the supreme ecclesiastical authority into a bureaucratic office, a sort of 'Ministry for the Affairs of the Orthodox Faith,' empowered to restrain and regulate the religious feelings of believing citizens."[122]

The initial declaration of the Christian Committee for the Defense of Believers' Rights (1976) extolled "the principle of freedom of conscience," particularly "the inalienable right of every man to believe in God and to live in accordance with his belief." Echoing the patristic strictures against religious coercion, Fr. Gleb also asserted that "any use of compulsion against people on the grounds that they are not Orthodox or belong to a different faith is contrary to the Christian spirit."[123] More than two decades later, Fr. Gleb sounded the same theme in his open letter to Gorbachev (August 1987), reminding the Soviet leader that it is "beyond dispute" that "freedom of conscience and freedom of confession" are among the "fundamental rights" guaranteed by a 1987 law governing all public discussions of issues of state.[124] The 1989 missive in which Fr. Gleb and others called for a "Church and Perestroika" movement proposed that the new movement "give legal help to believers, participate in the drafting and discussion of new legislation on freedom of conscience."[125]

It was only fitting that during the failed coup in August 1991, Fr. Gleb appeared on the balcony of the RSFSR parliament building with Boris Yeltsin and others. The dissident priest was willing to risk his life for freedom even in full sight of dozens of Soviet tanks with gun barrels trained on him. His latest foray into the battle for human rights —his role in the Russian parliament's special commission investigating the KGB files and the archives of the Communist Party—pits him against his original nemesis, the Patriarchate's leaders. At the previously mentioned press conference in Washington in March 1992, Fr. Gleb contended that Patriarch Aleksii II had attempted to thwart this research. A smear campaign against the priest's personal credibility seemed to be under way in Moscow and, with the help of some of the Patriarchate's most fervent American defenders, in the United States. While Fr. Gleb continues to insist that the Church must be restored to its proper prophetic role vis-à-vis the state, he harbors little hope that either Patriarch Aleksii II or the rest of the senior hierarchy of the Moscow Patriarchate will bring this to pass. Since June 1992, he has been declaring openly what he discovered months earlier in the KGB files: "They indicate that all the bishops were full-time KGB collaborators."[126]

Fr. Gleb continues to excoriate the bishops of his Church publicly even in the post-Communist era. In September 1993, for example, in the midst of a running battle with the Patriarchate over an amendment to the Law on the Freedom of Religions initiated by the patriarch himself, Fr. Gleb dismissed the hierarchy for its excessive "stagnation and conservatism."[127] Earlier that summer, on July 14, in an act of courage and defiance typical of this Orthodox prophet, Fr. Gleb cast the sole vote in the lower house of the Russian parliament against the proposed amendment: 167 "aye" votes to 1 "no." This legislation would have required foreign religious organizations and missionaries to obtain either the sponsorship of indigenous Russian religious organizations or "government accreditation." Although Patriarch Aleksii had, only a year earlier, assured a European journalist that "the Russian Orthodox Church does not seek to become the state Church," the proposed legislation would have granted to the Patriarchate (and to the other, much smaller Russian religious communities) a virtual veto power over potential rivals from the West.[128] Fr. Gleb denounced the restrictions as "discriminatory, anti-democratic and counter to international human rights."[129]

Just as the full legalization of the re-emergent Ukrainian Catholic Church will validate Russia's and Ukraine's commitment to religious freedom and democracy, so will the continued liberty and unhindered pursuit of the truth by Fr. Gleb, the foremost Russian Orthodox confessor of our time, signify the commitment of the Russian government and the Moscow Patriarchate alike to religious freedom and democracy on a personal level. Fr. Gleb was eventually vindicated in his opposition to the proposed legislative restrictions on foreign religious activity. President Boris Yeltsin refused to sign the bill and returned it to the parliament, and when he dissolved that body on September 21, the issue finally became moot. Ironically, as we have seen earlier in this chapter, this episode probably was the final blow to Fr. Gleb's active priesthood. But though he has been "defrocked" by the Holy Synod, Fr. Gleb is not about to fade into obscurity. The patriarch and the prophet will surely continue to wage their personal war.

THE PRICE OF PROPHECY

The Anglican scholar Trevor Beeson cautioned against attributing either vice or virtue to religious leaders in Communist lands, as if collaboration with and resistance to evil were clearly and easily distinguishable.[130] The caution is a valid one. Still I must conclude that the record of the Russian Orthodox Church in the Soviet era yields a remarkably sharp division into two camps. The behavior of most of the hierarchy of the Patriarchate and the behavior of the Orthodox "dissidents" in the struggle for religious freedom in the Soviet Union reflect not different ways of achieving common ends but conflicting values and apparently irreconcilable ways of construing the role of the Church in a hostile—specifically Communist—society.

The various modes of collaboration adopted by the patriarchs of Moscow after St. Tikhon and by most of the other prominent hierarchs displayed a spirit of servility that undermined the evangelistic mission of the Church and virtually reduced the Church of Christ to a propaganda tool of the Soviet state. To be sure, not all the collaborationist hierarchs consciously promoted Communist ideology or the "socialist" view of human rights with its unmistakably self-serving slant toward collectivism. But even those whose collaboration was of the interim or pragmatic sort pledged their loyalty to the regime, thereby fostering a distinctly untraditional spirituality of deception. Many were, and some still may be, willing to benefit institutionally from the persecution of other religious communities such as the Ukrainian Catholics.

The moral complexity of their motives notwithstanding, the public statements and actions of the Patriarchate's leaders on the whole promoted an agenda that is foreign to the Orthodox moral tradition. One may not consistently acquiesce in the suppression of religious freedom and nonetheless be deemed a defender of human rights or a faithful representative of the Orthodox doctrine of uncoerced religious belief.

Archbishop Khrizostom and **Metropolitan Kirill.** In this regard, Archbishop Khrizostom of Vilnius and perhaps Metropolitan Kirill of Smolensk may be the exceptions that prove the rule.

Khrizostom has emerged as a fearless defender of liberty. During the January 1991 Soviet crackdown in Lithuania, this Russian Orthodox archbishop apologized to the Lithuanians for the behavior of the Russian soldiers and protested the "forces that want to confirm Communist power in Lithuania," adding, "This is a shame for us Russians."[131] Archbishop Khrizostom is also the only bishop thus far to have publicly confessed that he was an agent of the KGB (codename "Restavrator")—for some eighteen years prior to 1990.[132] Ironically, he must have been recruited very soon after the Furov Report.

But even he seems unwilling to confront the enormity of his collaboration. In an interview published in the April 24, 1992, issue of *Russkaya Mysl'*, Khrizostom protested: "I cooperated [with the KGB], I signed things, I had regular meetings, I made reports. . . . But I was never an informer, I never denounced anyone." He also echoed the earlier self-justifications by Patriarch Aleksii by insisting that the bishops had to maintain contact with their political oppressors: "There was no other way."[133] There may be some merit to his fine distinction between superficial collaboration and betrayal of the Church. But Khrizostom proceeded in the same published interview to call dissident priest Georgi Edelshtein (whom he himself had ordained) a liar and to speak dismissively of Fr. Gleb Yakunin as "a politician," criticizing him for continuing to wear a priest's cassock and cross. Having demonstrated in this interview that he sometimes has feet of clay, Khrizostom nevertheless atoned for his collaborationist past and demonstrated his potential for genuine prophecy when confronted with the moral challenge of a lifetime in Vilnius.

Another relatively young bishop, one who arrived on the scene after the Furov years, may be the point man for a new generation of maverick bishops who have firm commitments to both the religious and the political establishment. Metropolitan Kirill Gundaev of Smolensk and Kaliningrad was the reputed author of the new Church *ustav* (law) passed at the June 1988 *sobor* and approved by the government of the RSFSR in a slightly different version (civil statute) in March 1991. Generally respected even within the Russian émigré community, Kirill by the late 1980s appeared to be beginning to exercise a prophetic ministry abroad as well as at home.

In an impressive essay on *perestroika* and ethics published in the World Council of Churches' *Ecumenical Review* in 1988, Metropolitan Kirill issued the familiar summons to "a new international moral order," a summons that may, amidst the appeals to natural law and absolute moral standards, have been little more than a faintly disguised call for world socialism.[134] But he concluded the piece by describing the final scene from a new film, *Repentance,* by the Georgian producer T. Abuladze. In this scene a woman, when told that there is no church on a particular street, laments: "What is this street for then, if it does not lead to a church?" Kirill went one step further:

> The film reminded us of the tragic events in the recent past of my country and helped many of us to realize that without the rejection of untruth, however painful that rejection may be, there cannot be change for the better either in the present or the future.[135]

A September 1990 "roundtable" discussion published in the Moscow journal *Dialog* included this pointed remark by Kirill: "We need a clear law so that we point our finger into the text and tell those [Soviet] officials, 'Do you see what is written in the law? All right, then, act in accordance with it!' "[136]

The trust that Kirill has cultivated among those devout Orthodox and others who have come to know him at ecumenical gatherings as a sincere Orthodox leader serves as a healthful reminder that the Patriarchate itself has never been beyond redemption. Metropolitan Kirill continues to sound an upbeat note: "[T]he Soviet state is changing; its relations with the Church are changing, and much is becoming different in the Church herself."[137]

Muddying the waters somewhat is the fact that in November 1989 Kirill was appointed chairman of the Patriarchate's Department of

External Church Relations. At the March 1992 press conference on the KGB files, Fr. Gleb said that the officials of this department in the Soviet era were usually those most trusted by the regime to advance its interests. Kirill's KGB code-name ("Mikhailov") was deduced by Russian journalists in 1992. It should come as no surprise that Kirill has thus far declined to confirm that charge.

Patriarch Aleksii II. The present patriarch remains an enigma. Despite an embarrassing history of obsequiousness to political authority second only in his generation to that of Patriarch Pimen, Patriarch Aleksii II finally emerged as his own man during the August 1991 coup attempt. For the first time since the saintly Patriarch Tikhon challenged the Bolsheviks at the dawn of the Soviet era, a Russian patriarch openly defied the power of the Communist Party, even with its military forces gathered to assert its political will.

But Aleksii still sometimes reverts to familiar ploys from his darker days. During his brief visit to the United States in November 1991, he pressed Undersecretary of State Arnold Kantor to make some changes in the Voice of America's Russian-language broadcasts. The patriarch complained specifically about the programs produced by Fr. Victor Potapov, a priest of the Russian Orthodox Church Outside Russia, charging him with undue bias against the Patriarchate.[138] The ramifications of this extraordinary intervention into U.S. governmental affairs—vigorously denied by the patriarch himself, according to Fr. Rodion Kondratick, chancellor of the Orthodox Church in America—were not lost on Fr. Victor's Orthodox jurisdiction, whose opposition to the patriarch is unrelenting. In a controversial decision announced in May 1990, the Russian Orthodox Church Outside Russia—already labeled "schismatic" by the Moscow Patriarchate and the Orthodox Church in America—had accepted under its "protection" several renegade Russian parishes from the Moscow Patriarchate and organized them into an alternative jurisdiction known as the "Free Russian Orthodox Church."[139] Soon after Patriarch Aleksii's visit to the U.S. State Department, the émigré Church published an epistle that claimed that some of the members of these dissident churches have been harassed by the secular authorities at the instigation of "representatives" of the Moscow Patriarchate.[140] The so-called schismatics are on the defensive in both Russia and the United States.

And yet Aleksii seems strangely intimidated by the sudden rise of the extreme right both in society and in the Patriarchate itself. Even so determined a defender of Aleksii as Dmitry Pospielovsky has publicly expressed his frustration over the patriarch's hesitance to distance himself publicly from the anti-Semitic ravings that Metropolitan Ioann Snychev of St. Petersburg and Ladoga has published in neo-fascist, or "Red-Brown," periodicals such as *Sovietskaya Rossiya*. Pospielovsky insists, correctly, that the patriarch must resolve "to take a stand, to condemn extremism, racialism, and ban dissemination of hatred by any groups within the Church."[141] Hoover Institution scholar John B. Dunlop suggests pessimistically that Aleksii "is unlikely to take action against an overtly racist metropolitan because at least some, and perhaps many, bishops share Ioann's views, and because his ideas are extremely popular in 'red-brown' circles in Russia."[142] Ioann has an additional mark in his favor: the secret Furov document in 1974 included Ioann among the third group of bishops, those mavericks who were the least dependable to the Soviet regime.[143]

But positive signs of the patriarch's renewed courage have appeared. Aleksii apparently has prevented Ioann from printing his accusations of an international anti-Russian Judaic-Masonic conspiracy and his feeble defense of the infamous *Protocols of the Elders of Zion* in the pages of the official organs of the Moscow Patriarchate. In an interview published in the April 17-24, 1994, issue of *Moscow News,* Aleksii finally declared that the position of Ioann "troubles many," that Ioann "cannot speak for the entire Church," and that the next meeting of the Holy Synod "will discuss how important it is for a church hierarch to weigh every word he utters." Aleksii also implicitly criticized Ioann's anti-Semitism: "The Russian Orthodox Church is free from racial prejudice — it should be clear to everyone that to fan the fire of inter-ethnic division in our very complicated times is insanity [*bezumie* in the original Russian]."[144] Unless he makes a cleaner break with Ioann, however, and actively attempts to quarantine the metropolitan's poisonous influence in the Church, Patriarch Aleksii II, erstwhile collaborator with the Communist left, may soon be perceived as a tacit collaborator with the neo-fascist right!

A Cloud of Witnesses. Among those Russian Orthodox who still maintain some ties to the Moscow patriarchate are vocal, nonconformist clergy and laity who, though diverse in their personal backgrounds and ways of witnessing, have a common devotion to the principle of religious freedom. Theirs is not merely a theoretical proposition. Every "dissident" who went public with his or her protest against Soviet oppression—and even some of those distinctively apolitical dissidents such as Zoya Krakhmalnikova—suffered grievously at the hands of the Soviet regime.

Their witness has been, on the whole, noble, courageous, prophetic, exemplary, and in accordance with the best that Orthodox Christianity has to offer on the question of personal religious freedom. Like the Christian martyrs and confessors in all ages, they have remained faithful to their prophetic calling, willing to pay the full price of prophecy in pursuit of the virtue of religious freedom—the loss of their own freedom.

3

The Romanian
Religio-Political Symbiosis

As the survivors sifted through the rubble of the toppled Communist regime in Romania, the magnitude of the evil that ended in December 1989 became clear. Nicolae Ceauşescu, whom the exuberant revolutionaries executed together with his wife, Elena, on Christmas day, was obsessed by a pathological, neo-Stalinist vision of nationalistic Communism. It was, however, a vision that drew upon a longstanding characteristic of Romanian political culture. Nationalism and politics have been two sides of the same coin in Romania since the birth of the modern state in the mid-nineteenth century, and perhaps as far back as the preceding centuries of Ottoman Turkish oppression. A fervent Romanian nationalism has always been a prerequisite for political success.

There is another essential ingredient in this political culture: religion. Before the Communists seized full control of the government in December 1947, the majority Romanian Orthodox Church and the state were so closely bound, the Orthodox ethos so integrated into the national culture, that the terms "Orthodox" and "Romanian" were virtually interchangeable. This kind of symbiotic harmony between Orthodoxy and popular culture was, if not unique, at least equal in intensity to that which prevailed in the neighboring Balkan states of Serbia, Bulgaria, and Greece.

Orthodox leaders, including clergy, monastics, and laymen, contributed greatly to the emergence of the modern Romanian state. They fought the Turks in the armies of St. Ştefan the Great in the fifteenth

89

century and Michael the Brave in the sixteenth century. They assisted in the unification of the principalities of Wallachia and Moldavia in 1859 and in the establishment of the independent Romanian state in 1877. Before the unification of Transylvania with the other Romanian provinces in 1918, some Romanian Orthodox nationalists such as Metropolitan Andreiu Şaguna of Sibiu fought valiantly for the rights of Romanians and promoted an independent Romanian culture under the oppressive Hungarians who ruled Transylvania within the Austro-Hungarian Empire. Şaguna's moderate mystical nationalism was rooted in the conviction that Romanian Orthodoxy was the religious expression of the "Rumanian soul" and hence the source of national progress.[1]

More virulent versions of mystical religious nationalism also appeared more often than most Romanian Orthodox Christians would care to admit. Though likely to extol the virtues of the ethnic Romanian, these were generally cast in the darker shades of xenophobia, and particularly anti-Semitism. The Legion of St. Michael the Archangel, an ostensibly religio-political movement between the two world wars in this century, represents the nadir of such neo-pagan nationalism.[2] Church-state relations under the Communist dictatorship perpetuated the trend.

Nicolae Ceauşescu, who came to power in 1965, capitalized on this remarkable symbiosis. He subjugated the leadership of the Romanian Orthodox Church more thoroughly than his predecessors. He also diminished the potency of Romanian religious nationalism by distorting his own personal significance beyond all measure and virtually destroying whatever national unity his people enjoyed.

Europe had not witnessed such an aggrandizement of personal power and cult of personality since the heyday of Adolf Hitler and Josef Stalin. None of the modern Romanian kings, including the power-hungry Carol II (1919-40), ever acquired the royal authority that Ceauşescu exerted over his people. Among recent world leaders, only Kim Il-sung of North Korea, who served as a model for the ambitious Ceauşescu, enjoyed a similarly forced national adulation.

The mythic proportions of this cult were evident in Ceauşescu's self-conscious identification with the great heroes of the Romanian past. Explicitly mentioned from time to time were the ancient Dacian kings Burebista and Decebal, who opposed the Roman legions; the medieval Christian princes St. Ştefan the Great and Michael the Brave;

and Prince Alexander Ion Cuza, who in 1859 became the first leader of the modern Romanian state. The officially sanctioned title *Conducător* ("Leader") may be traced back to the 1940s, when it was routinely applied to the fascist dictator Ion Antonescu. Other terms of praise for Antonescu that Eugen Weber has catalogued—namely, "visionary, philosopher, apostle, father, saviour, synthesis of Latin genius, personification of Daco-Roman tradition, and superman of dizzying simplicity"—were also commonly addressed to Ceauşescu.[3]

Nicolae Ceauşescu surpassed all his Romanian precursors in one respect: like a Romanian Bonaparte, he brought his entire family into the inner circles of political power. His crude, pretentious wife, Elena, emerged as second-in-command, presiding over the development of science and technology in Romania, although her credentials as a "scientist" apparently consisted only of numerous unearned "awards" and academy memberships that she coerced scientific and educational institutions into giving her.[4] Their son Nicu, a sadistic hedonist and ne'er-do-well, was secretary of the Union of Communist Youth and presumed heir to the Communist throne that his father had fashioned. Captured after his parents were executed by the revolutionary interim government known as the Frontul Salvarii Naţionale (FSN, or "Front for National Salvation"), he now resides alternately in prison and in a hospital in Sibiu. Numerous Ceauşescu relatives occupied other important positions in the Party or in the government. If Stalin tried to create "socialism in one country," a critic has observed wryly, Ceauşescu was busy promoting "socialism in one family."[5]

Even before his violent downfall, Ceauşescu's bubble had burst. The closet "liberal"—in the self-deluded minds of many Westerners—had at last been exposed as an old-fashioned Stalinist. His promise of "reform" after he assumed power had been as insubstantial as the myth that he was another Tito-like "maverick" in the Communist orbit. By the late 1980s the idol of a nation had become the target of an unrelenting volley of criticism from abroad and the butt of jokes—told secretly, of course—at home.

A New Dark Age

The *Conducător* had led Romania backward into a new dark age of cultural barbarism, political tyranny, and economic primitivism. But as the inexorable tide of democracy flooded Eastern Europe, finally in December 1989 the last reactionary hold-out in the Soviet bloc was washed clean. The people of Romania—first the Hungarian Reformed minority in Timişoara and subsequently the ethnic Romanian, generally Orthodox, majority—finally reached the limit of their patient servility to a government that freely massacred its people and even refused to allow the surviving relatives to bury their dead.[6]

Ceauşescu, like his reform-minded Soviet nemesis Mikhail Gorbachev, had launched a three-pronged program to "improve" his country's standing in the world. But unlike Gorbachev's troika of *glasnost', perestroika,* and *demokratizatsiya,* Ceauşescu's madcap scheme of "systematization," "modernization," and "civilization" forced Romania into a suffocating political and economic straitjacket.[7] Ceauşescu envisioned a wholesale reconstruction of the Romanian Communist way of life. Approximately 8,000 rural villages and hamlets, he announced in March 1988, were to be razed and their five to eight million inhabitants shunted into proletarian communities in high-rise apartment buildings; the remaining 5,000 to 6,000 rural settlements would be reorganized into some 550 "agro-industrial" centers under tight state control.

In addition, Ceauşescu planned to cut out the heart of old Bucharest to make way for a new civic center laden with monuments to himself and his accomplishments. This insane scheme—reminiscent of Nero's attempt to rebuild ancient Rome or Hitler's vision of a new Berlin for the Third Reich—together with construction of new modern industrial sites such as hydraulic works would have destroyed hundreds of cultural treasures and religious sites, including scores of Orthodox churches and monasteries. As a down payment on this modernized society, Ceauşescu announced in March 1989 that Romania had repaid its $21 billion foreign debt—the first Communist government ever to do so.

Industrialization and urbanization—twin staples in classic Communist ideology—thus secured in Ceauşescu a champion without peer. His proletarianism was an ideologue's dream but a nation's nightmare. To create virtually *de novo* his truly civilized Romania, Ceauşescu was prepared "to radically wipe out the major differences between towns and villages, . . . to more powerfully homogenise our socialist society, to create a single worker people."[8] This fierce, anti-rural obsession turned Pol Pot's equally maniacal anti-urban primitivism on its head. What the Cambodian and Romanian dictators shared, however, was a single-minded ruthlessness in constructing their socialist "civilizations."

Horror stories from Ceauşescu's Romania filled the Western media in the waning months of his regime. "Hundreds of thousands of urban property owners have already lost their houses," reported Dinu Giurescu in a book sponsored by the World Monuments Fund and published shortly before the December 1989 uprising.[9] The two-million-member Hungarian minority, mostly in Transylvania, suffered grievously from a "homogenization" policy that forbade public use of their native language. Rationing of food began in 1983, and after the downfall of the regime severe shortages persisted in this fertile land.[10] In June 1989 Communist Hungary accused Romania of building a wire barrier along a 188-mile section of the Romanian-Hungarian border[11]—an intra-Communist "iron curtain" at a time when the border barrier between Hungary and free Austria had been dismantled. What was once, to use Walter Bacon's apt metaphors, the Soviet bloc's "breadbasket and gas station" had become an economic basket case with an official ideology that had run out of gas.[12]

Perhaps the most shocking features of this pathetic society were revealed in American media reports in 1990. A January edition of ABC-TV's "20-20" disclosed that as many as a third of the babies born in hospitals in Bucharest and Constanţa during the last few months of the Ceauşescu regime had contracted the deadly AIDS virus, owing to repeated reuse of scarce medical supplies such as hypodermic needles. In June the *Washington Post* exposed the many state-run orphanages, where 15,000 to 30,000 abandoned children were living in sub-human conditions—again the product of Ceauşescu's draconian eugenics program.[13]

To describe Romania under Ceauşescu as a police state would be a grave understatement. Romania was caught in the iron grip of one of the most effective thought-control networks ever devised. If Ion Pacepa, the former chief of intelligence, can be believed, so pervasive was the Securitate (secret police) and so effective was its intelligence-gathering that virtually nothing—not even the sexual behavior of foreign diplomats and their wives—escaped Ceauşescu's or his wife's personal scrutiny. Instead of the anticipated "Prague spring" of socialist diversity and fuller personal expression, or Communism "with a human face," Ceauşescu plunged his people into a "Bucharest winter" of discontent, a fearfully inhumane society where the regime had, in Vladimir Tismaneanu's words, a "perpetual fixation on internal and external enemies as a basic driving force."[14]

Amnesty International described a "persistent pattern" from 1980 to 1987, wherein the regime imprisoned at least hundreds of persons "either for the non-violent exercise of their right to free expression or for attempting to leave the country illegally."[15] Only public speech and activities that advanced Ceauşescu's peculiar version of Communism—including his own cult of personality—were tolerated by the government. Dissidents of every stripe—religious believers, secular intellectuals, striking workers, Party members—were systematically searched and incarcerated. What remained in public forums was the obsequious cant of those who would survive the terror by praising the Ceauşescu regime. Historian Walter Bacon coined the term "sycophantocracy" to describe the political minions in Romania.[16] This word could apply equally, as this chapter will illustrate, to the behavior of most of the Romanian Orthodox hierarchy.

When the dam holding back the pent-up frustrations of the people finally gave way in December 1989, the Ceauşescu dynasty was swept away with dizzying speed. Virtually no one inside or outside Romania had thought such a change was possible. A nation that had been cowed into abject submission to Communist authority suddenly found its courage and managed to rid itself of a terrible curse.

To be sure, the shameful political and social legacy that Ceauşescu bequeathed to his native land may yet prove quite durable. The post-revolution Front for National Salvation government consolidated its power with a surprisingly massive victory in the national election in May 1990. But the election was not a wholly convincing example of democracy at work; it was at least in part the result of the FSN's pre-election intimidation of its chief political rivals and its monopoly of the national broadcast media. Seven months later, in a speech celebrating the first anniversary of the "December Revolution," President Ion Iliescu, a former Communist, praised the Church for its "important role" as "one of the factors of cohesion and spiritual regeneration of the Romanian society."[17] But such occasional speeches are hardly reassuring to most veteran human-rights advocates in Romania.

By the end of 1990, key members of the original 250-person FSN central committee such as vice-president Claudiu Iordache had resigned in frustration at the perceived incompetence of the government in reforming the crippled economy or to protest the hauntingly familiar tactics of suppressing dissent. When ex-king Mihai was swiftly "expelled" from his native land in December 1990, during a hastily arranged Christmas visit, diverse political groups in Romania lodged protests with the FSN.

Despite proud boasts by the Front that the dreaded Securitate has been eliminated, vestiges remain. The Securitate was officially dissolved on December 30, 1989, and replaced by the more innocuous-sounding Servicul Român de Informaţi ("Romanian Information Service"), or SRI. But pockets of determined and perhaps dangerous pro-Ceauşescu resistance remained. The ringleaders of the "coal miners" from the Jiu Valley who brutally suppressed a student-led protest in Bucharest against the FSN government in June 1990 were widely suspected within the Romanian-American community of being thinly disguised Securitate agents.

Romania's status as a "liberated" ex-Communist state remained in doubt through 1991 and 1992. Fear was widespread among distinguished former dissidents such as Doina Cornea of Cluj—president of the Antitotalitarian Democratic Forum—that their more or less spontaneous "revolution" had been "stolen" from the people by the ostensibly born-again "democrats" of the FSN, who nevertheless remained Communists at heart.[18] Another prominent reformer, Nicolae Manolescu, professor of literature at the University of Bucharest and a key leader of the Civic Alliance formed in November 1990, sounded a different alarm: "We are not very far from a fascist-style dictatorship," he said in 1991. Manolescu viewed the FSN as a group of bureaucrats and political hangers-on who were not committed to democracy and who feared a genuine transformation of society.[19]

Even the small steps toward democratization in the first half of 1992 proved short-lived. The local elections in February gave the opposition Democratic Convention Alliance 24 per cent of the national vote to the FSN's 33 per cent, and the *New York Times* a few weeks later quoted a spokesman for the U.S. State Department as saying that these elections conformed to "generally accepted international standards."[20] In March, Petre Roman, the former prime minister who had resigned the previous October when coal miners staged raucous protests in Bucharest, wrested control of the FSN from his archnemesis Iliescu at a national convention. President Iliescu then had to create a new splinter party of neo-Communists, which he named, unimaginatively, the Democratic Front for National Salvation (DFSN).

But the newfound hopes of democratic reformers were dashed in the national elections held on September 27, 1992, when Iliescu and his DFSN emerged with substantial pluralities. Iliescu himself easily prevailed in a two-man runoff election for president on October 11 with Dr. Emil Constantinescu, a professor at the University of Bucharest and presidential candidate of the Democratic Convention Alliance. The DFSN has since formed a surprisingly stable majority coalition government in the parliament with several of the smaller ultra-nationalist parties.

Iliescu's consolidation of power, however, has exacted a heavy toll from post-Communist Romania's fragile democracy. Public dissembling, extreme partisanship, and suppression of dissent seem, increasingly, to characterize the Iliescu-DFSN government. During a public interview at the Romanian Embassy in Washington, D.C., on April 20, 1993, Iliescu brushed aside my question whether his government was actively discriminating against religious minorities, particularly the evangelical Protestants. Every religious group, he insisted—contrary to reliable reports from the Romanian evangelicals themselves—was quite pleased with his national religious policy. In an interview with a Polish journalist on January 31, 1994, Iliescu offered a self-serving apologia for the continuing presence of ex-Communists in "the political and economic life" of Romania. "Almost the entire intellectual elite in Romania was in the [Communist] party," he claimed, so there was nothing to be gained by checking dossiers for erstwhile Communist affiliations.[21]

More alarming was the arrest of Nicolae Andrei, a Romanian journalist, in Craiova on February 14, 1994, reportedly for publishing two articles deemed personally offensive to President Iliescu.[22] Whether the president himself ordered this action or the Police General Inspectorate merely acted on its own initiative, the incident has had a chilling effect on freedom of the press in a country with no living memory of a truly independent fourth estate. Observers both in Romania and in the West still have every reason to wonder whether any real solutions to Romania's continuing political woes are in the offing.

The Church, together with the nation it serves, thus has to come to grips with a grievous political and moral legacy. As this chapter will demonstrate, the public moral witness of the Romanian Orthodox Church on issues of religious freedom and human rights during the past four decades compels us to hope that the past is not prologue.

Subjugation of the Orthodox Church

Western observers have sometimes viewed the behavior of the Romanian Orthodox patriarchs through rose-colored glasses. When Patriarch Justinian died in 1977 and was succeeded by Metropolitan Justin of Moldova, the highly respected Keston College quarterly *Religion in Communist Lands* said, "It is believed that he [Justin] would do well to follow the policies of his predecessor."[23] Admirers usually cite Justinian's role in preserving monasticism, improving the education of the clergy, establishing internationally respected theological journals, and generally maintaining the Church as an integral dimension of the lives of the vast majority of the Romanian people. He is cherished in the memory of most Romanians I met in Bucharest, Iaşi, and Cluj as the Orthodox leader who preserved the Church from the wrath of the Communists. His image is painted on the walls of several monastery churches and refectories, as if he had been canonized.

But the whole story of Church-state relations during Justinian's reign is far more sobering. Long before Nicolae Ceauşescu mounted his assault on traditional Romanian culture, his Communist predecessors succeeded with surprising alacrity in co-opting the hierarchy of the Romanian Orthodox Church. The post-war Communist regime turned the erstwhile symbiotic partner of the state into its abject slave.

The chronicle begins shortly after the Communist-dominated "Popular Front" (Blocul Partidelor Democrate) established a coalition government in March 1945. Patriarch Nicodim Munteanu encouraged the people to support the new government while the government took pains to emphasize the "Orthodox" lineage of several of its principals. Prime Minister Petru Groza (1945-52) was the son of an Orthodox priest and supposedly a practicing Orthodox Christian. The new minister of education was himself an Orthodox priest, and the minister of propaganda a professor of theology. Groza pledged more generous government subsidies to the clergy, provided they offered greater support to the government.[24]

By the end of 1947, the pressures upon the Church had become less subtle. Previously the membership of diocesan assemblies convened for the election of bishops had been determined by popular election within each diocese. Now a new law provided that members of the National Church Assembly (a membership carefully monitored by the government) and ministers of state and their undersecretaries who were also members of the diocese would constitute a *de jure* majority in the diocesan assemblies. The three episcopal elections in November 1947 accordingly produced bishops who had the regime's seal of approval; the Communist newspaper *Universul* acclaimed them "hierarchs of the people."[25] Then, in December, the priest-monk Ioan Marina was, with uncommon haste, consecrated metropolitan of Moldova and Suceava. This Church region, with its see in Iaşi, has become in the twentieth century the penultimate assignment for all the patriarchs except Patriarch Miron Cristea (1925-39); Marina was obviously being groomed for the highest Church post. In February 1948 Patriarch Nicodim died—allegedly poisoned by the Communists—and in May Justinian was "elected" patriarch, after Moscow reportedly insisted that no other candidate was acceptable. As we shall see, Justinian's enthronement address made it immediately clear why the new patriarch was favored by the Groza and Stalin regimes.

Meanwhile, the Popular Front had "collapsed," King Mihai had fled the country, and the People's Republic of Romania had been proclaimed on December 30, 1947. Within a month all clergy had been forced to take an oath of allegiance to the new Communist regime in the presence of the government's "minister of cults"—the cabinet-level position charged with supervision and control of religious bodies. The oath for bishops was virtually identical to that of the oath for state employees:

As a servant of God, as a man and a citizen, I swear to be true to the People and to defend the Rumanian People's Republic against its enemies abroad and at home. I swear to respect that I shall not allow my subordinates to undertake or to take part, and that I myself shall not undertake or take part, in any action likely to affect public order and the integrity of the Rumanian People's Republic. So help me God.[26]

The legal restructuring of Church-state relations proceeded apace. The Education Reform Act of August 1948 eliminated "all sectarian or private schools of whatever nature," replacing them with schools "organized exclusively by the State on the principle of unification of structure" and "based on democratic, popular and realist scientific principles." Any violator of this thorough secularization of education would be subject to a sentence of five to ten years of hard labor and "confiscation of all his property."[27]

Even more devastating was the Grand National Assembly's Decree No. 177, which established, also in August 1948, a "General Regime of Religion." This document prescribed detailed regulations of every aspect of religious life and organization, not with a view toward the "separation" of Church and state but rather to lend legitimacy to the state's stranglehold on the churches. The elastic clause that undermined any guarantee of religious freedom was the requirement that the religious bodies function in ways "not contrary to the Constitution, security, public order or morality." Accordingly, the state now insisted, for example, that hierarchs assume office only upon approval by the Communist presidium,[28] and that "clergy with an anti-democratic attitude may be struck off State pay-rolls, [temporarily] or for good."[29]

The inaugural year of the new social order was no honeymoon for the Church. Christian youth organizations were suppressed. The government seized ecclesial buildings, libraries, and equipment. Religious publications were restricted, and the name "Jesus Christ" was prohibited in government organs. The Orthodox welfare societies were displaced by strictly lay committees directly responsible to the regime. In October an entire denomination—the Greek Catholic, or "Uniate," Church—was, like its counterpart in Ukraine in 1946, dissolved at the behest of the regime; its twelve bishops were imprisoned, and its roughly 1.5 million faithful were forcibly integrated into the national Orthodox Church. The "Lord's Army"—a lay evangelistic movement within the Orthodox Church—was the target of an all-out attack by the government, reportedly with the cooperation of the Orthodox hierarchy.

The second full year of the regime brought complete victory to the Communists. When the winter term of the Orthodox Theological Institute in Bucharest began in January 1949, special "missionary courses" had entered the curriculum to steer future priests toward a Marxist-Leninist social outlook. In February, the government deposed fifteen Orthodox priests. When, in June, a conference of national religious leaders including Orthodox hierarchs issued the first public denials of religious persecution, the Romanian Orthodox Church obviously had reached the point of no return:

> Not one of the faithful, not a single priest, has been punished in the Rumanian People's Republic for his religious belief or for being loyal to his faith. Only those who have placed themselves in the service of the imperialist interests and have intrigued against the Republic, its independence and its sovereignty, have been punished.
>
> We shall not cease to carry on the work of enlightenment of our clergy and our faithful, urging them to place themselves in the service of the people and of the regime of the people's democracy.[30]

According to an estimate in a Romanian Orthodox émigré publication, from 1948 until the first general amnesty announced by Communist dictator Gheorghe Gheorghiu-Dej (1952-65) in 1964, more than a million Romanians suffered in Communist prisons or concentration camps, of whom at least 200,000 were murdered by government agents or died as a direct result of physical torture or exile. Included in the latter figure were thirty-three Orthodox bishops and priests who can be identified by name, twelve Greek Catholic clergy, and seventeen Roman Catholic clergy.[31]

From the early years of the Communist regime, the Romanian Orthodox Church, like its counterpart in the Soviet Union, had to endure periodic waves of persecution, the accommodationist policies of its patriarchs notwithstanding. Between 1958 and 1964—years roughly coterminous with Nikita Khrushchev's crackdown on religion in the Soviet Union—the government of Gheorghiu-Dej arrested some 1,500 clergy, monastics, and laymen and ruthlessly went after the Orthodox monasteries. The government closed the three monastic seminaries and at least half of the 200 monasteries. The

Orthodox hierarchs were compelled to send about 4,000 monks and nuns back "into the world" and to forbid persons under the age of 60 to enter monastic life.[32]

When Gheorghiu-Dej began in earnest to chart an independent course for Romania on the international scene, he relaxed the persecution of the Church and released most of the "political criminals" who had been arrested for religious reasons. The high-water mark in Church-state relations was reached under Gheorghiu-Dej's successor in 1968, when Nicolae Ceauşescu, seeking to consolidate his power as head of state (since 1965), officially received the leadership of the Patriarchate and acknowledged the positive role that the Orthodox Church had played in the development of the modern Romanian state. At the end of that year, the *Conducător* was photographed—for the first and only time in the history of Communist Romania—with the leaders of all the officially recognized religious bodies in Romania.[33] The funeral of Ceauşescu's father in April 1972 was conducted according to Orthodox liturgical tradition and announced to the nation by Romanian radio. Also auspicious for the Church was its inclusion in May 1974 in the Socialist Unity Front, a national "advisory" organization.[34]

But this respite proved short-lived. Widespread oppression of religion resumed in 1979 and gathered a formidable momentum from 1984 until the downfall of Ceauşescu. The dictator destroyed some three dozen old churches and monasteries in Bucharest alone, ostensibly in the name of "modernization." Orthodox clergy and lay dissidents, together with other religious believers, were regularly arrested, imprisoned, and usually banished from the country. The best known of these involuntary expatriates was Fr. Gheorghe Calciu-Dumitreasa, who arrived in the United States in August 1985 after enduring two prison terms that totaled twenty-one years. (We shall hear more of him later.) More subtle forms of oppression included a strict rationing of Bibles and liturgical books that kept the supply well below the ever-increasing demand; frequent interrogations of seminarians by government agents; the punitive reassignment of spiritually exemplary clergy; discrimination against Christians in higher education and certain careers; and the intimidating presence of government agents at meetings of the clergy.[35]

In short, the Romanian Orthodox Church enjoyed some privileges that the Greek Catholic Church obviously could not, as long as it remained officially non-existent and absorbed in the Orthodox Church. But the Romanian Orthodox Church as a whole had to endure its own Calvary in the Communist kingdom of Nicolae Ceauşescu.

FORGING A NEW SOCIAL ETHIC

Twenty-seven bishops currently serve some 19 million baptized faithful in the Patriarchate of Romania. Five of these bishops administer the five metropolitanates that comprise the territory of the nation. Most prominent is the patriarch, who serves also as archbishop of Bucharest and metropolitan of Ungro-Wallachia, the southeastern region of Romania. Second in prominence and historically the heir-apparent to the Patriarchal throne is the archbishop of Iaşi and metropolitan of Moldova and Bukovina, the northeastern region of Romania.

Two bishops are permanently assigned to archdioceses outside the country. These hierarchs serve the émigré Romanian communities in Western Europe and North America.

Furov's categories might seem irrelevant to the Romanian hierarchy. Only one bishop may be classified with confidence as a non-collaborator with the Ceauşescu regime: **Bishop Gherasim Cocosel**, who was summarily retired to a monastery long before the conflagration in December 1989.[36] Two others showed some degree of resistance. **Bishop Justinian Chira**, who was transferred to the see in Baia Mare in 1990, is held in high esteem by his own clergy for his unquestioned spirituality. The only other bishop from the Communist era who earned any measure of respect from the clergy and people for his challenge—albeit belated—to the Ceauşescu regime is **Metropolitan Nicolae Corneanu** of Banat.

During the early stages of the public protests in Timişoara beginning on December 16, 1989, Nicolae, whose diocese includes Timişoara, was visiting Jerusalem. When he returned to Romania on December 18—four days before Ceauşescu's ouster—he remained in Bucharest but was in "constant communication" with the clergy in his diocese. When I interviewed Nicolae in Bucharest in September

1990, he said that he had signaled his approval for his clergy and the laity to join the Timişoara demonstrations, which were orchestrated by the Hungarian Reformed community on behalf of their beleaguered pastor, Lazlo Tökeş. This decision involved considerable risk to Nicolae's own security and may be viewed as a singular act of courage.

Since then Nicolae has continued to demonstrate his new reformist perspective. He was the first Romanian Orthodox hierarch to return to the Greek Catholics church buildings they previously owned, including the cathedral in Lugoj. In November 1990 he officially endorsed the so-called Civic Alliance based in Bucharest, "being convinced," he wrote, "that it will support the values of faith, humanity and democracy" and "ensure the regaining of national identity and dignity."[37] Metropolitan Nicolae is also the only holdover from the Ceauşescu era who has publicly repented for his own moral compromises. In an interview published in the *Romanian Orthodox Church News* early in 1991, Nicolae said,

> Here I must confess that as a hierarch, I have witnessed for years many events repugnant to my Christian convictions, without however acting according to the promptings of my conscience. Regrets are obviously superfluous, yet the clear conscience of past guilt compells me at least not to fall again into such pitfalls.[38]

All the hierarchs, other than these three, who reigned during the Communist era collaborated to one degree or another, with no visible signs of resistance. Most of these would appear to be what we have called "ideological" or, at best, "pragmatic" collaborators.

The Principals

Four hierarchs played key roles in forging the official response of the Patriarchate of Romania to the Communist challenge. Another who was consecrated to the episcopate after the December 1989 uprising promises a fresh approach to Church-state issues.

1. **Patriarch Justinian**—*Apostle of Synthesis.* Though not well known in the Christian West, Patriarch Justinian, who reigned from 1948 until 1977, was one of the most innovative Church leaders in the twentieth century. Unfortunately for the spiritual integrity of the Ro-

manian Orthodox Church, his theological and pastoral creativity forged a unique synthesis of Marxist-Leninism and Orthodox Christianity.

Born into a peasant family in the Oltenia region in 1901, Fr. Ioan Marina served in village parishes after his ordination to the priesthood in 1924. Like the Catholic worker-priests in Western Europe and the theologians of liberation in Latin America decades later, Fr. Ioan was troubled by the poverty of the peasants, and he sought to involve the Church more deeply in the social problems of these people.

In 1930 he published an influential essay entitled *Cooperaţie şi Creşt-inism* ("Cooperation and Christianity"), which drew upon the moral witness of the Bible and the Church Fathers to justify efforts by the clergy to improve the material status of the people. Gradually he moved toward a full-blown socialist worldview, becoming a vocal critic of the socio-economic conditions in interwar Romania. He focused much of his ire on what he perceived as the concentration of wealth in a shrinking social elite and the corresponding impoverishment of the peasants and proletarians.[39]

Fr. Ioan had no qualms, therefore, about providing sanctuary from the right-wing pre-war government to the Communist Party chieftain Gheorghe Gheorghiu-Dej, even as his family was shielding another prominent Communist, Gheorghe Apostol.[40] It was hardly surprising when Fr. Ioan—who in 1945 took the monastic name Justinian— suddenly became patriarch of all Romania in 1948. Having been consecrated a suffragan bishop in 1945 and "elected" only two years later to the important metropolitanate of Moldova and Suceava, Justinian had risen with lightning-like speed to the pinnacle of spiritual authority in Romania, assisted by the grateful Communist whom he had sheltered and who had now seized control of the government.

Once entrenched on the Patriarchal throne, Justinian pledged his full support and that of the Church to the regime and its socialist ideology. Friendly publications describe his collaboration with the Communist regime variously as foresight, creative genius, prudent pragmatism, or genuine Orthodox *praxis* (pastoral practice). For example, an obituary in the Patriarchate's own *Romanian Orthodox Church News* exclaimed that Justinian "foresaw the reality of the historical moment"—a euphemistic convention for cooperation with the Communist regime—and directed the Church "on a new road, authentic Christian Orthodox."[41]

Perhaps his greatest legacy, aside from the monastic "reforms" he implemented at the insistence of the regime and the part he played in the sheer survival of the Church as a viable entity in Romania, was a twelve-volume collection of essays, speeches, and assorted documents spanning most of his exceptionally long (twenty-nine-year) reign. The collection is entitled *Apostolat Social*. The concept of "social apostolate" not only undergirded Romanian Orthodox theology and praxis in the Communist era but also denotes a radically modern worldview that attempted to synthesize Marxist-Leninist social analysis with Orthodox spirituality. It was a "theology of liberation" before that movement became popular in the West.

As the first Romanian Orthodox patriarch under the Communists, Justinian was the original apostle of the "social apostolate." He was an "ideological" collaborator par excellence, though at times "pragmatic" in his efforts to preserve Orthodox monasticism from extinction. He may be likened to Metropolitan Sergii of the Moscow Patriarchate in his struggle to achieve a *modus vivendi* with the new social order. But in another way he might be likened to Lenin himself, for both the first Soviet dictator and the first Communist Romanian patriarch were revolutionaries who successfully instituted their peculiar ideologies.

2. **Patriarch Justin**—*Leading Intellectual.* If Justinian was the Lenin of the Romanian Orthodox "social apostolate," his successor as patriarch, Justin Moişescu, served as the Leon Trotsky of the movement —the leading intellectual. Long before his comparatively short reign as Romania's fourth patriarch (1977-86), Justin had established his credentials as the foremost activist-theologian and ecumenical spokesman of the Romanian Orthodox Church.

A contemporary of Justinian, Justin was born in 1910, the son of a village schoolteacher in the South Carpathian village of Cindeşti. He was educated abroad, first at the Faculty of Theology of the University of Athens and then at the University of Strasbourg, France, receiving a doctorate from the Roman Catholic Faculty of Theology. Justin became a bishop in 1956, when he was consecrated metropolitan of Ardeal (Transylvania) in Sibiu, and was elected the following year to the metropolitanate of Moldavia and Suceava, thus becoming heir-apparent to Patriarch Justinian. His future loyalty to the Communist regime was foreshadowed in the late 1950s: when Patriarch Justinian balked at the regime's demand that the Church suspend 4,000 monks and nuns, Metropolitan Justin rushed to the fore as vice-president of the Holy Synod of Bishops and carried out the order.[42]

Justin's theological works include scores of New Testament and patristic studies and the routine "peace" essays incumbent upon any Romanian Orthodox hierarch or theologian during the Communist era. His personal leadership as an international promoter of the "social apostolate," however, was unequaled during his lifetime. He led the Romanian delegations at the various pan-Orthodox conferences in the 1960s and 1970s and at the general assemblies of the World Council of Churches at New Delhi (1961), Uppsala (1968), and Nairobi (1975). He also figured prominently at meetings of the Conference of European Churches and the Christian Peace Conference, especially the formative meetings of the latter in 1961 and 1964.

Patriarch Justin's contributions to the Moscow-dominated "peace" movement were duly noted in an obituary that appeared in the *Journal of the Moscow Patriarchate:* "His Beatitude Patriarch Justin was an eminent peacemaker and tireless preacher of the Christian ideas of peace."[43] In particular, he sponsored peace and disarmament conferences in 1980, 1984, and 1985; hosted a meeting of the International Secretariat of the Christian Peace Conference in Bucharest in 1981; and personally led the Romanian Orthodox delegation to Moscow in 1982 for a world conference of "Religious Workers for Saving the Sacred Gift of Life from Nuclear Catastrophe." In recognition of this yeoman service to Soviet and Romanian Communist peace ideology, Patriarch Justin was awarded a medal by the World Peace Council— the infamous Communist front organization.

When Moscow began its full-court press for nuclear "disarmament" in the late 1970s, Justin proved as enthusiastically compliant on this issue as on questions of religious freedom and national security. His moral positions and behavior were always predictable: the Communist regime's wish was his command.

3. **Patriarch Teoctist**—*Political Activist.* Patriarch Teoctist Arapaşu served only three years before his sudden resignation "for reasons of health" in January 1990, after some 200 disgruntled priests

demanded that he abdicate the Patriarchal throne.[44] However, as political events whirled around them in April, the bishops of the Holy Synod, in a state of confusion and disarray, invited Teoctist to return to the Patriarchal see. Although 136 religious and cultural leaders including Archimandrite Bartolomeu Anania protested this "defiance of the no-confidence vote of the faithful that made him to step down," the patriarch and the Holy Synod held their ground.[45]

The 78-year-old Teoctist is a contemporary of his two immediate predecessors, the last of the generation born before the First World War who will occupy the Patriarchal throne. His early life is typical of the pre-Communist hierarchs: monastic vows, undergraduate seminary, study at the Theological Institute in Bucharest, various teaching positions and episcopal sees. In 1977, when Justin became patriarch, Teoctist was appointed to the metropolitanate of Moldova and Suceava, where he devoted much of his time to improving monastic education and daily life. He has, as a bishop, been a tireless political activist, serving as a deputy in the Grand National Assembly, a participant in the congresses of the Socialist Unity Front, and a key member of the National Committee for Peace.[46]

Teoctist's published statements on peace, freedom, and security have closely followed the conventions established by his predecessors, Justinian and Justin. His primary talent during the *ancien régime* was his polished oratory on behalf of the "social apostolate" in official government circles.

4. **Metropolitan Antonie**—*Propagandist Extraordinaire.* Metropolitan Antonie Plămădeală of Transylvania (episcopal see in Sibiu), who is in his late sixties, has distinguished himself in ecumenical "peace" circles and is perhaps the best-known Romanian Orthodox prelate abroad. He is an accomplished theologian, having earned doctorates at the Roman Catholic Heythrop College in Oxford, England, and at the Orthodox Theological Institute in Bucharest. His dissertations at both institutions investigated the theme of the "servant church"—a biblical and patristic concept that Antonie subjected to a socialist metamorphosis in conformity to the "social apostolate" that has dominated contemporary Romanian theology.

For ten years, as assistant bishop to the patriarch after his consecration in 1970, Antonie was entrusted with the management of the

Department of Church Foreign Relations. During his tenure, the *Romanian Orthodox Church News* reported, this department "became a real embassy of the Romanian Orthodoxy, open to relationships with all Christian Churches and international Christian organizations, and to dialogues with other religions."[47]

The peripatetic, prolific metropolitan has enjoyed special prominence in the World Council of Churches. At the Nairobi Assembly in 1975 he was elected to the powerful Central Committee, a position he exploited to advance the interests of the Patriarchate and the Communist Romanian government. Owing primarily to his association with the WCC, but also as a result of a calculated decision by the Holy Synod of Bishops, Antonie became the most familiar Romanian Orthodox personage to the Western communications media. His considerable gifts as an articulate, trusted spokesman of the Patriarchate have been displayed in numerous interviews and articles.

For a while after the fall of the Communist regime and the temporary resignation of Patriarch Teoctist, Antonie kept an uncharacteristically low profile. When I interviewed him in Bucharest in September 1990, he seemed defensive and suspicious. He refused to comment on the political changes in Romania since the December 1989 uprising except to observe that the Church was "finally truly independent" and would begin now "to purify" its statutes from political "intrusions." Antonie's hold on his episcopal throne was weakened, at first, by the appointment of the young, widely esteemed, spiritual Bishop Serafim Joanta as his suffragan (assistant) in autumn 1990. Three years later, however, Antonie engineered Serafim's transfer to Western Europe, severely disappointing the reform-minded clergy in Transylvania. Antonie's participation as an official delegate of the Patriarchate at the international Orthodox–Roman Catholic dialogue in Balamand, Lebanon, in June 1993 testified further to his re-emergence as a powerful player in the internal politics of the Romanian Orthodox Patriarchate.

5. **Metropolitan Daniel**—*Progressive Realist.* A surprising development in June 1990 was the selection of the well-traveled theologian Daniel Ciobotea as the new archbishop of Iaşi and metropolitan of Moldova and Bukovina.[48] Only 38 when he was consecrated to the episcopacy, Metropolitan Daniel has led an active life as a scholar,

much of it away from Romania. After graduating in 1974 from the Orthodox Theological Institute in Sibiu, he proceeded to the University of Strasbourg in France, where he received a doctorate in theology in 1979. He began lecturing at the Ecumenical Institute in Bossey, Switzerland, in 1980 and did not return full-time to Romania until September 1988, when, having finally been ordained to the diaconate and priesthood, he became a Patriarchal counselor and a lecturer at the Orthodox Theological Institute in Bucharest. He has published well-received essays on Orthodox ecumenism and theology both in Romanian journals and in publications in the West such as the *St. Vladimir's Theological Quarterly*.[49]

Metropolitan Daniel's meteoric rise to the position of heir apparent to Patriarch Teoctist inaugurates a new generation of episcopal leadership untainted by overt collaboration with the Communist regime. One of Daniel's first acts as metropolitan was to insist publicly that religion must be taught in the schools of Romania. In an interview published in in June 1990 he declared, "Teaching religion in schools should be seen as a form of broadening one's horizons and improving one's knowledge, not as ideological indoctrination."[50]

A key member of the Reflection Group for Church Renewal, which sprang up in the wake of the December 1989 uprising, Metropolitan Daniel has carried this reformist vision into the episcopacy. When I interviewed him on October 1, 1990, in his episcopal headquarters in Iaşi, Daniel spoke with unexpected candor and animation. He cited as his greatest priority the need to combat the inertia and corruption within the Patriarchate that decades of collaboration with the Communists had wrought. This will, he said, require venturing into "new" areas that are quite familiar to Christians in traditionally freer societies: social work, youth ministry, and public education.

His sojourn in Western Europe has convinced Daniel that "democracy" may take root in diverse ways. Further, his realistic perspective would allow for the gradual implementaion of democratic structures and practices in Romania. The Church may play a profound role in teaching about virtues and fostering a sense of responsibility in a people grown accustomed to vice.

While denouncing Communism, as everyone else in the Church has done since the fall of Ceauşescu, Metropolitan Daniel eschews both socialism and free-market capitalism. Another of his insights is refreshingly unique: in the new era of free-market capitalism that seems to be dawning in Romania, he said, the Patriarchate may have to become a kind of "loyal opposition" on behalf of those who are not up to the task of competing in an economic and social free-for-all. The special role that the metropolitan in Iaşi envisions for his ancient Church is thus twofold: to provide prophetic criticism of new injustices as they arise, and to offer priestly consolation and encouragement to the vanquished.

With Metropolitan Antonie's star again in the ascendancy, Metropolitan Daniel may pose the only viable alternative to business-as-usual at the highest echelon of the Patriarchate's hierarchy.

The "Social Apostolate"

The role of the "servant" Orthodox Church in the Romanian nation-state is multi-faceted, according to the *apostolat social* propounded by Patriarch Justinian and the mainstream of the Patriarchate. Three aspects of this role as it was played during the Communist years relate to the public moral witness of the Church concerning freedom and human rights: (1) effusive praise for the regime and for Nicolae Ceauşescu personally; (2) operative definitions of freedom; and (3) the cosmocratic style of Church-state relations as expressed particularly through blatant support for "socialist," or more properly Communist, ideology.

1. *Paeans of Praise.* Liberal doses of Ceauşescu's speeches and Communist maxims appeared regularly in the publications of the Romanian Orthodox Patriarchate.[51] The paeans of praise for Ceauşescu would have been comical had they not been a tragic reflection of the personal indignities and moral ignominy that the Patriarchal leaders were willing to endure in their collaboration with the Communist regime. Each patriarch strained to surpass his predecessor in effusive praise of the *Conducător,* using officially sanctioned titles and accolades.

In 1974 Patriarch Justinian marveled at the "uninterrupted progress" of "all aspects of life" in "our present-day socialist Romania, wisely guided by her best sons under your [Ceauşescu's] leadership."[52]

In 1983 Patriarch Justin pledged the "unbounded patriotic love" of the Romanian Orthodox people for "the most beloved son of the Romanian people."[53] When Ceauşescu was "re-elected" as president of the Socialist Republic of Romania two years later, Justin expressed "the greatest joy" of the Church to the nation's "hardworking and unfatigued leader." The patriarch added that the first two decades of the Communist leader's rule had been christened "Ceauşescu's Epoch," supposedly "by a spontaneous manifestation of the consciousness of the country."[54]

In a statement in 1978, Patriarch Justin touched on all three themes of the present study. The occasion was the national leader's sixtieth birthday and forty-fifth year "of activity devoted to the progress of the Romanian people and motherland." Justin rendered "Homage" (the actual title) in these words:

> A great son of this nation, you came up from among the people and identified yourself with people's strivings giving life to the most passionate aspirations of our forerunners by rising [sic] ever higher the material and spiritual life of our socialist nation, by firmly asserting the principles of sovereignty and national independence, of justice and freedom, and also making worldwide known the desire of our country to live in peace and understanding with all peoples.[55]

Here is a succinct, albeit poorly translated, advocacy of peace, freedom, and security Romanian-style.

These more recent statements by patriarchs of the Romanian Orthodox Church followed a pattern established at the very beginning of the Communist regime. When the Communists seized power in December 1947, then Metropolitan Justinian hailed the new order as "the enthronement of social justice."[56] In his own enthronement address in June 1948, Patriarch Justinian rejoiced uncharitably at the expulsion of King Mihai, an Orthodox monarch with a German, specifically Hohenzollern, bloodline: "But all evils come to an end. The last pillar of the Caesarian Papacy and of imperialism in this part of the world, the last Hohenzollern, has abdicated."[57] Meanwhile, Justinian cultivated close working relations with the atheistic Communist leaders who supplanted the Orthodox monarchs of Romania and Russia. When Josef Stalin died in 1953, Patriarch Justinian honored the Soviet dictator as if he were an Orthodox prelate by ordering that the bells of all Romanian Orthodox churches and monasteries be rung for half an hour each morning for four days beginning at 11:15 — the precise time of Stalin's death.[58]

Patriarch Teoctist carried the praise of Ceauşescu to a new extreme. In 1988, on the occasion of Ceauşescu's seventieth birthday, the patriarch assured the national leader that the Church was "thinking of you with great appreciation, deep gratitude and unlimited love" — the last of which feelings was obviously misdirected from the Lord Himself. "Never before," Teoctist added, "has the Romanian people found a more perfect embodiment of their most noble strivings and aspirations than now, in the prominent personality of Your Excellency, the most brilliant son of this nation." The great oppressor of religion was credited with having guided the nation "on the way towards continuous economic and spiritual development." Ceauşescu was, indeed, a giant of world civilization: "You have excellently affirmed yourself on all occasions as an inspiring protector of rapprochement, good-will and peace between people and between nations," continually demonstrating "wisdom, abnegation and creative genius in serving the people, the country and the world."[59]

Immediately after the first mass protests in Timişoara on December 15, 1989, Patriarch Teoctist reaffirmed his support for the internal and foreign policies of the tottering Ceauşescu regime. A mere ten days later, as soon as the Communist dictator had been executed, Teoctist presented himself as a born-again democrat and friend of the people. "Freedom of church is indescribably important," he insisted. "Romanians lived all these years with their church, and now they realize how they escaped from a nightmare."[60] The ruler whom he had hailed the previous year as "an inspiring protector of . . . good-will and peace" Teoctist now denounced, invoking the odious biblical image of King Herod, murderer of the thousands of "holy innocents" in Israel at the time of Jesus' birth. "Ceauşescu was a follower of Herod," Teoctist declared. The recent upheaval in Romania, with the massacre of hundreds of civilians, especially children, was "a painful re-enactment of the Bible."[61]

While turning against his former patron, the patriarch also sought to whitewash his own role and that of the Patriarchate in the Communist era. "We were not collaborators," he protested. But then contradicting himself, Teoctist added, "We merely protected what was left of religion in Romania. In all honesty there is not a single Romanian adult who has not been affected by some form of collaboration with communism."[62]

2. *Freedom Romanian-Style.* The concept of religious freedom fared no better among most of the official leaders of the Romanian Orthodox Patriarchate in the Ceauşescu era than it did in the Moscow Patriarchate.

Patriarchs and other bishops frequently paid lip service to the freedom that was ostensibly guaranteed by the Romanian Communist regime. In a 1981 collection of essays edited by James E. Will, a United Methodist ecumenist, Bishop Vasile Tîrgovişteanul, assistant to the patriarch, proclaimed to Western readers the official party line of the Patriarchate: "Religious denominations in Romania are recognized by the law and can organize themselves and function freely."[63] In 1986, Metropolitan Antonie of Transylvania said in an interview with the Ecumenical Press Service, an arm of the World Council of Churches, that atheism was taught in the schools of Romania "no more than . . . in western countries," and that the "presentation is done decently, so that the feelings of those who believe should not be hurt." He also insisted, "Nobody is persecuted, nor is anyone subjected to any restrictions for one's belonging to any church." Antonie also assured Westerners, "We teach our faith freely in churches, during burials, marriages, and during our pastoral visits in homes."[64] Notably absent from this list was the freedom to teach the faith freely in schools of any kind for children and adults.

The same placebos were offered for domestic consumption. Patriarch Justinian liked to assure "the State Leadership" that the Church "enjoys complete religious freedom, enshrined in the constitution and guaranteed by the State."[65] Patriarch Justin often extolled Ceauşescu for "securing complete freedom to all religious cults in our country to carry out their activity among the faithful."[66] This "full freedom" mantra also found its way into the declarations of the present patriarch. For example, Teoctist's birthday "homage" to Ceauşescu in January 1988 thanked the *Conducător* for his "great understanding to the activity of the religions in the country, who enjoy full religious freedom."[67]

Coupled with these pro forma pronouncements of "untrammelled religious freedom" were explicit denials or justifications of persecution and other abuses of the law. When the *Wall Street Journal* reported that some 20,000 Bibles sent to the Reformed Church in Romania by the World Reformed Alliance had been seized by the government and converted into toilet paper,[68] Metropolitan Antonie vigorously denounced these "rumors" as "not only fantastic, but also absurd," and as "anti-Romanian propaganda."[69] In the same interview with the Ecumenical Press Service, Metropolitan Antonie downplayed the reports of massive destruction of church buildings in Bucharest in accordance with Ceauşescu's "renovation" of the capital: "The urbanization and modernization of the cities is a general and inevitable phenomenon. Unfortunately, this process requires, as everywhere, some sacrifices."[70]

Occasionally a Patriarchal document struck a chord familiar to genuine advocates of religious freedom and human rights. In an article published originally in 1967 in the *Ecumenical Review,* Patriarch Justinian argued in classic Western liberal terms that freedom is the foundation of justice and peace. The desire for freedom is innate in all human beings, he said. It allows them to choose among the various ways of asserting their existence, without, however, depriving others of *their* opportunities.[71] Similarly indisputable language characterized the official Romanian Orthodox witness at a human-rights colloquy in Bucharest organized in October 1982 by the Conference of European Churches. "By virtue of their mission," the Romanian delegation declared, "the Churches are called to involve themselves in the defence of human rights whenever and wherever they are violated."[72]

In reality, however, freedom and human rights Romanian-style were highly circumscribed by ideological conformity and bore little resemblance to what was taught by the Church Fathers or to the predominant models in modern Western societies. The *Journal of the Moscow Patriarchate* reported early in 1949 that the newly enthroned Patriarch Justinian wished to see "the freedom of the Church bound up with its responsibilities towards the new order in the State."[73]

In his contribution to a collection of "Faith and Order" essays published by the World Council of Churches, Metropolitan Antonie of Transylvania explained how the Church balanced its freedom with its duty to the state.[74] The statutory principles of the 1948 General

Regime of the Cults "provide for true and perfect religious freedom and rights for all religious beliefs and bodies in Romania," he said. The religious bodies, in gratitude for this opportunity, "have felt obliged to take part in the process of building socialism" and have ceded to the state the right to "impose certain natural limits" on the exercise of their religious freedom. Otherwise "the assertion of unlimited religious freedom" would tend to "interfere with the equal rights of all people within this freedom."

This argument effectively ordains the state — not the religious bodies themselves — as the final arbiter of what religious expressions are tolerable in the public arena. The free exercise of religion was supposedly guaranteed by the Communist state but only, explained Antonie, "provided that its exercise does not contravene the constitution, security, public order or morality . . . or state sovereignty." This slippery condition paved the way for the regime to restrict religious "liberty" for all kinds of political reasons.

Occasionally the dark underside of this twisted concept of religious freedom also came into full view. From the beginning of his Patriarchate, Justinian sought to expose and root out the "enemies" of the new social order and of the policies of the "social apostolate." In his enthronement speech he promised "to eliminate those [priests] who no longer correspond to their evangelical mission."[75] A couple of years later he threatened "to pluck out with resolution the weeds, the enemies concealed in the cover of night."[76] Justinian made it clear that religious "freedom" would be permitted only to those clergy who toed the party line.

3. *Socialist-Orthodox Cosmocracy.* The ideological content and political style of the "social apostolate" may be described as "socialist-Orthodox cosmocracy." Whether socialism or cosmocracy took precedence in this formula is not clear. One may argue plausibly that the Patriarchate viewed socialism as imposed by the Communists as a necessary condition for Orthodox life in the contemporary world and consequently adopted a cosmocratic mode of relating to the Communist regime. Conversely, the Patriarchate may be seen to be so historically and culturally inclined to support any regime in Romania that it loyally joined the "socialist" (read "Communist") bandwagon. If the latter is the more accurate interpretation, the Patriarchate may

be expected to adjust quite readily to the post-Communist government, whatever polity and ideology it eventually adopts. In either case,
cosmocracy was the formal principle, or structure, and socialism the
material principle, or content, of the Romanian religio-political symbiosis in the Communist era.

Representatives of the Patriarchate such as Metropolitan Antonie
of Transylvania frequently protest—correctly, in theory—that "the
Orthodox Church has never identified itself with any particular ideology or any political regime or social systems."[77] But the documentary evidence from the Patriarchate itself belies this claim in the case
of the Romanian Orthodox Church.

Patriarch Justinian sounded the keynote immediately upon his enthronement, when he announced, "Our people must be guided,
orientated and convinced of the social apostleship required by men
of the new times." Everything, apparently, had been made "new" by
the advent of the Communist regime in Romania. Monasteries would
have to be reorganized on "a new basis." Priests would acquire the
"new spirit" in order to assist the "new man" by preaching the Gospel
in "the new light."[78] Traditional Orthodox observers may have
wondered whether Justinian was about to introduce a "new" Gospel
to reflect the new fulcrum of modern Romanian history—the "anti-
fascist and anti-imperialist Revolution of social and national liberation" that began on August 23, 1944.[79]

Patriarch Justinian and his successors seemed truly to believe that
this political "revolution," facilitated, to be sure, by Soviet military
might, had ushered in a new era of social justice. In 1949 Justinian
asked rhetorically: "Can we not see in the present social order the
most sacred principles of the Gospel being put into practice? Is not
the sharing of goods, thus excluding them from the use of exploiters,
better?"[80] Bishop Vasile Tîrgovişteanul commemorated the fortieth
anniversary of the revolution in 1984 by saying: "It was then that the
most just social order was set up in Romania, in which all creative
forces of our people manifested themselves."[81] An unsigned editorial
in *Romanian Orthodox Church News* in 1988 went further in this official
exuberance for socialism. The August event "inaugurated the epoch
in which the people's ideals: social and national justice—for which
many generations of Romanians have sacrificed their lives—were to
be achieved." Subsequent "victories in the class struggle," the "con-

quering of the whole political power by the people," and successively "higher levels of material and spiritual development" have fulfilled "the possibility to edify in the country the justest social order: the Socialist order."[82]

The entry of the Romanian Orthodox Church into the Socialist Unity Front in 1974 provided an occasion for Metropolitan Justin of Moldova and Suceava to wax eloquent about the virtues of socialism. Justin observed that from the beginning of the new regime the religious communities in Romania "have supported the great reforms, and contributed with patriotic elan to the building of socialism in our country." The participation of the Church in the Socialist Unity Front signified "our communion with the social realities in the midst of which we find ourselves." But this was no mere accommodation to reality, for it reflected an ideal: "Our whole sacro-human work in the social field, is carried out to a certain purpose, i.e. in serving our socialist country; it is carried out here in the land of our forefathers even more in the stage of building up socialism."[83]

Under the new socialist Orthodoxy, monasticism in Romania could have become a matter of proletarians at prayer. Patriarch Justinian restructured the monastic life, imposing the new requirement of a "useful" trade. "I want an enlightened monasticism," he declared, "not an ignorant one."[84] Notwithstanding the obvious devaluation of prayer as not being "useful," this untraditional concept of worker-monks impressed at least one Western observer. Sr. Eileen Mary, S.L.G., remarked in a 1980 article in *Religion in Communist Lands* that this new "productive work" of monks and nuns had so enhanced their popular image that monasticism was "not regarded as an exotic anachronism unrelated to the life of modern Romania."[85] Fortunately, the spiritual strength of Romanian Orthodox monasticism has helped it endure this ideological assault. Monks and nuns everywhere in Romania are today some of the most joyous people in that land.

The more acerbic ideological flavor of the Patriarchate's socialist Orthodoxy can be sampled in the following paragraph from a 1951 issue of *Biserica Ortodoxa Română* ("Romanian Orthodox Church"), the primary informational organ of the Patriarchate. Reacting vociferously to the declaration of independence from Patriarchal control by the Romanian Orthodox Episcopate in America, the journal employed the usual Communist invective:

In the waters made turbulent by all kinds of passions, intrigues and personal interest, the capitalist exploiters and the new warmongers have started to fish. They have tried to catch the Romanians of America in the nets of their nefarious political propaganda and make use of them against the regime of popular democracy ruling presently in the Romanian People's Republic. They wish to make of these sons of our nation mercenaries employed in the service of their imperialistic interests and maneuver them to act against the legitimate interests of the Romanian nation.[86]

If socialism—that is, Marxist-Leninism, Romanian-style—served as the material content of the Patriarchate's vision of Romanian society during the Communist era, the justification for ceding to the state the initiative in enacting that vision derived from a cosmocratic mode of relating the Church to the state. Patriarch Justin announced simplistically on one occasion, "We have been charged by the Lord to serve with unswerving loyalty our homeland, Romania."[87] Far more subtle was a comment by Professor Constantin Galeriu of the Orthodox Theological Institute in Bucharest: "We are trying to train priests who are realists; . . . who do not get lost in speculative flights from reality. . . ."[88]

In contrast, the following statement by Patriarch Justinian constituted a carefully nuanced, sophisticated argument for collaboration between two ostensibly harmonious social entities:

The wisdom and realism of our state leaders, who interpreted in the most perfect way the will of the people, gave us the possibility to create a new legal position of equality, reciprocal respect, and harmonious collaboration among the religious bodies in our country. In Romania, there is no state religion, but no religious body is separated from the state. We live in full union and collaborate towards raising the material and spiritual standard and happiness of our people, being fully convinced that the prosperity of the country will have an impact upon our churches and other religious bodies. A perfect and permanent cooperation was set up between our state and the religious bodies, and we can say that the believers of all of them take part in solving the great problems with which our state is confronted, in working for a better and happier life for our people, because they are convinced that while they hold religious beliefs, they are also citizens of the country in which they live. . . . The Romanian Orthodox Church lives within the state and recognizes its authority. Our church is present and active within the state, not only because the members of the church are also members of the state, but also because a close natural relation was set up in the common interest of the members of the church and the citizens of the state: that of the state and the church.[89]

This argument "from above" attempted to justify collaboration with the Communist regime in terms reminiscent of the Byzantine concept of a *symphonia* between the Church and the Christian empire. Justinian thus christened the Communist regime, equating it to bygone Orthodox Christian empires and kingdoms. But the "full union" of the religious community with the atheistic state that he perceived was obviously illusory. The "natural relation" that he detected between churchmen and citizens was, at best, coincidental in a nation so overwhelmingly Orthodox by custom. The key to Justinian's argument, however, was precisely his identification of faith with citizenship. This premise led him to defer automatically to the state as the "most perfect" expression of "the will of the people." The state was, therefore, entitled to rule, and the Church was obligated to "cooperate." Thus was *symphonia* transformed into cosmocracy.

Metropolitan Antonie of Transylvania advanced an argument "from below" that based collaboration with the Communist regime on the "strict separation" that supposedly characterizes Church-state relations in Communist states.[90] His starting point was the Romanian religio-political symbiosis whereby the destiny of the Romanian Orthodox Church has, from the inception of that Church, always "merged" with that of the people it serves. The Church "has always stood side by side with the Romanian people, with the nation, in its struggle for national freedom and political unity," said Antonie. This identity as a "Church of the people" requires that the Church continually "adapt itself in accordance with the times," specifically "the new social, political, economic, cultural, and spiritual realities." Such adaptation includes "avoiding any interference in the secular field of the state."

Antonie rested this forfeit of social responsibility to the state on the familiar "render unto Caesar" passage in the Gospel of St. Matthew (22:21) to which advocates of "strict separation" usually resort. Since

Jesus did not deny the authority of the pagan Roman emperor, Antonie deemed this a suitable precedent for affirming "the civic duties of Christians" in whatever state they find themselves. But the metropolitan extrapolated from this tacit approval of given political realities that he detected in the gospel. "To render unto Caesar the things that are Caesar's," he argued, "does not mean being neutral and passive but, on the contrary, being active and contributing to Caesar's activity so that everything on this estate may go on well and the people be free, equal and happy."

Thus Antonie tried to have it both ways. On the one hand, he emphasized the "full autonomy" from the state of the religious bodies in Romania and "the separation of civic life from religious life" — that is, "a separation between the functions of the political power and those of the religious power." This "precise division" of powers replaced the confusion of the two that marked the regime before the Communist revolution. On the other hand, Antonie acknowledged the "full sovereignty of the state in internal and external affairs." Owing no "special obligation towards any religious body," the "state reserves the right to determine the kind of societies, organizations, and institutions which carry out useful activities, the kind whose activities are harmful to public order or morality." This state sovereignty enables the state to allow or to forbid a particular "society" (read "church") to exist.

Metropolitan Antonie constructed his case for collaboration from what purports to be a separationist perspective. But he, like Patriarch Justinian before him, actually proposed instead a cosmocratic political ethic.

In light of this dubious record, how the next generation of bishops, led by Metropolitan Daniel, will adapt to the post-Communist era in Romania should prove fascinating. Daniel clearly eschews the label *apostolat social*. When I spoke with him in Iaşi in October 1990, he contended that the label itself must be replaced, owing to its association with the old regime. Further, the concept itself ought, he insisted, to be developed in a radically new way: the Church should now practice genuine philanthopy, struggle for true justice in the face of the nihilistic materialism that may replace Communism, and actively instill in the culture the virtues of Orthodox Christianity.

THE BETRAYAL OF MINORITIES

The Romanian Orthodox Patriarchate has, like its counterpart in Moscow, displayed a disturbing tendency to exploit the plight of other religious and ethnic groups in Romania. Two prominent cases are Hungarians and Greek Catholics.[91]

The Hungarian Ethnic Minority

Roughly two million ethnic Hungarians live in Romania. Before the December 1989 uprising, the Communist governments in Bucharest and Budapest were engaged in a name-calling contest, and Romanian and Hungarian Church leaders had joined the fray.

On the Hungarian side, Cardinal Laszlo Paskai, the Roman Catholic primate of Hungary, rose to the defense of his fellow Hungarians, objecting in particular to the destruction of Hungarian villages under Ceauşescu's policy of "systematization."[92] Reportedly, Bishop Antal Jakab, Latin Rite Catholic bishop of Alba Iulia in Romania, cautioned Cardinal Paskai to refrain from speaking out publicly on the issue, lest it lead to still worse treatment of the Hungarian minority by the Romanian regime.[93]

On the Romanian side, the response of the Patriarchate was hardly forthright, certainly not prophetic. The point man was Metropolitan Antonie of Transylvania, the region where most ethnic Hungarians live. In an interview published originally in 1987 in a journal of the Ecumenical Patriarchate of Constantinople,[94] Antonie simply denied the charges and blamed "some irredentist circles in Hungary" for the tensions that had arisen between the neighboring countries. There were no complaints from within Romania, he contended, since the relations between the Romanian Orthodox Church and other religious communities, including the "Magyar Roman-Catholics" and "Magyar Reformed," were "based on equal rights." Antonie questioned the lack of specifics in the allegations and stressed the presence of "a Magyar church" in each of the Transylvanian towns inhabited by ethnic Hungarians.

Then, taking the offense, Antonie delved into history to find the real villains: the Hungarians themselves.

I can name more than thirty localities, only in my diocese, in which the Romanians were Magyarized by force during the dualist Austro-Hungarian regime (1867-1918) and, particularly, the Horthyist regime (1940-1944), when their names were changed and another religion imposed on them.[95]

Though undoubtedly true, this point obscured the fundamental moral issue. Whatever the injustices perpetrated upon ethnic Romanians when Hungary controlled Transylvanian territory, Orthodox Christians who wished to remain faithful to their traditional precepts of religious freedom and human rights could hardly countenance the violation of the civil rights of ethnic Hungarians by the Communist regime. But it is precisely this concept of rectificatory "justice" that has, for the most part, governed the attitude of the Romanian Orthodox Patriarchate toward the ethnic Hungarians and the Greek Catholics, as it also characterizes the feelings of many Russian Orthodox toward the formerly domineering and oppressive Poles and the Ukrainian Catholics of the Byzantine Rite.

Another tack is to avoid the issue altogether. Metropolitan Antonie endeavored to dissuade the Central Committee of the World Council of Churches from discussing the violation of the human rights of Hungarians and other ethnic minorities in Romania without additional information from Romanian members of the WCC. He warned the August 1988 session of the committee that he would leave if the committee continued its examination of this issue.[96]

Ethnic tensions in Transylvania remain high. The brutal beating of Hungarians by hooligans in Tîrgu Mureş in March 1990, whatever its genesis, has not been duplicated elsewhere, but it showed how easily the old bigotries can surface. And yet, in the May 1990 national elections the Democratic Union of Romanian Magyars garnered 29 seats in the 387-seat Romanian House of Deputies and 12 in the 119-seat Senate, which made this ethnic political party the nation's second largest after the FSN. In the February 1992 local elections, the Hungarian party captured the mayoralties of several Transylvanian cities, but the extreme right-wing Romanian National Unity Party (PUNR)—no friend of Hungarians—won the region's major city, Cluj.[97] Another ominous sign was the unexpected success of the National Unity Party's candidate in the September 1992 presidential election. Gheorghe Funar, the mayor of Cluj, got 10 per cent of the vote, placing third behind Ion Iliescu and Emil Constantinescu. To be sure, a politically enervating internal feud between Funar and PUNR senator Viorel Salagean suggests that this extremist party may have already peaked at the polls.[98]

These political and social developments will surely test the Patriarchate's commitment to freedom. An encouraging event occurred, however, on November 5-6, 1990, in Novi Sad, Yugoslavia, where Church leaders from Romania and Hungary met to seek reconciliation. A joint statement, signed by Metropolitan Nicolae Corneanu of Banat and Bishop Nifon Ploieşteanul on behalf of the Romanian Orthodox Church, expressed "sincere repentance" for "all our . . . failures and compromises" in "the recent past" and pledged resistance to "all kinds of national division and strife."[99]

The Greek Catholic Church

The fate of the "Uniates," or, in accordance with their own preference, the "Greek Catholic Romanian Church United with Rome" (or Greek Catholics, for short), was sealed in October 1948, when the new Communist regime pronounced it null and void. This followed the precedent established by the Soviet liquidation of the Catholic Church of the Byzantine Rite in Ukraine two years earlier. The response of the Romanian Orthodox Patriarchate to this event— indeed, its active participation—virtually duplicated that of the Russian Orthodox Patriarchate in the 1946 travesty.

To be sure, the Greek Catholic Church in Romania, like its counterparts in Ukraine and what is now the Czech and Slovak republics (also liquidated in 1948 by the Communists), owed its existence historically more to political and cultural opportunism than to a genuinely spiritual, grassroots demand for union with the Pope in Rome. Ever since the formal schism between the Orthodox Church in the Eastern Roman Empire and the Catholic Church centered in Rome, the pope had been regarded in the East as a heretic, and the Roman Catholic Church had been deemed guilty of doctrinal error, particularly concerning the Person of the Holy Spirit in the Holy Trinity.

Following the successful attempts at "reunion" resulting from aggressive proselytism directed toward Orthodox peoples, especially by

Polish Jesuits at Brest in Ukraine in 1596 and at Uzhorod in sub-Carpathian Rus in 1646, wealthy, powerful, Catholic Austria sent Jesuit missionaries to Romania at the end of the seventeenth century. Their mission was to "convert" the Romanian Orthodox in Transylvania, a region that had suffered economic and cultural stagnation under Turkish domination. In 1700 their efforts bore fruit when Bishop Athanasius of Alba Iulia led 1,548 Orthodox priests and some 400,000 faithful into submission to the papacy. In the following decades, hundreds of Orthodox loyalists were arrested and imprisoned by officials of the Hapsburg Empire. By 1762, Hungarian soldiers commanded by General Nicholas Adolf von Bukow, acting under direct orders from Empress Maria Theresa, had leveled some 200 Orthodox monasteries and hermitages that dared to resist the new religious order. Understandably, then, the Romanian Orthodox Church has always viewed the "Unia" as an act of ecclesial and political imperialism.[100]

A Church Abolished. When the Communist regime overturned this action—naturally for its own pernicious reasons—the Orthodox leaders finally had the opportunity to seek redress of their historic grievance. On October 1, 1948, thirty-eight Greek Catholic priests—a symbolic number duplicating the number of signatories at the Union of Alba Iulia in 1700—met in Cluj to declare their desire to sever all ties to the Vatican and to reunite with the Romanian Orthodox Church. These thirty-eight were among only 461 priests out of 2,340 Uniate clergy who had signed a similar declaration under severe pressure from Communist Party activists and the secret police. On October 3, the thirty-eight priests were formally and canonically received into the Orthodox Church by the Holy Synod of Bishops in Bucharest. Patriarch Justinian quickly proclaimed October 21 as a special religious holiday to celebrate "the re-integration of the Rumanian Church in Transylvania," and the cathedral in Alba Iulia was consecrated as the "Cathedral of Reintegration of the Rumanian Church of Transylvania."[101]

To overcome the stern resistance offered by many Greek Catholic bishops, priests, and laymen, the government expedited the "conversion" of local Uniate congregations by acting decisively. On December 1, 1948, the regime's Decree No. 358 abolished the 1.5-million-member Greek Catholic Church. The Decree maintained the fiction of the voluntary return of the Uniate parishes to Orthodoxy, as a result of which all Uniate institutions and organizations simply ceased to exist. The "entire property" of that denomination accrued to the state, which, the Decree concluded, "may allocate part of it to the Rumanian Orthodox Church, or to its various component parts."[102]

The six Greek Catholic bishops had to witness the dissolution of their Church and the confiscation by the new regime of approximately 2,500 church buildings, as well as seminaries, schools, and charitable institutions. They themselves subsequently were arrested and variously subjected to lifelong internment in an insane asylum, a political prison, or a restricted monastery. At least 600 of their priests also were imprisoned—roughly 200 in the Soviet Union—and only half of them survived the ordeal. More than 1,000 of their brothers became Orthodox, usually to minimize the hardships that their families would otherwise have to endure.[103]

Patriarch Justinian represented the official position of the Patriarchate on this issue when he seized the moment and welcomed the return of the Uniates to Orthodoxy, the brutally coercive circumstances notwithstanding. Fr. Mircea Păcurariu, professor of church history at the Orthodox Theological Institute in Sibiu, summarized this position in his monumental history of the Church: "A community was restored to the hearth of their ancestors' belief, . . . the fulfillment of a legitimate and secular desire of the Romanians of Transylvania"; "it constituted the reparation of an historic injustice that had caused the Romanian soil often to be soaked in blood."[104]

But not all the Romanian Orthodox clergy and faithful were party to this self-aggrandizing policy. As many as seventy-six priests suffered arrest rather than assume control over former Uniate churches.[105] Fr. Alexander Raţiu, a Greek Catholic priest who survived Communist prisons, credits "many Orthodox priests and faithful" with suffering imprisonment and torments in solidarity with their Uniate brothers.[106] In particular, he honors the memory of "Fr. John," spiritual director of the Orthodox monastery at Vladimireşti, who "wrote a memorandum to Patriarch Justinian" in which he "criticized the treachery of the unification program."[107] Bishop Flaviu Popan, a Greek Catholic hierarch who died in Austria in 1979, reported that many of the Orthodox faithful objected on moral grounds to the forced "reunion" of the Uniates with the Romanian Orthodox Church.[108]

A Church Restored. On December 31, 1989, nine days after the overthrow of the Ceauşescu regime, Dumitru Mazilu, vice-president of the FSN, assured a special papal envoy that both the Latin Rite and Greek Catholic Churches would be free to worship legally and to appoint bishops. Even more striking was the promise by Patriarch Teoctist in the days following the December 1989 uprising that the Romanian Orthodox Church would return to Roman control the Greek Catholic churches and properties that had been incorporated into the Orthodox Church since 1948.[109] By the spring of 1994 this pledge had been honored only piecemeal: 66 churches were again in Uniate hands, most prominently the cathedral in Lugoj in Metropolitan Nicolae Corneanu's region of Banat.[110] Nicolae also waxed irenic in an interview published in *Romanian Orthodox Church News:* the Greek Catholic Church, which had been "crucified," remains "wounded, bruised and scattered. Yet her members are our own brothers, although from a different pulpit."[111]

Disputes have arisen between the Orthodox and Greek Catholic hierarchies over how to determine which community ought to own specific properties. Such squabbling is an unfortunate distraction at a time when a united front toward the DFSN would better serve the religious interests of both communities.

The Romanian Orthodox Patriarchate prefers to subject the decision to a plebiscite in each disputed congregation. At least a generation of Greek Catholics-turned-Orthodox have lived and died in these churches since 1948. Whatever injustice was perpetrated then, the Orthodox bishops including Metropolitan Daniel of Moldova and Bukovina argue, the religious needs and preferences of the present generation ought to be respected. Let the majority in each case— whether Orthodox or Greek Catholic—"possess" the church property, while providing reasonable access to the minority until the latter can build its own facility. Some Orthodox bishops such as Metropolitan Antonie admit that they expect only about a third of the disputed churches to revert to Greek Catholic hands, simply because most of the former Uniates prefer to remain in the Orthodox camp.

The Greek Catholics approach the issue quite differently. In Sep-

tember 1990 I interviewed Bishop Gheorghe Guţiu in Cluj. A septu-
agenarian veteran of the notorious Jilava prison, Bishop Guţiu presented a strong case for *restitutio in integrum,* the return in full of church
properties to their proper owners—not immediately, to be sure, but
within a "reasonable" period of time. "We want an act of justice from
the Orthodox Church," he insisted: "to return to us what they took
by force." He rejected both the use of force to regain these properties
and the resort to plebiscites even as a transitional policy. After more
than forty years of manipulation of the people by the Communists,
he was skeptical of any "popular" means of justice. He said that already
some Orthodox priests were repeating the old canard that the Greek
Catholics in Transylvania, whose contributions to Romanian national
identity in the nineteenth and early twentieth centuries rival those of
the Orthodox, would agitate as irredentists to "deliver" the region to
Hungary. Further, he said, such referendums in the parishes would
lend moral legitimacy to an act of unjust coercion in 1948. Finally,
Bishop Guţiu contended that when the FSN abolished that 1948 act,
it also abolished its "effects."

On the Orthodox side, even the otherwise moderate Metropolitan
Daniel has shown little patience with what he regards as Greek Catholic intransigence on the property issue. In a statement drafted before
his consecration to the episcopacy, Daniel cited the "rebirth of Uniatism" as "proof of the religious freedom" that Romanians now enjoy.
But he also condemned "Uniatism" as an egregious offense against
Orthodoxy by Rome, implying that the Greek Catholic community
ought to be dissolved.[112] Relations between the sees in Bucharest and
Rome reached a new low in August 1991, when Patriarch Teoctist
urged all Orthodox churches in Romania to sever relations with their
Roman Catholic counterparts until Pope John Paul II ceases his
"propagation of Catholicism to the detriment of Orthodoxy in Eastern
Europe." Teoctist was especially offended by the reported comment
of the pope to the Romanian Catholic bishops in March 1991 that
Romanians had been Catholics until the Bulgarians converted them
to Orthodoxy in the Middle Ages.[113]

On the other side, Bishop Guţiu and his aggressive vicar general,
Monsignor Tertullian Langa, threatened in September 1990 to present
their case to the European Parliament and to the United Nations
through the good offices of Roman Catholics in the West, including

several U.S. senators. The purpose of this radical political act, the monsignor told me, would be "to show the whole world" that human rights in Romania do not extend to this religious minority.[114] The decision—born of extreme frustration—to resort so quickly to an overtly political "solution" would have called in question the good faith of these Greek Catholic leaders. But by spring 1994 they had not yet gained a hearing in such political forums.

Local Orthodox priests in Cluj claim that Bishop Guţiu's decision to celebrate Masses in an open-air square downtown is another case of Greek Catholic grandstanding. The bishop has spurned the offer of access to the Orthodox cathedral in that city at times other than the late-Sunday-morning period required by the Orthodox, although his clergy, influenced by their Latin Rite Catholic counterparts, may celebrate Sunday Mass at any time between Saturday evening and Sunday evening. Through these political maneuvers the Greek Catholics may curry favor among human-rights groups for now, but over time such tactics may, ironically, tilt the moral balance in favor of the Romanian Orthodox Patriarchate.

Further, the Greek Catholic community in Romania is still reeling from two unexpected events. First, a national census in January 1992 counted only a quarter of a million Greek Catholics—substantially below the 1.5 million souls claimed by the Uniates. Then, in June 1993, the international Orthodox–Roman Catholic dialogue in Balamand, Lebanon, rejected "uniatism" as a means of church unity between the Orthodox Churches and the Vatican. This generated a frantic letter of protest from Bishop Guţiu to Pope John Paul II.[115] Thus shrinking numbers and lukewarm support from the Vatican may yet do more to undermine the Greek Catholic position in Romania than the persistent disdain of the Orthodox.

DISSENTERS FROM THE PARTY LINE

The courageous refusal of hundreds of Orthodox clergy and laity to exploit the plight of their Greek Catholic brethren while their hierarchs justified such abuse should discourage any hasty, wholesale discounting of the public moral witness of the Romanian Orthodox Patriarchate on issues of religious freedom and human rights. Beyond doubt, collaboration with the Communist regime and the attempt to forge a new social ethic in complete harmony with socialist ideology characterized the official policy of the Patriarchate and perhaps the practice of even the majority of Romanian Orthodox Christians during forty-two years of Communist rule. But a portion of the Church always remained faithful to the Orthodox understanding of religious freedom. This "faithful remnant," to use an honored biblical term, constituted the prophetic voice of the Romanian Orthodox Church during the Communist era.

The paucity of Romanian dissidents, however, especially of those who professed their faith publicly, contrasts immediately to the historical waves of dissidents in the Soviet Union. The names of only a few Orthodox dissidents reached the West in the Ceauşescu era.

Several living dissidents deserve mention as survivors of that unholy regime. The layman **Gheorghe Braşoveanu** is a retired economist and distinguished proponent of human rights who was confined in a psychiatric hospital by the Ceauşescu regime several times. In July 1978 he was the only Orthodox founder—together with twenty-five Baptists and one Pentecostal—of the Romanian branch of the Swiss-based organization Christian Solidarity International, popularly known as ALRC after its Romanian name, Asociaţia pentru Libertatea Religioasă Creştină ("Christian Committee for the Defense of Religious Freedom").[116] **Fr. Alexandru Pop** sent an open letter in 1986 to Radio Free Europe in Munich decrying the persecution of the Church by the regime. For his courage as a solitary witness in behalf of religious freedom he was deported by the government.[117] An anonymous group of priests from the deanery of Lugoj in the diocese of Timişoara sent a similar open letter to the West during the Paschal season in 1988. These clergy defended their colleague, **Fr. Marian Ştefanescu**, who had "borne the consequences of an unjust decision" by Metropolitan Nicolae of Banat. The priests hoped "to inform international public opinion of this case" and serve notice to the Romanian Orthodox hierarchy that the truth about religious persecution would "come out into the light."[118]

Fr. Gheorghe Calciu-Dumitreasa. The most celebrated Romanian Orthodox dissident undoubtedly was Fr. Gheorghe Calciu-Dumitreasa, who, prior to his forced emigration from Romania in June 1985, earned the reputation of a modern-day confessor of the faith.[119] His outspokenness and willingness to risk imprisonment for his beliefs rank him with Fr. Gleb Yakunin as one of the most prophetic voices in the contemporary Orthodox world.

Fr. Gheorghe's early years before ordination to the Romanian Orthodox priesthood in 1972 are, notwithstanding his own unpublished memoirs, somewhat obscure. He was arrested in May 1948 as a 23-year-old medical student, apparently on charges of neo-Fascist activity. The nature and extent of his political activity are unclear. He contends that his arrest was merely one aspect of a massive purge of high school and university students by the new Communist regime.[120] He survived for fifteen years in the notorious Jilava and Piteşti prisons before his release in 1963, having vowed in the meantime to enter the Orthodox priesthood in gratitude for divine protection.

Denied the right, as a former political prisoner, to become a priest, he began in 1964 to study the French language and soon became a professor of French. In 1968, however, he convinced Patriarch Justinian, whom he continues to revere to this day, to allow him to study theology in secret and to be ordained. Appointed professor of French at the Orthodox Theological Institute in Bucharest in 1972, Fr. Gheorghe was ordained at last later that year.

In autumn 1977 Fr. Georghe publicly protested the demolition of the Enei Church in Bucharest and the Domneasca Church at Focşani. In a sermon at the Patriarchal cathedral in January 1978, he denounced atheism as a "philosophy of despair." In his Lenten sermons at the Bucharest seminary in 1979 he mentioned both themes, the destruction of churches and the nature of atheism, to groups of students numbering as many as 600. In particular, he contrasted "the fullness of the Gospel life" to "the lies of the materialistic doctrine and the communists' ideology of hate."[121] Soon afterward the director of the seminary silenced Fr. Gheorghe, and a month later Patriarch Justin suspended the popular priest from his teaching position, reassigned him to the central administration of the Patriarchate, and finally enjoined him from the exercise of his priesthood.

Fr. Gheorghe had experimented with open seminars at the seminary in which students freely discussed religious and moral problems in Romania, particularly the plight of the Hungarian and German-speaking minorities and the need for a free trade union. The formation of this trade union under Fr. Gheorghe's academic tutelage gave the government a reason to go after him on political grounds, and in March 1979 he found himself under arrest again for the same alleged offense — "neo-Fascist activity." He was sentenced to ten years' imprisonment.

The year before his arrest Fr. Gheorghe had sent letters to the newly elected Pope John Paul II and to the Committee of Intellectuals for a Free Europe (CIEL) in Paris. In the former he expressed hope that the Polish pope would attend to the cries of the suffering faithful in Romania: "We are not the official church. We are not visited by the brotherly ecumenical delegations. Our brothers do not bend over our injuries. Their ears are only hearing the denigrating words uttered against us."[122] In his letter to CIEL, Fr. Gheorghe detailed his "struggle for man's religious rights." He had demanded "the freedom to preach with no restrictions" and insisted "that the priest should no longer be forced to disseminate political programmes from the pulpit, since for us, who are priests, there is only one single theme for preaching, Jesus Christ." He had protested the demolition of churches. He had insisted that seminarians be exempt from conscription into the military, that religious youths not suffer discrimination, and that free access to the monastic life be available to anyone at any age. Fr. Gheorghe concluded this open letter with an appeal to conscience:

> We demand an end to persecutions! Let there be an end to the violation of human rights and religious rights! We appeal to all international associations to defend human rights and protect us! For there is only one struggle that is just and worthy for all Christianity: the struggle for man's freedom and dignity.[123]

Some of his fellow clergy joined the government in vilifying Fr. Gheorghe. In an English-language letter sent to Keston College, a committee of five Romanian Orthodox priests from the Orthodox Theological Institute in Bucharest, led by Fr. Dumitru Popescu and purporting to represent "all the priests of our country," denounced their colleague as a member of the Fascist "Iron Guard" during his years as a medical student and, more recently, "an unbalanced man and a megalomaniac" who attempted "to poison the souls of the seminarians with fascist ideas."[124] Even after the demise of the Ceauşescu regime, some of his former professorial colleagues were still critical of Fr. Gheorghe. Fr. Dumitru Radu, vice-rector and professor of moral theology at the seminary, told me in an interview in Bucharest in September 1990 that Fr. Gheorghe "preferred his own ideas to those of Orthodox Tradition."

In August 1984 Fr. Gheorghe was released from prison with half of his sentence unserved. But the archdiocese of Bucharest "defrocked" him in October, apparently executing the will of the regime against the recalcitrant priest. This decision was confirmed and Fr. Gheorghe's appeal denied by the Holy Synod, the highest governing authority of the Romanian Orthodox Church, in April 1985. The synod cited Fr. Gheorghe's "disobedience and insubordination to the ecclesiastic authority and his infringing the Regulations in force in the Orthodox theological schools."[125]

His early release was as politically motivated as his "defrocking." International advocates of religious freedom and human rights had exerted considerable pressure on the Romanian regime on Fr. Gheorghe's behalf. But what probably turned the tide was a direct appeal to the regime from sixty-four members of the U.S. Congress at the same time that the U.S. government was beginning to reexamine Romania's "Most Favored Nation" trade status.

Release from prison, however, only thrust Fr. Gheorghe into another sort of confinement, in which he was shadowed crudely by the Securitate and shuttled from place to place to keep him from potential visitors. Fr. Gheorghe and his family endured this virtual house arrest for several months. Then, realizing that they would not be able to have any kind of normal life and ministry in their homeland, they emigrated to the United States in August 1985.

Fr. Gheorghe currently serves as a pastor of a small Romanian Orthodox Church in northern Virginia, under the spiritual and canonical authority of Bishop Nathaniel Popp of Detroit, a hierarch of the Orthodox Church in America. The "defrocking" of Fr. Gheorghe by the Patriarchate obviously carries little weight among the American Orthodox bishops. Although the Patriarchate has reversed the defrockings of dozens of clergy that it now claims it was forced by the regime to impose, by spring 1994 it had not yet reversed that of Fr. Gheorghe.

Since his arrival in the United States, the expatriate has witnessed vigorously on behalf of religious freedom by providing broadcasts in

Romanian for Radio Free Europe, organizing financial assistance for Romanian refugees in the West, and publicizing the plight of persecuted Romanian believers, Orthodox and non-Orthodox alike.

Fr. Georghe maintains a distinctive perspective on ecumenism, particularly the public moral witness of the World Council of Churches. In 1977, he had appealed to the WCC as well as to the U.N.'s UNESCO to intervene to stop the destruction of historical Romanian churches by the Ceauşescu regime. Receiving no response from either organization, he concluded that "official ecumenism" effectively "collaborates with the political system" in Romania.[126] He wrote in his memoirs:

> I have come to the conclusion that we must distinguish between official ecumenism and real ecumenism. Official ecumenism I also call "banquet ecumenism," where important churchmen and theologians get together in elegant palaces, study long years about abstract problems, express their differences, make subtle theoretical formulations that do not touch the flesh-and-blood reality of Christ in his members, then eat well together and go home with nothing accomplished for the faithful, for the real, suffering church. That official ecumenism, the World Council of Churches, for example, never did anything to help me or other persecuted Christians in the East Bloc, or to help the real church in Romania.[127]

Fr. Gheorghe's departure from Romania, however forced and reluctant, left a huge void in that country's prophetic Orthodox witness. Fortunately, the incredible events that began in December 1989 have begun to fill that void. It may be only a matter of time before Fr. Gheorghe returns to his native land to continue his lifelong struggle for freedom and human rights.

THE PRICE OF PROPHECY

It is difficult to conceive of a more repressive regime than the fallen Communist government of Nicolae Ceauşescu. Only Albania under Enver Hoxha, North Korea under Kim Il-Sung, mainland China under Mao Zedong, or the Soviet Union in Stalin's heyday *may* have been worse. If so, it was not for lack of effort on Ceauşescu's part:

those four regimes served at different times as models for the grandiose schemes of the Romanian *Conducător*.

It is also difficult to conceive of a more sycophantic group of Church leaders than the Romanian Orthodox Patriarchate during the Ceauşescu era. So eager to please the regime and so compliant with its intrusive demands, despite its brutal oppression of their Church, the Patriarchate's leaders may be said to have perfected the art of collaboration. To be sure, the unique religio-political symbiosis that has characterized Romanian Church-state relations for at least a century facilitated the relatively harmonious cooperation between the Orthodox Church and the Communist state. For some collaborators, the substitution of commissars for king and court left the equation essentially unchanged—as long as the commissars were Romanian.

The highest echelons of the Church, beginning with Patriarch Justinian Marina in 1948, surpassed their Russian counterparts in developing a synthetic response to the social, political, and moral challenges posed by the "new" order. The patriarchs and most of the other hierarchs seem to have been, by and large, genuinely socialist at heart, quite willing to accommodate Communist social policy, and sincere about promoting the *apostolat social*, the "social apostolate." This new ethic attempted to blend traditional Orthodox spirituality and moral concerns with the exigencies of modern industrial society as viewed through Marxist-Leninist spectacles. It purported to represent a necessary updating of the Orthodox theological perspective, a seminal change in the Orthodox worldview. In their most grandiose hopes, Justinian and the other hierarchs may have likened their achievement to St. Augustine's baptism of Plato or Aquinas's christening of Aristotle. The architects of the "social apostolate" rendered the same retroactive service to Karl Marx and Vladimir Ilych Lenin.

The "social apostolate" was little more than radical social reform based on classic Marxist social analysis, draped, however, in traditional biblical appeals to justice on behalf of the poor and oppressed. It was a kind of "liberation theology" before that theology became popular in the seminaries in Western Europe, North America, and Latin America. The Romanian "social apostolate" required the same obsequious paeans of praise for the regime and its dictator that besmirched the public moral witness of the Moscow Patriarchate in the pre-Gorbachev era.

The "social apostolate" also entailed the same socialist view of religious freedom and human rights that prevailed in the Moscow Patriarchate, but with a twist. In Ceauşescu's Romania, the bishops also brazenly maintained to the bitter end the fiction of complete religious freedom and denied all charges of religious persecution. Led by that articulate purveyor of disinformation, Metropolitan Antonie of Transylvania, the Romanian hierarchy calmly circumscribed religious freedom in accordance with the overriding demands of "state sovereignty." This was done with a particular vengeance to the troublesome minority communities of Hungarians and Greek Catholics: rather than link arms in solidarity with these fellow oppressed Christians, the Romanian Orthodox Patriarchate shamelessly exploited the government's persecution of them to its own aggrandizement.

The "social apostolate" produced, in the name of socialism, a systematic rationale for cosmocratic domination of the Church by the Communist regime. It is difficult indeed to find genuine Orthodox strands in this ideological quilt.

If Metropolitan Daniel of Moldova and Bukovina can persuade his fellow bishops that this concept deserves burial, perhaps the Patriarchate may be able to extricate itself from one of the last generation's worst legacies. There is no longer any apparent ideological pressure from the political authorities. The current DFSN secretary of state for "cults," Gheorghe Vladuţescu, told me in an interview in Bucharest in September 1990 that the post-Communist government would maintain a very low profile in religious affairs. Persistent complaints by Romanian Protestants suggest, however, that the majority Orthodox may actually be "favored" by the DFSN. A draft religion law presented to the Romanian parliament in autumn 1993 drew sharp protests from Romanian Baptist leaders for its exclusive designation of the Romanian Orthodox Church as "National Church."[128] To be sure, by spring 1994 the parliament had not yet enacted this law.

If the Patriarchate's leaders allowed themselves to become exponents of the political propaganda that once emanated from Communist Bucharest, the handful of known Orthodox dissidents cast their fate to the wind and often found themselves swept right out of Romania. In the former Soviet Union, persistent religious-freedom and human-rights movements finally achieved miraculous victories, but Romania never had such a "movement" under Ceauşescu. The price of prophecy in matters of religious freedom and human rights in Romania was, in recent decades, extremely high. To maintain a prophetic Orthodox witness usually meant forfeiting at least one's citizenship and quite possibly one's life.

Now for the first time in a generation there are real prospects for genuine religious freedom and perhaps even governmental protection of human rights in Romania. The opportunity is golden for the Romanian Orthodox hierarchy and the former dissidents to work together to rebuild their nation and to reshape their Church in accordance with Orthodox moral traditon. Patriarch Teoctist has, indeed, finally begun to exercise a genuinely prophetic ministry independent of and even properly critical of the new regime. One extraordinary sign of renewed confidence and moral rebirth was a January 1994 "open letter" of the hierarchy that appealed to the government to halt the reputed 1.5 million abortions in Romania each year.[129]

If Teoctist and his successor continue to confront Iliescu's government vigorously on an expanding range of moral issues, if the dissidents such as Fr. Gheorghe Calciu adopt a conciliatory attitude toward their former ecclesial nemeses, and if the democratic opposition to the DFSN maintains its vigil for freedom despite repeated defeats at the polls, Romania and its Orthodox Church may be on the verge of a spiritual, ethical, and political renaissance. That would represent a most happy development in the enduring Romanian religio-political symbiosis.

4

Parochial Human-Rights
Concerns in America

To the casual observer, the various Orthodox communities in the
United States may appear as a crazy-quilt of rival, predominantly
ethnic churches. The Orthodox themselves tend to be uncertain about
their proper identity in the American religious mosaic, in which Protestants are dominant and the Roman Catholic and Jewish minorities
enjoy considerably greater visibility.

In an influential study entitled *The Naked Public Square,* the then
Lutheran scholar Richard John Neuhaus dismissed the Orthodox as
negligible contributors to the debate about religion and public policy.[1]
Although there are two-thirds as many Orthodox Christians as there
are Jews in America—approximately four million compared to six
million—and the Orthodox considerably outnumber some of the
very visible Protestant denominations such as the Episcopal Church,
the Orthodox "influence upon the general culture escapes detection,"
said Neuhaus. He attributed this, correctly, to a long-term identity
confusion among the Orthodox in North America. They have not yet
officially decided whether they are an *Eastern* Church in exile from
the mother Churches overseas, merely another American denomination alongside the plethora of Protestant and Roman Catholic communities, or *the* Church pure and simple.

It isn't as if they were newcomers to the American scene. In September 1994, Orthodox Christians in America concluded a year-long
celebration of the bicentennial of the first permanent Russian Orthodox community in Alaska. A shrine in St. Augustine, Florida,

commemorates the arrival in 1768 of the first Greek Orthodox colonists in what is now the United States. And yet Neuhaus is right —their collective moral witness to American society, and especially in public policymaking, has, until quite recently, been negligible.

A turning point may have occurred with the *amicus curiae* brief filed by the "Holy Orthodox Church" in the 1989 U.S. Supreme Court case *Webster* v. *Reproductive Health Services*.[2] This collective action by almost all the Orthodox Churches in the United States propelled the Orthodox community—heretofore content to issue occasional ad hoc resolutions and encyclicals on a rather limited range of social and moral issues—to the forefront of the abortion debate, if only for a season.

A Disorderly Diaspora

Though professing to be the one, holy, catholic, and apostolic Church in America, the Orthodox Churches are pluriform. This continent was initially for them the scene of a *diaspora*—a "dispersion" of peoples who are most concentrated in Eastern Europe and the Middle East. The United States, in particular, has attracted Orthodox immigrants seeking religious freedom, economic opportunity, or both. Only during the last three decades have some segments of the Orthodox community viewed the United States as a fertile—and permanent—mission field.[3]

As Orthodoxy approaches its third century on this continent, and its second since the first great wave of immigration from Eastern Europe that commenced in the 1880s, this religious community is still marked by distinctive, often overwhelming ethnicities. This has been altered somewhat by the influx of converts with Western European and, to a lesser extent, African and Asian ancestries that began in earnest in the 1970s. Certainly the popular perception of this faith group identifies it more as "Eastern" than as "Orthodox."

The identity problem is compounded by the lack of administrative unity among the various ethnic Churches. Although they have a common faith, including doctrinal traditions, moral and spiritual practices, and liturgical life, the various groups are virtually independent, inclined to guard their own flocks jealously, often competitive rather than cooperative, and sometimes even suspicious of one another. This situation is clearly uncanonical, a violation of the ancient Orthodox practice of identifying the Church with the people of the empire or nation and of having one bishop in each metropolis. In the United States, major cities like New York or Chicago or Pittsburgh may have as many as four Orthodox bishops. Certain jurisdictions may find their canonicity questioned and may, in turn, challenge the claims of other jurisdictions to be authentic Orthodox Churches. A particularly troublesome aspect of this ecclesial fragmention is that sometimes conflicting, even mutually exclusive statements on public-policy issues emanate from the various jurisdictions.

Given this confusing institutional context, any attempt to categorize the jurisdictions may appear unavoidably subjective. Nevertheless I propose the following typology, patterned after one suggested by Fr. Paul Schneirla[4]. Statistics are based on the official claims of the jurisdictions reported in the 1994 edition of the *Yearbook of American and Canadian Churches,* which is published under the aegis of the National Council of Churches.[5]

1. The **Constantinopolitan Connection**. Largest, richest, most financially stable, and most administratively efficient among the jurisdictions is the *Greek Orthodox Archdiocese of North and South America* (GOA). Headquartered in New York City, the Greek Archdiocese is led by the most recognizable Orthodox personage in American history, Archbishop Iakovos Coucouzis. This group was formally and canonically organized in 1922 by the Ecumenical Patriarchate of Constantinople after the Russian Revolution disrupted the paternal oversight of the Russian Orthodox Patriarchate of Moscow over all the Orthodox in America. The Greek Archdiocese claims some 2 million members in 535 parishes.

A member-communion of the National Council of Churches (NCC) for forty years, the Greek Archdiocese, as noted in chapter 1, initiated the temporary suspension of Orthodox participation in the NCC in June 1991. But nine months later it pressed for the return of the five prodigal Orthodox jurisdictions in the Standing Conference of Canonical Orthodox Bishops in the Americas (SCOBA) to "provisional" member status in the NCC. In 1994, the Greek Archdiocese supported this ecumenical organization to the tune of $5,000 (after a two-year hiatus pending the extension through 1995 of SCOBA's "provisional status" in the NCC), for which it was entitled to send ten voting delegates to the semi-annual meetings of the NCC's General Board (formerly called the Governing Board).[6]

Closely affiliated with the Greeks are several satellite jurisdictions that, though theoretically tied directly to Constantinople, actually function as dependencies of the Greek Archdiocese under Iakovos as exarch (head of a province) of the Patriarchate. These are the *American Carpatho-Russian Orthodox Greek Catholic Diocese* (18,600 members in 72 parishes), the *Ukrainian Orthodox Church of America* (5,000 members in 27 parishes), and tiny *Albanian and Byelorussian dioceses,* currently without their own bishops. In 1990, the *Ukrainian Greek Orthodox Church of Canada,* a historically "independent," maverick jurisdiction headquartered in Winnipeg, with 120,000 members in 258 parishes, was formally received by the Ecumenical Patriarchate and granted canonical status. This surprising turn of events enhanced not only Archbishop Iakovos's ecclesial empire in North America but also Constantinople's historic interest—and canonical claims—in the Ukrainian Church centered in Kyyiv.

2. The **Autocephaly Axis**. What has been known since 1970 as the *Orthodox Church in America* (OCA) began its mission in 1794 as an outreach of the Church of Russia on this continent through the "back door," as it were, of Alaska. It was formerly known as the Russian Orthodox Greek Catholic Metropolia—a cumbersome designation, to be sure—because most of its faithful earlier in this century came from Greek Catholic churches of the Unia. The OCA received its "autocephaly," or independence as a self-governing national Church, from the Moscow Patriarchate in 1970. It now claims some 600,000 members in 700 parishes and missions.

Despite internal disagreements among the ancient Orthodox patriarchates, particularly Constantinople, over the canonical propriety of this action, the OCA has drawn into its orbit three previously independent "ethnic" jurisdictions. These Romanian, Bulgarian, and Albanian groups function in the OCA as special dioceses under their own bishops, who serve as full and equal members of the OCA's Holy Synod of Bishops under the current primate, Metropolitan Theodosius Lazor, Archbishop of Washington and Metropolitan of All America and Canada.

To cite only one of these three special dioceses, the *Romanian Orthodox Episcopate of America* (ROEA), headed by Bishop Nathaniel Popp of Detroit, has 73,600 members in 50 parishes in the United States and Canada. It was organized in 1929 as an autonomous diocese of the Romanian Orthodox Church, but the majority of its leaders and churches severed all ties with the mother Church in 1951, when it became clear that the Communist domination of the Patriarchate was irreversible. In 1960, the Episcopate affiliated with the Metropolia, and it reaffirmed this covenant with the new OCA in 1971.

The OCA was, in its former role as the Metropolia, a founding member-communion of the NCC in 1950, but it has maintained an erratic witness in that ecumenical body. Its financial contribution in 1990, for example, amounted to $2,000, all of it earmarked for the NCC's administrative office for Europe/U.S.S.R., then directed by an OCA deacon, Michael G. Roshak. According to the OCA's chancellor, Fr. Rodion Kondratick, the NCC requested $4,000 in 1993 but had to "settle" for $2,000. Nevertheless, the OCA sent its full allotment of five delegates to the General Board each year, and one of these, Fr. Leonid Kishkovsky, was elected NCC president for a two-year term from January 1990 through December 1991. Critics of the NCC within the OCA (particularly the clergy and laymen of the Diocese of the South, headquartered in Dallas, and the Diocese of the West, based in San Francisco) contend that Fr. Leonid squandered the opportunity that election to this prestigious—albeit largely ceremonial—office afforded him by following the familiar left-leaning political agenda.

The OCA remains an active member-communion of the World Council of Churches, which it joined in 1954.

3. An **Antiochian Alternative**. The flagship of this extraordinarily evangelistic Orthodox community is the *Antiochian Orthodox Christian Archdiocese of North America* (AOCA), a missionary outreach since the 1930s of the Arabic-speaking Patriarchate of Antioch, headquartered in Damascus, Syria. Metropolitan Philip Saliba serves as exarch, presiding over 250,000 members in 160 parishes from his headquarters in Englewood Cliffs, New Jersey. Waves of Arabic-speaking immigrants from Lebanon and Palestine have, in the last decade, radically altered the demographics of this heretofore aggressively English-speaking jurisdiction.

A member-communion of the NCC since 1966, the Antiochian Archdiocese, in its efforts to promote the Palestinian cause, has wrestled mightily with the NCC's predominantly pro-Israel Protestant majority. In 1991, the Archdiocese contributed $1,000 to the NCC and was allowed to send five delegates to the General Board. Like its sister jurisdiction, the OCA, the AOCA maintained a separate membership in the World Council of Churches from 1954 until 1975, but it made only token financial contributions to that body.

The Western Rite Vicariate, a distinct subgroup within the Archdiocese, consists of a dozen or so parishes that use liturgical rites derived from the 1928 Book of Common Prayer of the Anglican Communion or the Roman Rite in force before the Second Vatican Council (1962-65). In 1986, a group of some 2,000 Protestants known collectively as the "Evangelical Orthodox Church" converted *en masse* to Orthodoxy and was placed under Metropolitan Philip's authority by the Patriarchate of Antioch. For four years they functioned as a distinct national diocese known as the Antiochian Evangelical Orthodox Mission before being integrated into the Antiochian Archdiocese. These evangelistic coups may yet push Metropolitan Philip —a "third" force to be reckoned with in American Orthodoxy—into prominence as a potential arbiter between the Greek Archdiocese and the OCA in their dispute over primacy in North America.

4. **Old World Colonies**. A fourth dimension of Orthodoxy in America is provided by a congeries of comparatively small churches that have not yet cut the umbilical cords to their mother Churches in Eastern Europe. The *Serbian Orthodox Church in the U.S.A. and Canada* (SOC) was organized in 1921 and now comprises four dioceses with 67,000 members divided among 68 parishes. Texas-born Metropolitan Christopher Kovacevich of the Diocese of Midwestern America, whose chancery is in the environs of Chicago, usually serves as spokesman in public forums for the four bishops, who, though full members of the Holy Synod of the Patriarchate of Serbia in Belgrade, Yugoslavia, have all along maintained a fierce independence from the once powerful Communist government there. Having joined the NCC in 1957, the SOC is entitled to send a four-person delegation to the meetings of the NCC's General Board, although financial constraints limit actual participation. (For example, only one delegate,

Fr. Rastko Trbukovich of Lackawanna, New York, attended the General Board meeting in Baltimore in November 1993.) According to Metropolitan Christopher, the Serbian Orthodox contributed the requested $600 in 1993.

The Serbian Orthodox community in the United States reached a milestone in April 1991, when Metropolitan Iriney of the rival "Free Serbian Diocese," claiming some 30 churches with headquarters in Grayslake, Illinois, recognized Patriarch Pavle as true head of the Serbian Orthodox Church. (The 78-year-old Pavle, a deeply spiritual man who survived physical abuse by Albanian irredentists in his Kosovo diocese, was elected to the high post in December 1990.) Then in February 1992 the two fractious Serbian Orthodox jurisdictions in North America officially healed their 29-year-old schism at a Divine Liturgy concelebrated by all the bishops. Iriney's diocese, now known as the New Gracanica Metropolitanate, was expected to be fully integrated into the SOC by 1995.

Other jurisdictions in this category include the *Romanian Orthodox Missionary Archdiocese,* an arm of the Patriarchate of Romania in Bucharest, with about 15 parishes; the *Bulgarian Eastern Orthodox Church,* a colony of the Patriarchate of Bulgaria in Sofia, 1,100 members in 9 parishes; and the so-called *Patriarchal Parishes of the Russian Orthodox Church in the U.S.A. and Canada,* an assemblage of 38 U.S. and 24 Canadian parishes (with 9,800 and 7,000 faithful, respectively) still administered directly by Moscow's representative in North America, currently Bishop Pavel Ponomarev of Zaraïsk (based actually in New York City). This Russian group shows no signs of merging into the OCA, as originally planned in 1970. The Patriarchal Parishes have secured a firm foothold in ecumenical organizations such as the National Council of Churches, which they joined in 1966, four years before the mother Church granted autocephaly to the OCA. Although their financial contribution in 1987 was zero, the Patriarchal Parishes maintained a four-person delegation to the NCC.

5. **Quasi-Canonical Communities**. The final category of Orthodox jurisdictions in the United States may be described, delicately to be sure, as "quasi-canonical." Included under this rubric are those jurisdictions that either are not recognized by the "canonical" Churches—especially the ten that constitute SCOBA, chaired by

Archbishop Iakovos—or simply do not care about maintaining close contacts with them.

Largest among these groups is the *Ukrainian Orthodox Church of the U.S.A.* (UOC), based in South Bound Brook, New Jersey. Metropolitan Constantine Buggan of Philadelphia presides over 107 churches with 87,000 members. The first bishop of this jurisdiction arrived in 1924, five years after Ukrainian immigrants organized their Church, with a dubious claim to apostolic succession. Bishop John Teodorovich had been consecrated by renegade Ukrainian Orthodox priests who had "consecrated" themselves in a controversial rite in Kyyiv.[7] A subsequent "reconsecration" of Bishop John and his colleagues during the Second World War by Ukrainian bishops of unquestioned canonicity in Poland has not, curiously, allayed the doubts of the jurisdictions in SCOBA.

Another quasi-canonical community is the *Russian Orthodox Church Outside Russia* (ROCOR), also known as the "Russian Synod Abroad," which regards itself as the free, authentic, continuing part of the Russian Orthodox Church in exile. Organized in 1920 among Russian émigrés in Bulgaria who had fled the new Communist regime during the Russian Civil War, this group moved its headquarters to New York City in 1950. It is relentlessly anti-Communist and sharply critical of modern ecumenism. ROCOR, currently led by Metropolitan Vitaly Ustinov, last released membership statistics in 1955. The figure of 55,000 members in 81 parishes is undoubtedly outdated, particularly in the wake of an internal schism in 1986.

As we saw in chapter 2, a new dimension was added in May 1990 when ROCOR blessed the formation of an alternative jurisdiction to the Moscow Patriarchate (on Russian soil) officially known as the *Free Russian Orthodox Church*.

To get a sense of the positions of these many bodies on issues of freedom and human rights, we shall consider the encyclicals and resolutions of the most active jurisdictions in each of the five categories sketched above.[8]

GREEK ORTHODOX ARCHDIOCESE

The Greek Orthodox Archdiocese did not begin in earnest to promulgate positions on moral and social issues until Archbishop Iakovos's encyclicals in the early 1960s and the resolutions of the seventeenth biennial clergy-laity congress in 1964. Only isolated expressions of concern had emanated from Iakavos's predecessors. Archbishop Alexander Demoglou (1922-30), for example, sent a letter to the U.S. secretary of state in 1921 concerning the persecution of the Greek Orthodox community in Turkey. Similarly, Archbishop Michael Konstantinides (1949-58) appealed to the secretary of state in 1950 on behalf of the persecuted Greek Orthodox on the island of Cyprus, and he interceded again in 1955 for the oppressed Patriarchate, confined since the 1920s to a ghetto of Constantinople known as the Phanar.[9]

With the advent of Iakovos's reign in 1959 the Archdiocese veritably burst onto the public-policy scene. The archbishop himself has a unique record of public involvement in moral issues and ecumenical activities. Moral and social themes recur frequently in his encyclicals to his flock, especially on two occasions each year: May 25, Greek national independence day, as well as the ancient Feast of the Annunciation; and October 28, "Ochi Day," which commemorates Greece's *"ochi,"* or *"no,"* to Italian dictator Benito Mussolini's surrender demand in 1940. These encyclicals issued by Iakovos have often inspired the clergy-laity congresses—the penultimate decision-making body, consisting of clergy and elected lay representatives from each parish—to issue similar statements and resolutions. No single event better illustrates the archbishop's dedication to human freedom and justice and his willingness to act on his convictions than his dramatic participation in the legendary civil-rights march in Selma, Alabama, on March 15, 1963, alongside Dr. Martin Luther King, Jr., labor leader Walter Reuther, and a host of national religious leaders from many denominations and faith groups.

We shall consider a representative sampling of statements on human rights, freedom, the so-called Turkish problem, and other international concerns. The Archdiocese also has strong records on other human-rights issues—namely, abortion (unequivocally pro-life) and civil rights (firmly against racial discrimination).

Human Rights and Freedom

Archbishop Iakovos sounded the keynote for a broad concern for "human rights" in his 1977 Ochi Day encyclical. The Greek Orthodox, as "law-abiding citizens," ought to exhort their political leaders not to "undermine our nation's struggle for human rights or damage her prestige both here and abroad."[10] The scope of such "rights" became clearer the next year, when SCOBA, at Iakovos's prompting, marked the thirtieth anniversary of the Universal Declaration of Human Rights by the United Nations Organization. The bishops urged all Orthodox Christians to pray "for those whose human rights are being denied and/or violated," specifically for their religious beliefs or in their pursuit of "justice, food, shelter, health care and education." The bishops also urged public support for President Jimmy Carter's efforts to persuade the U.S. Senate to approve the U.N. International Covenants on Economic, Social, and Cultural Rights, and on Civil and Political Rights.[11] By so doing, the leading Orthodox bishops in America subscribed to a comprehensive definition of human rights, which includes material "rights" in addition to the classic Western liberal emphasis on liberty.

Long before 1978, however, the clergy-laity congresses of the Greek Archdiocese had professed similar beliefs. A resolution in 1966 called for "the protection of individual human rights, particularly in such areas as employment, housing, education and hospitalization."[12] The 1968 resolution on "The Dignity of Man" expanded these rights: now included in "the divine birthright of every human being" were "the opportunity and right of earning a living, of raising his children in decent surroundings, and seeing them obtain the finest education possible."[13] The 1978 congress offered "our unreserved support to our President [Carter], who has courageously and strongly demanded from the governments of all nations respect for human rights."[14]

Finally, the 1980 congress produced a lengthy resolution on human rights (reissued almost verbatim at the 1988 and 1990 congresses) that defined the term as broadly as possible: "those conditions of life that allow us fully to develop and use our human qualities of intelligence and conscience to their fullest extent, and to satisfy our spiritual, social and political needs." The "political needs" encompass three of the freedoms cited by President Franklin D. Roosevelt in his famous "four freedoms" speech in 1940—namely, (1) freedom "of expression," (2) freedom "from fear, harassment, intimidation and discrimination," and (3) freedom "to participate in the functions of government and to have the guarantee of the equal protection of law." These freedoms are meant to be exercised freely in every country "by all citizens, regardless of racial or ethnic origin, or political or religious espousal."[15]

The 1990 clergy-laity congress added to the list of human rights another one especially relevant in the last decade: "freedom from terrorism."[16]

Archbishop Iakovos ranks freedom "above every other human right."[17] It has a theological as well as a political import: "Freedom . . . is not an accident of history, but rather the natural state of God's children."[18]

Referring in 1972 to "our three identities as Orthodox Christians, descendants of Hellenes and citizens of America," Archbishop Iakovos has woven a curious tapestry of American patriotism and Hellenism in his often exuberant declarations on freedom.[19] In the halcyon pre-Vietnam days of 1963, he extolled the unique role of the United States as a defender of liberty, peace, and justice in the world.[20] In a Fourth of July encyclical in 1966, he waxed patriotic about "those champions of American liberty"—the president, government, and soldiers, "who are the defenders of our freedom."[21] But "the best kind of American patriotism," the archbishop declared in 1965, was manifested "by the youth of this great American nation in far-away South Viet-Nam"; this kind was similar to the best kind of Greek patriotism as exemplified by the "brave Hellenic sons and daughters" who fought for their freedom in the Greek war for independence in the 1820s, against the Fascists in the 1940s, and against the continuing Turkish oppression in Cyprus. What the two kinds of patriotism shared was "the love of freedom," "those purposeful ideals of freedom for which Christ died," "the real meaning of wholehearted giving."[22]

Fortunately for the Orthodox Church, Archbishop Iakovos does not allow his fervent Hellenism—the "vision of Eternal Greece"[23]—to obscure his appreciation of the fundamentally Christian legacy of freedom. It was clearly symbolic, not coincidental, that Bishop Germanos of Old Patras issued his clarion call to revolution in 1821 on the Orthodox Feast of the Annunciation—which the bishop called a divine "summons out of bondage, a call to freedom and a new life." The revolt would be not only against slavery and the violation of human dignity but also "against faithlessness and against those who blasphemed the faith," in the name of a "freedom that rejects all compromise with political, social or religious untruth." The virtue of freedom to which these two events—the Annunciation and the Greek revolution—bore witness is, the archbishop concluded, "our greatest and most precious inheritance from Christianity and Hellenism."[24]

The clergy-laity congresses in 1980 and 1984 produced general statements on religious freedom. The 1980 statement noted "growing persecution of Orthodox Christians because of their identity, faith and religious practice." But this declaration was not merely parochial in its appeal. The delegates also urged the Orthodox who live in freedom to cooperate with all others who value freedom in helping any persons who are persecuted for their beliefs. The first paragraph laid the foundation for this truly catholic perspective:

> All people have the God-given right to be free from interference by government or others in (1) freely determining their faith by conscience, (2) freely associating and organizing with others for religious purposes, (3) expressing their religious beliefs in worship, teaching and practice, (4) and pursuing the implications of their beliefs in the social and political community.[25]

The Turkish Problem

Not surprisingly, the Greek Archdiocese reserves a considerable portion of its concern for human rights and freedom in the world to situations involving the government of Turkey. For nearly four hundred years, from the fall of Byzantium in 1453 until the emergence of the modern Greek nation-state in 1821, the Greek people chafed under Turkish political and religious oppression. Although the Greek peninsula is now free, the Ecumenical Patriarchate of Constantinople remains tightly restricted by the Turkish government in the Phanar ghetto in Istanbul (the modern name for the city of St. Constantine the Great). The Greek-speaking majority on the ancient island of Cyprus in the eastern Mediterranean south of Turkey has, especially since the sudden Turkish invasion in 1974, suffered the ravages of war, and those living in the Turkish-controlled section of the island have reported repeated human-rights abuses, including violations of their religious freedom. The pattern of centuries of Greek-Turkish animosity shows no signs of dissolving.

In 1964 both Archbishop Iakovos and the clergy-laity congress began their ongoing public moral witness on the Turkish problem. The July congress issued "A Protest Regarding the Persecution of the Ecumenical Patriarchate and Greek Minority in Turkey."[26] An encyclical by Archbishop Iakovos in August lamented the unjust expulsion of more than one thousand Greek Orthodox from Istanbul and the horrible effects of napalm raids on Cyprus by the Turkish Air Force.[27] His advent encyclical in November reported increased pressures on the Greek minority in the Phanar and renewed Turkish agitation on Cyprus against the Greeks, "who are engaged in the sacred struggle for their self-determination."[28] A news release from the Archdiocesan headquarters two days later cited a *New York Times* editorial that characterized the deportations from the Phanar as "violations of human rights."[29]

The Turkish problem was the focus of resolutions at the congresses in 1980, 1984, 1986, and 1988. The 1988 resolution "On Human Rights in Cyprus and Northern Epirus" (or southern Albania) bewailed the virtual elimination of "the civil liberties of the Orthodox minorities" in the areas under Turkish military occupation.[30] The preceding congress (1986) had issued a more coherent ethical rationale for a political solution to the problem:

> In keeping with the traditional and historic principles of the United States in safeguarding justice, freedom, respect for human rights and the rule of law, we earnestly request and urge that the government use its influence and good offices with the government of Turkey to remove its occupation troops from Cyprus and moderate its intransigence so that an honorable and fair compromise solution to the Cypriot problem may be achieved with the human and civil rights of both Greek and Turkish Cypriots guaranteed and protected, the historic ethnological character of the island maintained, and the freedom of the Cypriot people and the territorial integrity of the Republic of Cyprus secured under effective international guarantees with security and justice for all its inhabitants.[31]

This appeal was obviously directed primarily at U.S. public officials —hence the lack of any explicitly Orthodox theological content. Similarly, the resolution "On Relations with Turkey" urged the governments of Greece and Turkey to "develop means of peaceful co-existence based on principles of fairness, justice and mutual respect" as promulgated in the U.N. Charter and the Helsinki Accords on Human Rights—not in the Bible or through religious revelation.[32] Another resolution at that congress addressed the plight of the Patriarchate. The delegates pledged their loyalty to Constantinople and appealed to the United Nations, to the governments of "all freedom loving nations," particularly the United States and Canada, to the World Council of Churches and the National Council of Churches, and to all Christian and Jewish religious leaders to use "their good offices with the Turkish government" to allow the Patriarchate to function freely.[33]

In his encyclicals Archbishop Iakovos has assumed the mantle of chronicler of the persecution of the Greek Orthodox on Cyprus and in the Phanar. His tone, however, has, on the whole been more plaintive than polemical. In his Ochi Day encyclical in 1964, the year he first broached the Turkish problem, Iakovos exhorted his fellow Greek Orthodox in America to be objective on the matter:

> We therefore appeal to your hearts and consciences, dearly beloved brethren, to do your utmost to enlighten American public opinion with the true facts of this great cause [self-determination for the Greeks in Turkey and on Cyprus], through the modern media of press, television and radio, and through public lectures and personal discussions. We denounce no one and accuse no one. Our entire effort in this vital matter should be characterized by objectivity and motivated by a well intentioned patriotism. For we know that public opinion in this land of ours is most sensitive and receptive to the objective truth.[34]

The archbishop's subsequent statements on this problem have sometimes taken a vituperative tone instead of the dispassionate "objectivity" he called for. In October 1965, for example, Iakovos suggested that "the nation of Turkey . . . does not comprehend and even scorns the meaning of freedom."[35] And in 1974, in the wake of an unsuccessful attempt to pressure the U.S. Congress to impose an arms embargo on Turkey, the archbishop bitterly railed against "political leaders who accept expediency as a basis for their actions, rather than rooting themselves in the self-evident truths, principles and traditions that made our Country the champion of all freedom-loving peoples throughout the world."[36]

In March 1992, however, Archbishop Iakovos waxed hopeful on this issue. In an encyclical to all parish councils of the archdiocese, he lamented that "the major powers seem to have forgotten Cyprus." But he also expressed his confidence in President George Bush's personal efforts to restore human rights to the divided island. Iakovos specifically urged all faithful elements of his Church to send to the White House a telegram drafted by the Cypriot organizations in America that commended the president for acting as "a catalyst for a just and early solution of the Cyprus problem," and that urged him to intensify his efforts to assist in the implementation of U.N. Resolution 716, which the United States had co-sponsored in 1991.[37]

The Greek Archdiocese has been surprisingly successful in persuading the National Council of Churches to take up the cause of the Greeks in Turkey and Cyprus. A 1955 NCC resolution on "Destruction of Churches in Turkey" complained that "extreme violence and outrage were unleashed against Greeks and other minorities in Turkey."[38] The NCC Governing Board next expressed to the U.S. government its concern that the Turkish government was about to expel the Ecumenical Patriarchate from Istanbul ("Threat to Patriarchate in Turkey," May 2, 1957). A resolution on "Religious Freedom in Turkey" (May 9, 1979) warned about "increasing pressure on Christians" in that country and sought to alert President Jimmy Carter and the U.S. State Department to this "issue of human rights." A resolution on "Missing Persons in Cyprus" (November 5, 1981) noted the ill effects of "the Turkish invasion of Cyprus in July 1974."

The NCC's record on these issues, however, is not solely critical of Turkey. A resolution on "The Cyprus Situation" (October 12, 1974) lamented "the unwarranted intervention of both Greek and Turkish governments into the affairs of the sovereign Republic of Cyprus." And in "The Ecumenical Patriarchate and the Turkish Government" (November 8, 1985) the NCC commended the Turks for their cooperation in rebuilding a Cypriot church destroyed by the Nazi German invasion in 1941.

Other International Concerns

The 1980 clergy-laity congress was held in July in Atlanta, Georgia —the home state of President Jimmy Carter, then in a titanic struggle with Senator Edward M. Kennedy (D.-Mass.) for renomination to the presidency by the Democratic Party. A "Statement on Morality in International Relations," like the location of the congress itself, signified support for the administration of President Carter, particularly his approach to human rights. The previous congress (1978) had sent the president a letter praising his human-rights policies and pledging support for them.[39] No president before or since the Georgian has enjoyed such warm public support from Archbishop Iakovos. Only in 1988, with the highly politicized ecclesial activities surrounding the ill-fated presidential campaign of Michael Dukakis, did the Greek Archdiocese take a more visible stand in support of a political figure. (To be sure, the Clinton presidency may yet prove the most cordial to the Greek Archdiocese.[40])

The 1980 resolution demanded consistency instead of ideology in the condemnation of armed aggression and violations of human rights. But the congress approached "the so-called great or super powers of the world" from the vantage of what Jeane Kirkpatrick has described as "moral equivalence"—that is, both the Soviet Union and the United States were presumed guilty of more or less equivalent abuses of "small and defenseless nations and racial minorities of the world" simply to advance "what they believe to be their interests or the interests of their allies." There followed a list of human-rights cases that were said to serve only as "useful and valuable pawns in their [the superpowers'] political chessgame":

> The Blacks in South Africa; the Thais and Tibetans; the Georgians, Ukrainians, Latvians, Esthonians [sic] and Lithuanians in the Soviet Union; the Afghans and Kurds in both Iran and Turkey; the Greek Cypriots in Cyprus, the Greeks in Northern Epirus, the Armenian and Greek minorities in Turkey. . . .[41]

Aside from the Turkish problem, the range of international concerns of the Greek Orthodox Archdiocese has been rather circumscribed. Not a single critical comment was recorded—even at the 1968 clergy-laity congress in Athens—concerning the human-rights abuses of the right-wing junta that governed Greece from 1967 until 1974. Nations other than Cyprus and Turkey received scant attention prior to 1980, when, besides naming human-rights abuses in the above list, the congress affirmed "the moral and social responsibility of the more prosperous nations of the world to share their bounty with the deprived in an honest and sincere effort to reduce the disparity and to alleviate their poverty and suffering."[42] Another statement in 1980 urged that Jerusalem "be declared a free city entrusted to the care not only of one tradition, or one faith, but to all three major faiths who collectively shall be charged with the awesome responsibility and task of preserving the free city concept."[43]

The 1986 congress introduced a few new areas of concern. One resolution demanded "absolute respect for the Greek character of Macedonia," thus taking sides in a long-standing nationalistic controversy involving the nations or governments of Serbia, Bulgaria, and Greece.[44] A resolution on "The Greek Orthodox in Albania" suggested that the peace terms between the governments of Greece and Communist Albania include the release of "those who are imprisoned without specific accusations for violations of penal law" and the restoration of free communication between Greek Orthodox outside Albania and their relatives inside the country.[45] Two resolutions addressed the violation of human rights in the Republic of South Africa by condemning apartheid and urging the government there "to free political prisoners" and "begin a dialogue with all those involved in an effort to guarantee basic human rights" for all inhabitants of that country.[46]

Finally, two 1980 resolutions concerned the Middle East. A resolution condemning international terrorism expressed "indignation to the governments which support this terrorism or cover it up." The concluding paragraph mysteriously shifted to the "Palestinian Problem," urging the U.S. government to intensify its efforts to resolve that problem as soon as possible. In a resolution on "the political and military unrest in Lebanon," the delegates proposed as a solution "the reestablishment of political order and the creation of a secular state with a governing system that guarantees civil and human rights and religious freedom to all faiths including the Orthodox."[47] A similarly inoffensive resolution on the Middle East came out of the 1988 clergy-laity congress. This one resolved to set aside a day of prayer for all those suffering from any source in that region of the world and encouraged the U.S. government "to assist in all appropriate ways and in a consistent manner" the process of peace and reconciliation.[48]

Archbishop Iakovos has, like his clergy and laity, devoted relatively little attention to abuses of freedom and human rights in areas other than Cyprus and Turkey. One other region that *has* drawn his moral indignation, however, is the Soviet Union. Early in 1975, in an extraordinary collaborative effort with Metropolitan Ireney Bekish, primate of the OCA, and Metropolitan Filaret Voznesensky, primate of the Russian Orthodox Church Outside Russia, Archbishop Iakovos took part in a joint appeal "to all Christians in the world who cherish the dignity of man" on behalf of the dissident Orthodox journalist Vladimir Osipov, who had been unjustly arrested and imprisoned by the Soviet government.[49] Similarly, in July 1978, the archbishop sent a "telegram of outrage" to President Carter and Soviet leader Leonid Brezhnev protesting the "denial of basic human rights" to three Soviet dissidents: Anatoly Scharansky (Jewish), Aleksandr Ginsburg (Russian Orthodox), and Victoras Pyatkus (Lithuanian Catholic).[50] Earlier that year in his March 25 encyclical, Archbishop Iakovos vigorously repudiated the "slogans and banners of so-called socialist republics," which engage in the systematic "subjugation and oppression of man" through "mind control."[51]

In April 1990, during a surprising controversy in Jerusalem over the questionable occupation by a group of militant Jewish settlers of a building owned by the Greek Orthodox Patriarchate of Jerusalem, Archbishop Iakovos effectively mobilized his brother bishops in SCOBA. Just a week after the international news media displayed scenes of Israeli officials tear-gassing Patriarch Diodoros and other Christian protesters, SCOBA sent a message of "brotherhood and solidarity" to Patriarch Diodoros, assuring him that "we stand ready to render any support in these trying times." To U.S. Secretary of State James Baker the SCOBA bishops expressed their concern over these violations of religious freedom and requested a meeting with Baker (which was not granted). SCOBA also sent a telegram to Chaim Herzog, president of Israel, protesting the violent occupation of the Greek Orthodox property and calling for "the prompt and just solution to the problem by the removal of the settlers and the return of the property to the Patriarchate."[52] Rarely has SCOBA acted so quickly and decisively as it did in this controversy.

Archbishop Iakovos also added his considerable spiritual weight to the battle over the proper name of a little breakaway republic from the former Communist state of Yugoslavia. In a statement issued in

March 1992 he objected strenuously to the "anti-Hellenic propaganda orchestrated over the years by the communists of Skopje"—that is, the self-proclaimed Republic of Macedonia. "They have usurped," he railed, "the historic Greek names of 'Macedonia' and 'Macedonian' in order to be given more attention and at the same time promote claims over territory, which is not theirs." The statement continued in this vein for several paragraphs, heaping indignation upon the republic for this "outrageous" abuse, while praising the "measure and prudence" demonstrated by the Greek government in the controversy.[53] On Sunday, May 31, 1992, the archbishop led a protest demonstration in Washington, D.C., near the White House, that drew more than 50,000 supporters of the Greek cause.[54] Again, on January 16, 1993, Iakovos spearheaded a four-hour rally at Dag Hammarskjold Plaza across from the United Nations building in Manhattan. The archbishop voiced his "righteous indignation" over the U.N. Security Council's apparent willingness to acknowledge the new ethnic republic under the convoluted name "Former Yugoslav Republic of Macedonia" (FYROM).[55]

But Archbishop Iakovos reserved his greatest ire for his own government in February 1994, after the Clinton administration announced its intention to grant diplomatic recognition to FYROM. In an official announcement issued on February 9, Iakovos expressed his "outrage" at Washington's "political conformism and alignment with the sinful European Balkan policy." The archbishop elaborated on this "sinful" policy in a personal message sent the same day to President Clinton, Secretary of State Warren Christopher, and National Security Advisor Anthony Lake. Recognition of a breakaway republic of the former Yugoslav state, Iakovos protested, would constitute "sanctioning the de facto and openly anti-democratic action of Communist ruler Tito"—an oblique reference to Marshall Josef Broz Tito's cynical nationalities policy that created ersatz Bosnian and Macedonian "nations" to check the presumably more dangerous nationalism of the Serbs and Croats. Upholding the banner of the Greek nation-state, Archbishop Iakovos concluded his message: "We feel betrayed in our hope that our Government would outrightly refuse to ally herself with Germany and those European nations who have little regard for the rights of an Allied nation that bravely stood and fought for the prevalence of justice, democratic principles and practices in this agonizing post-Communist world."[56] His profound frustration with President Clinton, however, did not prevent Archbishop Iakovos from trying one more time to dissuade the U.S. president from his errant policy. On March 9, he and several other Greek-American leaders including U.S. Senator Paul Sarbanes (D.-Md.) met with Clinton at the White House. The result was impressive: Clinton promised not to establish formal diplomatic relations with FYROM for a while.[57]

It is safe to say that Archbishop Iakovos's preoccupation with what many outside the Balkans might regard as a tempest in an ethnic teapot, or a political issue with little religious resonance (the population of Macedonia, too, is predominantly Orthodox Christian), reveals Iakovos at his best as ethnarch of the Greek (Orthodox) community in America.

ORTHODOX CHURCH IN AMERICA

The public moral witness of the Orthodox Church in America necessarily suffers in any comparison to that of the larger, better organized, and more politically attuned Greek Archdiocese. The primates of the OCA have issued far fewer encyclicals on moral and social themes than their counterpart, Archbishop Iakovos, and the seven All-American Councils prior to 1986 passed only a handful of resolutions on issues of freedom and human rights. In 1986 and again in 1989, the councils finally produced an output roughly equivalent to that of their parallel institution in the Greek Archdiocese, the clergy-laity congress.

The 1989 council considered some two dozen resolutions, but, owing to poor time management by the organizers, the delegates were unable to vote on most of them. That may have been a blessing in disguise, since most of the proposed resolutions, such as one condemning Zionism, were highly politicized. The OCA's Holy Synod of Bishops—the primate and the ten diocesan hierarchs, who reserve the right to approve, reject, or modify any resolutions passed at the council—had to sift through these texts at their semi-annual meetings in October 1989 and March 1990 and eventually issued only a handful of decrees.

Hierarchical Statements

Metropolitan Ireney Bekish, who reigned from 1965 until 1977, was the first primate of the OCA after Moscow granted autocephaly to the former Metropolia in 1970. Publicly, at least, he seemed concerned only with events in the Soviet Union, the ancestral homeland of the vast majority of his flock. As noted previously, he appealed jointly with Archbishop Iakovos and Metropolitan Filaret on behalf of the imprisoned Russian Orthodox dissident Vladimir Osipov.[58] In November 1970, Ireney also intervened in the unusual case of a Lithuanian seaman, Simas Kudirka, who, when he attempted to defect, was handed over to Soviet authorities by the U.S. Coast Guard. Metropolitan Ireney sent a stong letter of protest to President Richard Nixon, in which he concluded:

I consider it to be my duty, on behalf of myself and my flock, to respectfully request that every possible measure be taken by you, Mr. President, to avoid the reoccurence of such deplorable incidents. The moral and spiritual dignity of the American democracy is at stake.[59]

Kudirka was not Orthodox, but Ireney's sense of justice was offended nonetheless.

The current primate of the OCA, Metropolitan Theodosius Lazor, is emerging as an impassioned defender of human rights in all political contexts irrespective of ideology. Earlier in his primacy, which began in 1977, he issued the usual fervent appeals on behalf of persecuted Orthodox Christians in Communist countries, such as the popular Russian preacher Fr. Dmitri Dudko[60] and "the Orthodox people in Yugoslavia."[61] The Holy Synod also produced at its October 1983 session a ringing denunciation of "the man-made and state-controlled famine of 1932-33" in the Soviet Union. The bishops, led by Metropolitan Theodosius, professed their solidarity with the worldwide Ukrainian communities on the occasion of the fiftieth anniversary of that atrocity, grounding their witness in an absolute principle of human rights. "We oppose the reduction of the human person to the condition of a means toward an end," they declared. "We believe in the dignity of every human life, and insist on the dignity of every human death before God."[62]

After a few years as primate, Metropolitan Theodosius began to adopt a more even-handed approach to human-rights abuses. After the 1986 council, broadening the scope of a 1985 decree of the Holy Synod concerning Christians,[63] proclaimed October an annual month of prayer for the persecuted and oppressed, the metropolitan remarked, "We're trying to keep a balance on human rights and not just point a finger behind the Iron Curtain or focus on Orthodox being persecuted. Others are persecuted, too, and have to be given support."[64] In an address to a symposium on religion in Communist lands in May 1987, Theodosius quipped, "Solidarity is not persuasive when it comes à la carte." A proper commemoration of the forthcoming millennium of Christianity in Kievan Rus, he continued, would preclude religious leaders and communities from "speaking and acting selectively" about human rights.[65] The metropolitan amplified that message in November 1987 in a letter to the National Council of Churches. Theodosius proposed the "model of a *shared affirmation of solidarity*" with "our brothers and sisters in the human family who are oppressed by the powerful . . . whether the *oppressors* are on the 'right' or on the 'left' of the political spectrum, and whether the *oppressed* are Christians, or Jews, or Muslims, or Buddhists, or Hindus, or anyone else."[66]

Conciliar Resolutions

Since the OCA received its disputed autocephaly in 1970, the All-American Councils have passed twenty-eight resolutions on issues of freedom and human rights. Eight of these reaffirmed the traditional Orthodox moral and political opposition to abortion, often calling for specific actions such as congressional approval of a "human life amendment" to the U.S. Constitution.[67] The 1975 council pronounced against euthanasia (without, however, specifying "active" or "passive") as "an act of murder which cannot be justified for any reason."[68] A hotly debated resolution against capital punishment was approved at the 1989 council in a close vote.[69]

Some resolutions have addressed the special concerns or needs of constituencies within the OCA. The 1986 council was relatively prolific in this regard. One resolution supported "the right of the Pribilof Aleuts to harvest the fur seal in a traditionally responsible way and to

sell them to a world market."[70] Another resolution pertaining to
Alaska exhorted Church members to "use all appropriate means to
effect Congressional action"—even political lobbying, if necessary—
to safeguard the possession in perpetuity by native Alaskan peoples of
certain lands, resources, and properties conveyed to them by Congress
in 1971.[71] Other resolutions deplored anti-Arab racism and anti-
Russian bigotry in America, particularly prejudice and discrimination
against persons with Russian or Arab ancestry as expressed in facile
associations of Russians with Soviet Communism or Arabs with international terrorism.[72]

Several resolutions have addressed other human-rights concerns
familiar to Orthodox Christians in America. The 1975 council expressed "profound indignation" at Soviet actions against the pilgrims
to the Monastery of Pochaev and at the closing of the historic cathedral
of the Dormition of the Virgin Mary in Vladimir.[73] The 1983 council
appealed to President Hosni Mubarek of Egypt "for the immediate
release of Pope of Alexandria Shenouda III from exile and the restoration to the Pope of the full and free exercise of his authority as head
of the Coptic Orthodox Church," and "for justice for the Coptic
Orthodox Church and all her clergy and lay people."[74] The same
council protested the imprisonment of leaders of the Orthodox religious revival in the Soviet Union, naming Deacon Vladimir Rusak,
Fr. Gleb Yakunin, Aleksandr Ogorodnikov, Vladimir Poresh, and Zoya
Krakhmalnikova. That resolution called on the Soviet government "to
release these prisoners of conscience who are imprisoned for the
expression of their faith" and, since "freedom is indivisible, . . . to
keep faith with its own pronouncements on the religious rights of its
citizens."[75] A third 1983 resolution lamented the systematic violations
of the human dignity and civil and religious rights of Orthodox Christians in the Middle East. Four examples were cited: Turkey, Cyprus,
Lebanon, and "the Holy Land," where Orthodox were caught in the
crossfire between the state of Israel and the Palestine Liberation Organization.[76] Resolutions condemning human-rights abuses in Romania, Lebanon, and Israel/Palestine were presented to the resolutions
committee of the 1989 council, but the delegates never had an opportunity to discuss them.

Some resolutions seemed motivated, at least in part, by American
patriotism. The 1980 council, which convened a week after the elec-

tion of Ronald Reagan as president of the United States, commended the U.S. government under President Carter "for its diligence in pursuing the safe release of those American hostages presently being held in Iran."[77] The 1986 council anticipated the bicentennial of the U.S. Constitution and its "principal [*sic*] of religious freedom" by instructing churches to ring their bells on September 17, 1989, and encouraging members and member institutions of the OCA to participate in appropriate local, state, and national celebrations of the Constitution.[78] A similar resolution celebrated the centennial of the Statue of Liberty in New York Bay as "a great symbol of the freedoms" enjoyed by U.S. citizens, particularly "the liberty to worship God in an Orthodox manner."[79]

Support for freedom and human rights in principle, however, has characterized the councils since 1973. The council in that year called for "a national effort to cultivate freedom and responsibility, honesty and love as means of overcoming the erosion of moral ideals in America."[80] The 1975 council affirmed a traditional theological proposition— namely, "that true human liberation can never be achieved without the spiritual and moral values given to man by God."[81] The 1977 council pledged "continued effort on behalf of the human rights and religious freedom of all."[82] The 1980 council proposed the establishment of a Church task force on human rights to monitor "the activities of all organizations concerned with religious freedom and violations thereof throughout the world."[83] This task force has not met.

The most comprehensive statement thus far on human rights emerged from the 1986 council, held in Washington, D.C.[84] The delegates voiced their solidarity with everyone who suffers persecution for religious reasons "as well as economic, social, racial, and political oppression." Anticipating Metropolitan Theodosius's phrasing, the council eschewed expedient "considerations of political ideology and political strategy" and explicitly cited human-rights abuses by governments on both the "right" and the "left" of the political spectrum. The litany of condemnation, which reads like the annual report of Amnesty International (an organization that is praised by name in the statement), mentions the Republic of South Africa, the Soviet Union, Ethiopia, Egypt, Cuba, Guatemala, "all countries dominated by Marxist ideology," Turkey, Lebanon (where "the large Orthodox population" has been left "defenseless" in the religious warfare between

Muslims and Roman Catholics), Albania, Bulgaria, Czechoslovakia, Poland, Yugoslavia, Afghanistan, Angola, Chile, Mozambique, Nicaragua, and "countless other countries." This list is breathtaking in its scope and unprecedented in Orthodox circles in America. A reader may wonder, however, which factions in the civil wars in Nicaragua and Angola the delegates were implicitly accusing of perpetrating "genocide" and "terror."

There was no vagueness in the list of persecuted Orthodox Christian confessors whom the 1986 council commended to the congregations for intercessory prayer: Fr. Gleb Yakunin, Aleksandr Ogorodnikov, Lev Timofeev, Zoya Krakhmalnikova, Felix Svetov, Pavel Prozenko, and Vladimir Zelinsky in the Soviet Union; the monk Ilarion Argatu and Frs. Romulus Bipart, Gavrila Ştefan, Marian Ştefanescu, and Alexander Pop in Romania; and Patriarch Dimetrios I of Constantinople in Turkey.

Aside from promising prayerful support for the victims of oppressive governments, the council could only resort to moral suasion in this extrordinary resolution. "The States and Governments responsible for the acts of repression and terror," the resolution concluded, "must be publicly exposed and called to change their policies."

Ecumenical Statements

The contribution of the OCA to the resolutions on religious freedom and human rights issued by the NCC and the WCC has been minimal. The pronounced leftward drift in the moral witness of these ecumenical organizations since the late 1960s has been amply chronicled by critics such as K. L. Billingsley and Ernest W. Lefever.[85] Before that time, the NCC frequently condemned Communist violations of human rights in the Soviet Union. By 1969, however, perhaps in response to the role of the United States in the Vietnam War, the delegates began to mix criticism of Soviet and Soviet-inspired abuses with verbal assaults on "right-wing" regimes such as Chile and South Africa and reminders of American culpability in various international affairs. A bellwether resolution on the 1968 Soviet invasion of Czechoslovakia (January 23, 1969) bewailed the continued oppression there at the hands of the Soviets but added with unwarranted aplomb that "our country itself has been guilty of oppression."

The tendency to soft-pedal the systematic violation of religious liberty in the former Soviet Union and its Eastern European satellites reached its apogee in an NCC-sponsored documentary broadcast by NBC in 1985. "The Church of the Russians" was a two-hour program hosted by the Rev. V. Bruce Rigdon, a Presbyterian minister and NCC official with a personal interest in Russian Orthodoxy. This rosy view of the Russian Orthodox Church failed, incredibly, to address the problems of Soviet domination of religion. No formal protests were lodged with the NCC by the OCA or any other Orthodox member jurisdiction. In a conversation with me in October 1990, however, Rigdon contended that primary responsibility for this one-sided picture lay with the network's producers and editors, who had had the last word in the project.

The role of the OCA in the World Council of Churches has been virtually negligible. The Church's delegation is continually dwarfed by the much larger and more determined delegation of the Moscow Patriarchate. But, though forced by circumstances to play David to Moscow's Goliath, the OCA has not been coerced into public silence. At the 1983 WCC Assembly in Vancouver, for example, when the leadership prohibited any open discussion of problems in the Soviet Union, Fr. Leonid Kishkovsky, Archbishop Iakovos, and the Orthodox layman A. Koulouris of Greece joined more than eighty other delegates in a direct appeal to Soviet leader Yuri Andropov. They expressed gratitude for the permission to emigrate granted to two Pentecostal families and requested amnesty or permission to emigrate for Andrei Sakharov, Fr. Gleb Yakunin, Zoya Krakhmalnikova, several others by name, and "all other prisoners of conscience."[86]

Similarly, Fr. John Meyendorff, the late, widely respected OCA theologian and dean of the OCA's St. Vladimir's Seminary in New York, did not mince words in his preliminary evaluation of the WCC's 1983 Vancouver Assembly.[87] He noted "the radical turn 'to the left,' away from the traditional ecumenical search for Church unity and towards solidarity with radical movements seeking to change society and the world," that had marked the 1968 Assembly of the WCC in Uppsala, Sweden. He also criticized the "flagrant partiality and unbalance" of the Vancouver Assembly's resolutions on public moral issues, particularly the "WCC's silence on the segregation and repression of religion in the communist countries." These serious defects notwithstanding, Fr. John suggested that perhaps the Vancouver Assembly had introduced a change for the better, and that, in any case, the Orthodox could hardly withdraw from the organization in "self-righteous isolationism."

Post-Communist Russia

As Russia began to emerge from under the rubble of seven decades of Communist domination, the position of the OCA on the role of the Moscow Patriarchate took an ominous turn. Once openly critical of the interference of the Communists in the life of the Church in the Soviet Union, OCA spokesmen seem determined to support the Patriarchate unwaveringly, even to the point of attempting to squelch any criticism of its past collaboration with the regime.

Metropolitan Theodosius and Patriarch Aleksii II have established a profound personal friendship that, nevertheless, may threaten the already disputed claim of the OCA to be a truly autocephalous national Church. On virtually every intra-Orthodox issue in which the Moscow Patriarchate has a vested interest, Theodosius and the national OCA leadership predictably side with the mother Church. In November 1993, for example, Metropolitan Theodosius hosted Metropolitan Volodymyr Sabodan of the Ukainian Orthodox Church—that is, the "autonomous" branch of the Moscow Patriarchate based in Kyyiv. The national OCA newspaper duly observed that Volodymyr "heads the only Ukrainian Church recognized by the Ecumenical Patriarchate and world Orthodoxy" (the same recognition, ironically, that the OCA itself has not yet received!), thus committing the OCA to Moscow's side in the three-way schism among the Orthodox in Ukraine.[88]

Theodosius and his chancery in Syosset, New York, have also worked feverishly to channel U.S. foreign aid to Russia through the Moscow Patriarchate; their efforts finally bore fruit on July 1, 1993, when the U.S. Department of Agriculture and the new International Orthodox Christian Charities (IOCC), based in Baltimore, Maryland, concluded a $15 million agreement to provide 10,700 metric tons of food items for distribution to Russians by the Moscow Patriarchate and other charitable organizations in the Russian Republic.

But Metropolitan Theodosius clearly squandered a unique opportunity to witness prophetically on pressing domestic moral issues such as abortion or "gay rights" when he and thirty-seven other Orthodox and Protestant leaders met on March 24, 1993, with the new, politically liberal president of the United States, Bill Clinton. Theodosius opted instead to carry water for Patriarch Aleksii and the Russian Church. "The Church is deeply concerned," he declared before introducing Bishop Pavel of the Moscow Patriarchate, "that a resurgence of former communist hardliners could catapult religious life in Russia back to the Khrushchev era."[89]

This "re-Russification" of the OCA, in the words of some frustrated OCA priests, also has an unmistakably dark side. An otherwise excellent resolution on "The Collapse of Communism" at the tenth All-American Council in Miami in July 1992 was marred by a mean-spirited antagonism toward the perceived rivals of the Moscow Patriarchate. After rejoicing at the liberation of Orthodox brothers and sisters from Communist oppression, honoring the thousands of confessors and martyrs, mourning the millions of victims of the Communist terror and genocide, affirming "the freedom of conscience and religious freedom of all peoples," and noting the current conflicts, obstacles, and challenges confronting the Orthodox Churches in "the former USSR, central and eastern Europe and the Balkans," the 400 or so clergy and lay delegates resolved to "affirm and support the Orthodox churches (such as those of Russia, Romania, Serbia and Georgia) which appealed for peace and tolerance."

The resolution turned negative, however, when the delegates also declared in nuanced language their "solidarity with all Christians and people of goodwill who censure those who use the tragic and chaotic conditions in these parts of the world for self-serving political, ideological, ethnic, economic and religious purposes." Lest there be any doubt as to who these enemies of the Moscow Patriarchate are, the delegates added "that the Orthodox Church in America . . . especially deplores the actions of émigré Orthodox groups, Western and Eastern-rite (Uniate) Roman Catholics and various Protestant denominations and sects which have shown themselves guilty of unscrupulous behavior in these newly-liberated countries."[90] Such boldness in naming competing religious bodies is perhaps the most striking feature of the last section. But more disturbing is the thinly veiled attack on the Russian Orthodox Church Outside Russia under the rubric of "émigré Orthodox groups." *Moral* resolutions of this variety are not usually given to jurisdictional bickering.

The role of Professor Dmitry Pospielovsky at the March 1992 press conference on Capitol Hill in which Fr. Gleb Yakunin spoke about the Russian Parliament's investigation of KGB archives may presage a more concerted effort by Patriarch Aleksii II's loyalists in North America to discredit the sharpest critics of Moscow. Brought down from the University of Western Ontario by the OCA chancery to rebut Fr. Gleb, Professor Pospielovsky directed one carefully worded question to the Russian priest at the press conference. He challenged Fr. Gleb—a cleric of the Moscow Patriarchate itself—to explain the apparent inconsistency between his simultaneous criticism of the collaboration of the Russian hierarchy and his personal support, as a member of the Russian Parliament, for former KGB agent Oleg Kalugin's candidacy for a political post in Russia. Fr. Gleb responded that the onetime murderous Kalugin, unlike the patriarch himself, had repented profusely and publicly. At a discussion later that evening at St. Nicholas OCA Cathedral in Washington, D.C., Professor Pospielovsky publicly criticized those who had organized and participated in the press conference for airing "dirty linen" before the nation; this, he averred, would only serve the interests of nonOrthodox churches that wish to proselytize the vulnerable Russian Orthodox people.

This sharp disagreement in tactics—and not ends, if one may charitably presume honor on both sides of this internal dispute—should not obscure the damage to its credibility that the OCA may inflict on itself as a Church if some of its most prominent scholars and clergy continue to attack dissident prophets such as Fr. Gleb Yakunin and Fr. Georgi Edelshtein. The OCA's filial loyalty to the mother Church in Russia may be laudable as long as it does not reduce the OCA to a vassal Church or turn a blind eye to the dangers still lurking within the leadership of the Moscow Patriarchate.

The Romanian Episcopate

The Romanian Orthodox Episcopate of America warrants special attention in light of chapter 3, which is highly critical of the Episcopate's mother Church. As a distinct albeit "ethnic" diocese of the OCA, the ROEA may issue its own moral and social resolutions, and the bishop may, on his own behalf as an apostolic archpastor and on behalf of his flock, proclaim the morality of the Church as long as he is faithful to Orthodox tradition.

Devotion to freedom and human rights has characterized this jurisdiction from its inception as an independent religious body. Since 1951, when the Church Congress in Chicago revised the articles of incorporation and severed all filial ties to the Communist-dominated Romanian Orthodox Patriarchate in Bucharest, the ROEA has had to fight for its ecclesial life. For almost three decades, the competing Romanian Orthodox jurisdiction in North America, with its direct ties to Bucharest, waged a war of attrition against the ROEA, challenging its canonical legitimacy and fighting it in the courts for control of churches and other Episcopate property.[91] In June 1993, however, a joint commision of the two jurisdictions proposed the restoration of "normal ecclesial relations . . . as between any other two canonical dioceses in America."[92] The clergy-laity bodies of the two episcopates subsequently adopted this proposal, thus ending a long and painful estrangement. In May 1994, for the first time in more than forty years, Bishop Nathaniel led a small ROEA delegation to Romania, where the Patriarchate's gracious hospitality further cemented the renewed ties between the erstwhile rival jurisdictions.

Owing to its strong immigrant consciousness, and in the face of the now mercifully terminated religious guerrilla war inspired by Bucharest, the ROEA has dedicated most of its moral witness to the abuse of human rights by the former Communist regime in Romania. The first hierarch of the newly independent ROEA, Archbishop Valerian Trifa, was a tireless advocate of religious and political freedom in his native land. In 1970, for example, he explained to U.S. Secretary of State William Rogers why he could not participate in any events intended to honor Nicolae Ceauşescu during the Romanian dictator's visit to the United States. "The Romanian people," then Bishop Valerian wrote, "are denied their God-given right to choose by their freely expressed will the government they want and the social and economic system to which they aspire." He observed that the Communist government denied "freedom of movement" to its people, particularly the right to emigrate to America and to be reunited with émigré family members. Valerian also said that "Romanian officials often use their presence in the United

States to interfere in the life of our American churches and fraternal organizations."[93]

In one of the supreme ironies in the history of the Orthodox Churches in North America, Bishop Valerian himself became the target of a "human rights" movement, when various individuals and organizations pursuing ex-Nazis in America fixed their sights on him. The Ceaușescu regime and the ever-pliant Patriarchate of Romania joined this witch-hunt, as the Romanian Communist defector Ion Pacepa revealed in 1987. Valerian's enemies in Romania spread wild rumors and disinformation through Securitate agents and other false witnesses, including the late chief rabbi of Bucharest, Moishe Rosen.[94] Although the most serious accusation against him—namely, that as a layman Viorel Trifa had committed atrocities against Jews in Romania in 1940-41—was never proved (and, in fact, was conclusively disproved by the historian Gerald Bobango[95]), Archbishop Valerian was deported from the United States in August 1984 on the grounds that he had supplied false information at his initial immigration hearings in 1955. He died in Portugal in January 1987.

Bishop Nathaniel Popp, Valerian's successor as bishop of the Episcopate, has continued this legacy of public moral witness on the Romanian problem, meeting with U.S. congressmen and other government officials and regularly issuing encyclicals on the subject. In 1989, Bishop Nathaniel and the ROEA were instrumental in securing an open letter signed by 119 members of the U.S. Congress that urged President George Bush to devise a new policy toward the Romanian government, one that would take into account the regime's egregious violations of human rights. Bishop Nathaniel followed this action with his own missive to the president, which the annual clergy-laity congress of the Episcopate had unanimously approved in advance. Nathaniel outlined the precarious situation of the Romanian people in the throes of the systematic material, intellectual, and spiritual destruction at the hands of "a government which intends to remake man in its own image and likeness of total sub-human existence." The Romanian-American community, he said, though neither large nor wealthy nor politically powerful nor socially distinctive, was all that the persecuted 23 million souls in Romania had to speak on their behalf against "the harshest of regimes."[96]

Bishop Nathaniel did not propose any specific U.S. policies. Similarly, a resolution approved at the 1989 congress vehemently condemned the planned destruction of some 7,000 villages and churches by the Communist regime in Romania but did not offer concrete policy options. The delegates appealed, "in the name of our Orthodox faith and for the humanitarian goal of preserving our culture and heritage," to the U.S. and Canadian heads of state, representatives of the governments and churches in North America, and "people of good will" simply "to stop this genocide-like action directed against our Church and the legacy of the Romanian people."[97]

This cautious approach suffered what one hopes will be a temporary setback at the 1992 congress. Outraged by the military conflict in eastern "Moldova"—the former Soviet Republic carved out of Romanian Bessarabia by Josef Stalin after World War II—the delegates approved a resolution deploring and condemning the alleged atrocities committed by the 14th Russian (formerly Soviet) Army and demanded its removal from Moldova by the Russian government in Moscow. This one-sided moral statement made no mention of atrocities against Russians and Ukrainians in the disputed lands committed in retaliation by the Romanian majority. Nor did it include a positive appeal to both of these warring, predominantly Orthodox peoples to resolve their political differences as fellow Christians. A few dissenting voices kept this angry resolution from being approved by acclamation.[98]

More recently, Bishop Nathaniel exercised a more traditional role as moral intercessor, when he appealed directly to Patriarch Aleksii II of Moscow in a December 14, 1993, letter on behalf of the "Tiraspol Six." Three Romanians in the "Transnistrian Republic"—that portion of the former Soviet Republic of Moldova carved out by pro-Russian forces—had been sentenced to death five days earlier, Nathaniel asserted in concert with the International Human Rights Law Group in Washington, D.C., "for the mere reason of having stood up for their own national identity" as Romanians. The wives of these three men also had been "dismissed from their jobs, . . . having been accused of being 'the wife of an enemy of the people.'" Bishop Nathaniel respectfully implored his brother bishop to "use your high office to intercede" with the pro-Russian government in Transnistria on behalf of these six "poor souls." Nathaniel also sent a similar letter on December 22, 1993, to President Clinton. Within two weeks,

Nathaniel received a positive response from the Moscow Patriarchate. Six months later he had still had no response from the White House.[99]

The lack of specific policy recommendations in most of the ROEA documents may, in the long run, prove more of a boon than a bane. Bishop Nathaniel and the ROEA have managed, for the most part, to speak directly and forcefully on issues of both parochial and universal concern, while avoiding the pitfalls of proclaiming empirical error, risking politically infeasible actions, or identifying too closely with ideological interests in partisan struggles. Now that the Communist regime of Nicolae Ceauşescu has fallen, Bishop Nathaniel and the ROEA are providing millions of dollars in humanitarian assistance and lobbying the U.S. Congress and the executive branch, sometimes in tandem with the Bishop Louis Puşcaş—the now retired ordinary of the Romanian Byzantine Catholic Rite in the United States—on behalf of additional governmental assistance. They are also poised to assist the "mother Church" in its struggle to develop a genuinely independent, authentically Orthodox moral identity vis-à-vis the post-Communist state, particularly on the controversial issue of abortion.

ANTIOCHIAN ORTHODOX ARCHDIOCESE

If the Greek Orthodox Archdiocese seems preoccupied with the plight of the Greek Orthodox (and non-Orthodox Greeks) in Turkey and Cyprus, the Antiochian Orthodox Archdiocese has, since the Six-Day War in July 1967, sounded a constant drumbeat of support for the Palestinians under Israeli rule and for the Christians in war-torn Lebanon.

This interest in human rights in the Middle East apparently does not extend, at least publicly, to Syria, the Muslim homeland of the ancestors of many of the Antiochian Orthodox in America. They have not lodged a single word of public protest with the restrictive Syrian regime, widely suspected of having fomented acts of international terrorism. The Antiochians have even welcomed representatives of the Syrian government and other political operatives to their biennial clergy-laity conventions.(The conventions were annual through 1979.) The 1981 convention, for example, featured Abdallah Saadeh, who was identified as a "representative of the Lebanese National Movement in the Arab People's Congress and of the leadership in the Syrian Social Nationalist Party." Saadeh used this opportunity to spout crude anti-Judaic slogans (the Zionists are "the sons of this Devil") and to promote, on behalf of the Antiochians' "Moslem co-patriots," a strange interfaith ecumenism ("Islam is not in contradiction with Christianity")—all without any disavowals or rejoinders from Metropolitan Philip or the assembled delegates.[100] (Of course, this Syrian connection may appear somewhat less odious in view of President George Bush's "temporary" alliance with that government in the Persian Gulf War.)

One may quickly dismiss as groundless, however, the charge made in 1977 by the late Rabbi Marc Tanenbaum of the American Jewish Committee that Metropolitan Philip and Dr. Frank Maria, chairman of the Archdiocese's Standing Committee on Near East and Arab Refugee Affairs, were "Arab propagandists . . . known to be subsidized by Arab governments to carry out anti-Israel and pro-Arab propaganda" within the National Council of Churches.[101] To be sure, Maria, in his own report to the 1972 convention, described a meeting in January 1968 between the metropolitan and "all the Arab diplomatic representatives" where Philip "told them that Arabs had lost two wars by fighting with words and . . . [that] an effective campaign to bring the truth of their cause to the American public would cost $10,000,000, a pittance to the oil-rich nations." Maria hastened to add, however, that Metropolitan Philip refused to lead such a "campaign" himself. Philip volunteered his own efforts in support, but stressed to the Arab representatives that he could not "divert the resources of the Church to politics or allow them to be wasted against superior forces."[102] Even in the light of these questionable dealings, it seems clear that Rabbi Tanenbaum confused sincere ethnic loyalty with sinister foreign intrigue.

Human Rights Outside the Middle East

The Antiochian conventions since Metropolitan Philip was consecrated in August 1966 have approved thirteen resolutions (and tabled or defeated two) concerning freedom and human rights in countries outside the Middle East. These have been interspersed among scores of resolutions on Lebanon, Palestine, and the plight of Arabs elsewhere.

Occasional resolutions on human-rights issues in the United States reflect inconsistent political views. On the one hand, the 1989 convention bucked a liberal trend in other Orthodox jurisdictions by tabling a proposed resolution that would have denounced capital punishment as "contrary to the fundamental values presented in the Gospel."[103] On the other hand, a 1979 resolution recited an ambitious litany of material "rights" supposedly possessed by children, including the right to "experience affection, love and understanding both in the home and in society; . . . to adequate nutrition and medical care; . . . to opportunity for play and recreation; . . . to a name and nationality; . . . to special care, if handicapped; . . . to develop their God-given talents; . . . to be brought up in a spirit of peace, freedom and love."[104]

The Antiochian conventions have, like their Greek and OCA equivalents, assumed a special moral obligation for the Orthodox victims of oppressive political systems throughout the world. A resolution on Cyprus in 1974 condemned the "flagrant external aggression" against the Republic of Cyprus (by unnamed Turkey), which the Antiochians likened to "the tragedy of the Palestinian people," and called for the "restoration of constitutional government" on that war-torn island.[105] The 1978 convention exhorted "President Carter and the heads of all civilized states to support the freedom of the Throne of Constantinople to meet its religious responsibilities."[106] A lengthy resolution in 1983 intervened on behalf of the persecuted Coptic Orthodox Church in Egypt—a non-Byzantine or "Oriental" Orthodox body with which many Eastern Orthodox feel an increasingly closer kinship. The delegates decried the hostility toward the Copts shown by the radical "Islamic Brotherhood" and the persecution of Pope Shenouda III himself, whom the Egyptian government had illicitly arrested and internally exiled; they set aside two days of prayer "as an expression of our solidarity with the Coptic Orthodox faithful" in their struggles to restore their hierarchy and clergy to their rightful positions. The resolution also appealed to the heads of state of the United States, Canada, and Egypt to restore immediately the "legitimate human rights of the Christian minority in Egypt."[107]

Human-rights abuses by Communist governments captured the attention of several conventions. In 1979 the Antiochians adopted a resolution on the "Plight of the Boat People" of Vietnam that excoriated "the callousness and insensitivity of the Vietnamese government and various other Asian governments" toward those Vietnamese who had been forced onto the high seas by the Communist regime. The delegates also criticized the U.S. and Canadian governments for their "inadequate policy" and urged them to alleviate the disaster through economic and medical aid and increased immigration quotas for these Vietnamese displaced persons.[108] More recently, two resolutions protested the mistreatment of religious believers, particularly dissidents, in the Soviet Union. In 1985 the Antiochians lamented the imprisonment or exile of several Orthodox dissidents—Fr. Gleb Yakunin, Aleksandr Ogorodnikov, Vladimir Poresh, Zoya Krakhmalnikova, and Felix Svetov—and petitioned the Soviet authorities "to release these prisoners of conscience" in accordance with "the Helsinki Final Act and other international covenants of which the U.S.S.R. is a signatory."[109] The 1987 convention, anticipating the celebration of the millennium of Christianity in Kievan Rus, broadened its concern and requested that "the Soviet government extend a general amnesty to all religious dissidents currently being held in prisons, labor camps, special psychiatric hospitals and serving terms of internal exile."[110]

The violation of human rights in the former white-minority Republic of South Africa also has vexed the Antiochians. The 1978 convention made a passing reference to "blacks in South Africa," together with "Palestinians and other peoples of all races, color, and creed throughout the world who have been and continue to be persecuted and exterminated without display of concern or outrage from the international community."[111] Seven years elapsed before another convention broached this subject. In 1985 the assembled delegates refused to join the chorus of churches lionizing the sometimes violent rebel groups committed only to the overthrow of the repressive white regime and not to its reform. They tabled a resolution that would have denounced the policy of apartheid and would have beseeched the government to treat all of its people with justice and racial equality, convinced by a priest who had served for many years as a missionary in the region that even this seemingly righteous and innocuous position would have focused unfairly and hypocritically on injustices perpetrated by the South African government alone. As its last item of

business, however, the convention did approve another resolution that
had been hurriedly prepared. The delegates resolved simply to "go on
record deploring the violence in South Africa, supporting all efforts
to restore peace and to bring racial equality to all its citizens."[112]
Although one might wish that the word "peaceful" had been inserted
before "efforts," this statement reflects a commendable attempt to
avoid politicizing a moral issue.

Focus on the Middle East

The Antiochian Archdiocese has been relentless in its advocacy of
the political and moral causes of the Arabs in Palestine and Lebanon
and unrestrained in its criticism of the state of Israel and "Zionists"
everywhere.

The pro-Arab activities of the Antiochian leadership span a
breathtaking variety of organizations, institutions, and media outlets.
Within the Archdiocese itself, Metropolitan Philip's "messages" to the
conventions often invoke the Arab cause. A special Committee on the
Near East and Arab Refugee Problems has, since 1968, served a dual
role. A source of information for the Archdiocese, it is also a combination communications arm and political pressure group. Both Frank
Maria, who heads this committee, and the metropolitan have witnessed to, or lobbied, the U.S. State Department and U.S. presidents
beginning with Lyndon Johnson in August 1967. Maria and the
metropolitan have also granted numerous interviews with the mass
media, issued press releases, and pushed a pro-Arab line at meetings
of the Governing Board (now the General Board) of the National
Council of Churches and, more naturally perhaps, the Middle East
Council of Churches.

Metropolitan Philip has forged a unique alliance among the "Bishops in the American Eastern Christian Church," to use the strange
ecumenical language of a resolution from the 1972 Antiochian convention.[113] Philip also was instrumental in forming a Standing Conference of Lebanese Christian and Muslim Religious Leaders of the
United States, which, early in 1989, issued a statement that ostensibly
sought a peaceful settlement among "all warring factions in Lebanon."
But these leaders revealed a not-so-hidden political agenda by insisting
on the complete withrawal of all Israeli forces from southern Lebanon

"as a first step toward the withdrawal of all non-Lebanese forces" —
an oblique, perhaps craven reference to the Syrians who had illegally
taken up residence in the Bekaa Valley.[114]

In 1978 Metropolitan Philip and Fr. Paul Schneirla of the Archdiocese prevailed upon SCOBA to issue a terse but politically charged
statement on "Peace in the Middle East." The bishops appealed to
President Carter and Secretary of State Cyrus Vance to (1) persuade
Israel to abide by the solutions to the Arab-Israeli crisis proposed by
the United Nations, (2) "guarantee the right of self-determination to
the Palestinian people living in the occupied territories" (that is, since
1967, the West Bank and the Gaza strip), and (3) enforce declared
U.S. policy "that economic and military aid not be given to any nation
which violates human rights."[115] The last point was directed rather
transparently at Israel. But the language was mild compared to what
emerged regularly from the conventions of the Antiochian Archdiocese.

After the first year of his tenure as primate of the Archdiocese,
Metropolitan Philip set the tone of his subsequent activities on behalf
of the pro-Arab cause. "Although we are not a political party by any
means," he cautioned the 1967 convention, "we could not remain
silent in view of the moral principles involved in this struggle since
1947."[116] The Antiochians have indeed proclaimed loudly and
frequently their solidarity with the Arab peoples in the Middle East
in clashes with non-Arab Orthodox and Israelis alike. The 1993 convention, for example, declared its "solidarity with the majority ethnic
Arab constituency within the Patriarchate of Jerusalem" and chided
Patriarch Diodoros I, an ethnic Greek, for "meddling in the affairs"
of the Patriarchates of Constantinople and Antioch.[117]

No fewer than forty-eight moral resolutions on Arab-Israeli problems were approved at the nineteen conventions from 1967 through
1993. Of these, fourteen dealt with the Palestinian problem and eleven
with Lebanon. Among the rest, nine sought to bring about a more
"even-handed" U.S. Middle East policy—perceived as heavily pro-
Israel—by including a request that the United States "suspend all
military and economic aid to Israel" pending its compliance with
international human-rights agreements.[118] Four resolutions complained about unbalanced and unfair coverage of the Middle East in
the American major media; Dr. Maria's report to the 1979 convention

referred to "our 'modern St. George crusade'" to educate the religious communities, media, and government of the United States about the "truth" of the Middle East problem.[119] Three resolutions insisted on an independent, internationally guaranteed status for Jerusalem. Two suggested appropriate assistance for Arab refugees from Israeli territory. One resolution strongly condemned the "irresponsible, lawless and unprovoked attack" by Israel on a nuclear reactor in Iraq in 1981.[120] Another commended Senator Charles Percy of Illinois for his support for the Arab cause. Still another resolution thanked President Hafez Al-Assad and the government of Syria "for their gesture of peace and friendship to the American government and people" in helping to secure the release in June 1985 of the hijacked crew and passengers of TWA Flight 847.[121] In addition to these forty-eight moral resolutions, others with a humanitarian thrust have pledged financial aid and medical supplies for Lebanon, moral and financial support for Balamand Theological Seminary in Beirut, and ecumenical cooperation and dialogue with Muslims, particularly in the Middle East.

These resolutions display a penchant for vitriolic condemnation of the government of Israel—and its "Zionist" fellow travelers, never clearly identified—as the primary, if not sole, cause of all the political ills and military conflicts in the region. And yet the Antiochians profess repeatedly an objectivity supposedly rooted in a universal Christian concern for freedom and human rights.

Resolutions on Lebanon. The resolutions on Lebanon illustrate this contradiction. At the 1978 convention the delegates adopted unanimously a statement moved by Dr. Maria that read in part:

> The Antiochian Orthodox Archdiocese of North America, many of whose parishioners are of Lebanese descent, restates that its position on Lebanon is non-partisan. The Archdiocese has repeatedly deplored the on going bloodshed in Lebanon and has repeatedly reaffirmed its support for the independence, integrity, sovereignty, and unity of Lebanon. It will continue . . . to impress on the U.S. Government the need for a comprehensive and just solution to the chronic Arab-Israeli conflict which has contributed to and aggravated the Lebanese tragedy. The Archdiocese definitely decries the media's erroneous reporting and the Zionists' false

portrayal of the strife in Lebanon as a Christian-Muslim conflict rather than what it is: a social-economic and political struggle aggravated by external forces.[122]

This statement began harmlessly enough but degenerated into a thinly veiled attack on Israel by shifting most of the blame for the violence from the principals in Lebanon itself—all of whom are Arabs, whether Christian (of several varieties), Muslim, or Druze—to the long-standing Arab-Israeli conflict south of the border.

In 1985, in the wake of the controversial incursion/invasion of Lebanon by Israeli military forces in pursuit of the Palestine Liberation Organization, the Antiochians acknowledged that the "on-going fratricide has been precipitated basically by domestic issues." But the convention delegates escalated their verbal assault on Israel. Declaring the Israeli military action a "violation of the UN Charter," they called for "the complete and unconditional withdrawal of Israel's occupation forces from South Lebanon in accordance with the UN Charter and resolutions" and for "the dissolution of all Israel's proxies in South Lebanon"—perhaps a veiled reference to the Christian Falangists, a violent Fascist political party. Further, the Antiochians reaffirmed "the right of the Lebanese people to resist occupation by all means at their disposal"—a remarkably blank check—"until all Lebanese territory is liberated from Israeli occupation and that of its proxies."[123] This wholesale blaming of Israel is also remarkable for its utter silence about the presence in Lebanon of Syrian military occupation forces. Not only did the Antiochians refuse to criticize the Syrians prophetically: the same convention also passed the resolution mentioned above that praised Assad and the Syrian government for their supposed role in the release of American airline passengers held hostage by an Islamic terrorist organization!

The two most recent resolutions have revealed just how close are the ties between the Archdiocese and Damascus. The 1991 convention pledged support for the Syrian-backed government of Elias Hrawi, who was installed after Syrian forces quietly occupied the rest of Lebanon during the Persian Gulf War over Kuwait.[124] The 1993 convention turned its ire against the U.S. Congress for passing Senate Concurrent Resolution 28 on June 19, 1993, which, the Antiochians complained, "interfered in the internal affairs of the Republic of

Lebanon by unilaterally calling for the withdrawal of Syrian forces from Lebanon, a subject which is officially a matter solely between the governments of Lebanon and Syria." The same Antiochian resolution, however, approved of U.N. Security Council Resolution 425, which unabashedly sought on March 19, 1978, to interfere in a matter between the governments of Lebanon and Israel by calling for the immediate withdrawal of Israeli forces from "all Lebanese territory."[125] Besides serving as an unofficial voice of Damascus in North America, the Antiochians resolved at their 1993 convention to lend their considerable ecclesial weight to Lebanese commerce. The delegates urged the United States to "lift the travel restrictions and permit United States airlines to serve Lebanon and Lebanese airlines (MEA) to serve the United States."[126]

Resolutions on Palestine. This extraordinary politicization of the Antiochian Archdiocese's public moral witness on issues of freedom and human rights is evident in all the resolutions on Palestine from the beginning of Metropolitan Philip's primacy. In the immediate aftermath of the Six-Day War in June 1967, the Antiochian convention unanimously urged the U.S. president and Congress to take "immediate action to see that the conquered territories are returned to Egypt, Jordan and Syria."[127] In that war, it should be recalled, Israel launched a preemptive strike on three fronts when its military intelligence service disclosed Arab plans for an imminent attack. The 1970 convention urged the U.S. government to affirm a moderate U.N. General Assembly resolution dated December 10, 1969, that recognized "the inalienable rights of the Palestinian people," particularly their right to self-determination.[128] And the 1974 convention presented a reasonable goal: "to secure for the Palestinian people those human rights and national aspirations which we as Americans regard as essential to human integrity and individual freedom."[129]

But in another resolution at the same convention the Antiochians recommended—in what could only be interpreted as a partisan political move—that the U.S. and Canadian governments "recognize the PLO [Palestine Liberation Organization] as the only legitimate spokesman for the Palestinian people wherever they may be" pending free, uncoerced elections "under neutral auspices."[130] The precise role that the PLO, under the leadership of Yasir Arafat, has played in acts of international terrorism during the past two decades is, at best, uncertain. One of Arafat's lieutenants, George Habesh—the late head of the affiliated Popular Front for the Liberation of Palestine (PFLP) —was Greek Orthodox by upbringing but, according to a recent critical study, "nonpracticing by all accounts."[131]

The same alloy of virtuous rhetoric and passionate prejudice surfaced the following year in a resolution praising tempestuous Lebanon as "a peaceful country" that had "opened its heart to the Palestinian victims of Zionist aggression." Further: "We, as Orthodox Christians deplore all forms of violence, whether by individuals, private groups, or governments, but we consider the premeditated act of technological terror by a government as the most deplorable of all."[132] Here the universal value of the stand against violence is quickly undermined when delegates choose as "the most deplorable of all" the one kind of violence that might be said to characterize the behavior of Israel in the Middle East; this effectively excludes from attention terrorist actions by non-governmental groups such as the PLO or the various tribal factions, Christian or otherwise, in Lebanon.

The Antiochian conventions in 1979 and 1981 proposed additional politically colored conditions for the resolution of the Palestinian problem. "The establishment of an independent and sovereign Palestinian state," the delegates asserted in 1979, is "the only just and lasting solution" to the problem.[133] Even the celebrated Camp David Accords between Egypt and Israel, which President Carter had engineered in September 1979, were, as far as the Antiochians were concerned, inadequate as a peace initiative and as a precursor of a just settlement of the Palestinian problem. The 1981 convention claimed that the treaty had "exacerbated Israeli aggression against the Palestinians and other states in the Middle East area" and hardened the Israeli refusal to recognize the Palestinians' "right to self-determination and statehood in their historic homeland." The delegates consequently urged the U.S. government to begin negotiations with the PLO to resolve the Middle East conflict and "to cease all economic and military aid to the state of Israel until the said state recognizes Palestinian national and human rights, and agrees to abide by international law in its relations with its neighbors."[134] These U.S. foreign-policy proposals were patently unrealistic: neither the Carter nor the nascent Reagan administration would have considered them seriously. By proposing such highly partisan measures, the Antiochians had fixed their rudder in a very tempestuous Middle Eastern sea.

A Turn for the Better. More recently, however, the political course in Israel and its additional territories has taken a dramatic turn for the worse, and the tone of the Antiochian response seems to have taken a turn for the better. Since September 1987, the restriction of political freedoms and the use of excessive force by the Israeli military in the West Bank has generated an increasingly violent insurrection among Palestinians known as the *intifada.* At their 1987 convention on the eve of the *intifada,* the Antiochians produced a resolution on Palestine that criticized in detail the "restrictions of freedom"—especially interference with "freedom of opinion and expression" and "non-violent political activity," "town arrest," and "denial of due process" —imposed on the Palestinians by the government of Israel through its Defense Emergency Regulations and Security Provision Orders.[135] The political and military conditions in the West Bank appear infinitely complex. Perhaps the Antiochians should be commended for their intrepid spirit in seeking to engage that complex scene prophetically. Or perhaps they should be chided again for choosing sides in a political-ethical controversy where experts dare not reach firm conclusions. In any event, the 1987 resolution was conspicuous for its dispassionate tone and its moderate proposal to communicate the Archdiocese's objections to Israeli authorities. It gave reason to hope for a shift in the style of the Antiochian Archdiocese's public moral witness on freedom and human rights in the Middle East.

The 1989 resolution on Lebanon toned down the harsh anti-Israeli language of the 1985 resolution and reverted to earlier appeals that the United Nations make Israel withdraw its military forces as "a first step" toward the removal of all non-Lebanese forces. But this resolution also continued the one-sided condemnation of Israel for exploiting Lebanon for imperialistic purposes.[136] Furthermore, the Antiochians sounded a new ominous note in their 1989 resolution on Palestine by referring provocatively to Israel's "holocaust against the Palestinians."[137]

In contrast, a hopeful sign appeared in September of that same year in the Peace Proposal generated at a meeting of the Standing Conference of Lebanese Christian and Muslim Religious Leaders of the

United States at the headquarters of the Antiochian Archdiocese in Englewood, New Jersey. This time, instead of requiring that Israel make the first move, the group called for "the withdrawal of all non-Lebanese armed forces from Lebanon and the assertion of Lebanese sovereignty over all parts of Lebanon." More significant in terms of human rights, these religious leaders, headed by Metropolitan Philip, added another new dimension to their moral witness with a blanket condemnation of "terrorism in all its forms," including "the taking of hostages by any group or any state."[138]

The dramatic accord between Israel and the PLO on September 9, 1993, may yet prove to be a watershed event for the Antiochian Archdiocese as well as the entire Middle East region. After decades of mutual hostility and atrocities, Israel and the PLO finally agreed to recognize each other diplomatically, thus enabling Israel to grant limited Palestinian self-rule in the Gaza Strip and the West Bank. Four days later, on the White House lawn, Israeli Prime Minister Yitzhak Rabin and PLO Chairman Yasir Arafat signed a "Declaration of Principles" in the presence of U.S. President Bill Clinton. With the stroke of a pen, the PLO became the recognized representative of the Palestinian people, and Arafat, his dubious past notwithstanding, achieved instant credibility as a national leader among the governments of the world. At this writing in spring 1994, it was not yet apparent whether the Antiochian Archdiocese viewed the September 1993 accord as a vindication of its staunch support for the PLO. The next biennial convention is scheduled for summer 1995. By that time the present euphoria may have evaporated, and renewed tensions over the continuing carnage by both sides in the Israeli-occupied territories may once again frustrate what President Clinton called the "great yearning for the quiet miracle of a normal life."[139]

Ecumenical Statements. The pro-Arab activities of the Antiochian Archdiocese in the NCC and WCC have been necessarily moderated by the neutrality both ecumenical organizations ostensibly endeavor to maintain toward the principal adversaries in the Middle East. In its first two decades the NCC supported the Israeli position on the Middle East conflict, but a policy statement issued in May 1969, "On the Crisis in the Middle East," adopted a more even-handed approach to the plight of the Palestinians, asserting in particular that "neither justice nor peace is set forward by being simply 'pro-Arab' or 'pro-Israel.'" A subsequent policy statement signaled perhaps a more fundamental shift toward the Palestinian cause. The November 1980 "Policy Statement on the Middle East" declared for the first time that the PLO was "the only body able to negotiate a settlement" on behalf of the Palestinians.

The Antiochian Archdiocese still regards the NCC's record on the Middle East with suspicion. Fr. Paul Schneirla, chairman of the Archdiocese's Department of Inter-Orthodox and Inter-Faith Relations, reported to the 1983 convention of the Church that the Archdiocese's participation in the NCC "has fluctuated from nominal to intense."[140] Although he had reminded the 1978 convention that "we are not, and have never been, a 'one issue' member of the NCC," the Antiochians have been clearly preoccupied with the Middle East even in ecumenical circles. In his 1978 report Fr. Paul had pointed to the need for a special responsiveness to this issue:

> There is until now, no diminution of Zionist provocation and our membership in the NCC has found us on the front line. As a long-time participant in ecumenical affairs and member of the NCC General Board, I do not welcome the Zionist issue, but I cannot in justice and fairness—to the Jewish community before anyone else—placidly tolerate the ruthless and immoderate propaganda of these would-be spokesmen for world Judaism.[141]

Such wariness of potential "Zionist" influence in the NCC has led the Antiochian delegates to assume a watchdog role in the General Board's deliberations on the Middle East. In 1976, for example, Metropolitan Philip instructed Fr. Paul to protest an official summons by NCC general secretary Claire Randall to the member communions to join Roman Catholic and Jewish leaders in a "three-faith prayer weekend" for the persecuted Jews of Syria.[142]

The Antiochians have also secured significant victories in the NCC. In his report to the 1981 Antiochian convention, Fr. Paul credited Frank Maria, the Archdiocese's special troubleshooter on the Middle East, with having "largely influenced" the NCC's 1980 recognition of the PLO. Fr. Paul also claimed that an NCC resolution in 1983 calling for the withdrawal of all foreign influences from Lebanon had been "inspired by Metropolitan Philip."[143]

SERBIAN ORTHODOX CHURCH

The Serbian Orthodox Church in the United States and Canada (SOC) has, since its inception as an immigrant diocese in the 1930s, nurtured a strong identity as an "old world colony." Even after the wrenching schism in 1963—indeed, perhaps because of the challenge to its "Serbianism" from the former breakaway faction—this branch of the Patriarchate of Serbia (based in Belgrade) maintained a staunch public moral witness regarding the Communist regime in Yugoslavia. As the free voice of the captive Serbian Orthodox Church in the homeland it used every opportunity and means to promote the religious freedom and fundamental human rights of the Serbian people. In the maelstrom of enmity and violence that has engulfed post-Communist Yugoslavia, Serbian Orthodox leaders, in the motherlands and in this country alike, profess unqualified support for the lives and liberties of Croats and Muslims as well as Serbs, though not always with equal fervor. We shall defer detailed discussion of the civil war in the former Yugoslavia until chapter 5. Here we shall focus on SOC documents and activities that touch on issues of freedom in the recent past.

National and Diocesan Resolutions

To be sure, SOC resolutions occasionally have addressed other human-rights issues. The clergy-laity *sabor* (Serbian for "council") in 1980 expressed solidarity with "all of the American people for the American hostages who are still being held captive in Iran."[144] The same *sabor* condemned "the arrest and inhuman treatment by the Soviet authorities toward the priests of the Russian Orthodox Church, Fr. Dimitri Dudko and Fr. Gleb Yakunin, as well as toward other fearless fighters for principles of freedom."[145] The 1980 *sabor* also issued a strong resolution endorsing "the right to life principle" and condemning abortion as "a mortal sin and murder."[146] The 1984 *sabor* produced a more detailed moral statement against abortion, which regarded "as morally intolerable the practice of, public support for, and public funding of abortions" and advocated "an amendment to the U.S. Constitution prohibiting abortion."[147]

The four local dioceses have also pronounced on such issues. In

November 1982, for example, during a national recession, the Diocese of Eastern America acknowledged the problem of unemployment in North America and confessed a collective responsibility to help the unemployed by sharing resources and job opportunities.[148] Since this resolution did not propose any particular *public* policy, it represented a refreshingly unusual moral exhortation by the diocese to its own membership instead of another demand on the public treasury.

But the SOC in North America has focused on one objective in its pursuit of freedom and human rights. The public moral witness of the SOC entails a complex mix of resolutions at the triennial national *sabors* and annual diocesan assemblies, occasional proclamations by the four diocesan bishops in North America (sometimes joined by the Serbian Orthodox bishops in Western Europe and Australia), and intense personal lobbying in the halls of American government dedicated to alleviating the perennial plight of the Serbs in the old country. The Serbian Orthodox hierarchs, clergy, and faithful have unflaggingly pressed their concern for the dignity of Serbs and their freedom from religious persecution, whether by the Communist regime in Belgrade, the restless Albanian ethnic majority in the regions of Kosovo and Metohija controlled by the Serb-dominated government in what is left of Yugoslavia, or the ostensibly democratic government in the new nation-state of Croatia.

Appeals to American principles of liberal democracy have been curiously blended with invocations of the time-honored Serbian slogan "Holy Cross and Golden Freedom." The latter dates from the Battle of Kosovo in A.D. 1389, in which the last medieval Serbian Orthodox tsar suffered an overwhelming, one-sided defeat by the Ottoman Turks instead of submitting pacifically to Muslim suzerainty. The Battle of Kosovo is the most cherished event in Serbian national history, and this blood-soaked territory is prized as both the "cradle" of Serbian Orthodoxy and the gravesite of Serbia's most heroic medieval martyrs. Kosovo symbolizes the uniquely Serbian blend of a fierce, militaristic spirit of independence and pride in their national legacy of suffering and persecution—by the Ottoman Turks for four and a half centuries, the Croatian Fascist state during the Second World War, and, after 1945, the Communists under Josip Broz Tito and his successors.

National resolutions against the human-rights abuses of the Communist regime date from 1970, when the second *sabor* after the schism of 1963 convened. The *sabor* announced that it

> stands for the uncompromising fight of Serbian Orthodox people in the United States of America and Canada against the Godless communist regime in Yugoslavia and atheist communism wherever it appears, which with its dictatorship deprives its peoples of the basic liberties of democracy so cherished in our beloved America and Canada.[149]

The next *sabor,* which met in 1980, upped the anti-Communist ante by resolving

> to forbid the admittance of communist representatives of Yugoslavia to church functions, gatherings, and festivities, and even to the use of church properties, as well as forbidding the presence of church representatives at any gatherings of a communistic character in the free world.[150]

The 1984 *sabor* specifically condemned "the unwarranted arrest and persecution of Serbian Orthodox clergy and seminarians" such as Dragan Stepkovic, "as well as the efforts of the government to intentionally and maliciously belittle and degrade the clergy and faithful of the Serbian Orthodox Church."[151]

A resolution at the 1984 *sabor* that commemorated the approximately 1.2 million victims (mostly Serbian Orthodox Christians) of the "Holocaust of Jasenovac" from 1941 to 1944 was also turned against the current Communist regime. The *sabor* delegates noted that "the efforts of the Yugoslav government to thwart, diminish and minimize the significance of Jasenovac and the consecration of this memorial church [of St. John] have met with failure." The *sabor* also applauded "the appearance of the Patriarchal flag on the Jasenovac Memorial Church" and commended the young Serbian Orthodox "who without fear, and with home-made Serbian [national] flags, participated in the consecration procession."[152] The support of the Church for such overt gestures of Serbian patriotism directed against the Communist Yugoslav state may seem routine in light of the explosion of anti-Communist or anti-Soviet nationalisms in the former Soviet Union and elsewhere in Eastern Europe since 1989.

But in 1984 these activities in Yugoslavia were unique, and the position of the Serbian Orthodox Church there and in North America was quite radical.

Unrelenting in its opposition to the Communist (now "Socialist") regime in Belgrade, the SOC has generally blamed the Communist authorities, more than the ethnic Albanian majority, for the rampant abuses of the religious and civil rights of the Serbian minority in Kosovo and Metohija—a part of the full story of the raging religio-ethnic conflict in the former Yugoslavia that the Western media seem either unaware of or determined to ignore. Militant Muslim, some-time Communist, and revanchist Albanians have forged a working political alliance there on the basis of their common antipathy to the Slavic government and the Serbian people in particular. The most violent activists among this Albanian-speaking majority appear to be irredentists who seek a territorial realignment of the Kosovo region with the neighboring post-Communist state of Albania.[153]

The 1984 *sabor* of the SOC protested the mistreatment of the Serbian minority in this region, calling it a systematic religious per-secution by ethnic Albanians with the self-serving cynical connivance of the government they despise. The *sabor* complained bitterly about the relegation of the Serbian Orthodox Church "to the status of a sub-class, particularly in the region of Kosovo and Metohija," where the Serbian Orthodox "have been subjugated to inhumane and de-grading treatment" and their religious shrines, artifacts, and even cemeteries subjected to desecration, "while the civil authorities blatantly condone, ignore and/or continue to overlook the basic rights of these faithful."[154]

A resolution approved as long ago as the 1982 annual assembly of the Diocese of Eastern America fired equal broadsides at the Yugoslav government and at "elements within Yugoslavia"—that is, the mili-tant ethnic Albanians. First, the clergy and lay delegates addressed the Albanian problem by condemning

[t]he anti-Serbian and anti-Christian campaign being conducted by Albanian nationalists in the Kosovo and Metohija regions of Yugoslavia. As the Yugoslavia government stands idly by, Serbian bishops and priests are physically attacked; Serbian nuns are threat-ened and raped; Churches and Church properties are vandalized

and desecrated; and Serbs from all walks of life are threatened, attacked, and even murdered, which is forcing large numbers of Serbs to flee from their historical and spiritual homeland.[155]

Second, this diocesan resolution scored the "anti-Church actions of the Yugoslav authorities." It mentioned the harassment of Orthodox clergy and laity in Bosnia and Hercegovina simply "for their religious and private activities"; the persecution of Orthodox believers who tried to establish formal programs of religious education for the youth of the Church; the continuing obstructionism of the government toward completion of the monumental St. Sava Church on the site in Belgrade where in 1594 the relics of the patron saint of Serbia were burned by the Muslim Turk, Sinan Pasha; and the government's reported anti-religious intimidation of Serbian citizens residing in North America, including the "denial of visas to visit families, lengthy questioning, and detainment when applying or visiting."[156] The assembly delegates concluded by calling upon the Yugoslav government "to abide by its own constitutional guarantees of religious freedom and national equality."[157]

What makes this multi-part diocesan resolution especially significant is the written response it drew from the U.S. State Department. This letter, signed by Robert W. Farrand, acting director of the Office of Eastern European and Yugoslav Affairs, was remarkable for its sensitivity to each of the points raised in the resolution. The letter attributed the disturbances in Kosovo to ethnic Albanians—a positive concession, especially, as we shall see, in light of later developments in the U.S. Congress. But Farrand said the State Department thought the Yugoslav government was in fact attempting diligently to protect Serbian lives and property. Although State had no evidence concerning the other charges in the resolution, he said, "we would act quickly were we to receive proof of intimidation or harassment of residents of the U.S. by officials of any foreign government."[158] The Kosovo issue quickly faded from view in March 1989, however, when the Socialist regime of Slobodan Milosevic, cynically exploiting Serbian national sentiment in Kosovo and in Serbia proper, threatened military force to coerce the regional parliament in Kosovo to revoke its own constitutional autonomy. This act launched a campaign of oppression against the Albanian majority and its aspirations of increasing autonomy from Belgrade.

The two most recent SOC *sabors* turned instead to the Serbs' historic archrivals. In November 1991, a special *sabor* convened in Chicago in response to the inter-ethnic war between Serbs and Croats in Croatia that followed Croatia's declaration of independence from Yugoslavia in June. The delegates tried to mobilize the faithful—and U.S. policymakers—on what was deemed a matter of life and death in the Serbian homelands. A special resolution invoked memories of the genocide against Serbs during the Second World War[159]:

> It is with alarm that we also recognize that this history is beginning to be repeated in those same areas [in Croatia]. Ethnic Serbs are again being subjected to the same kinds of terror and atrocities as occurred fifty years ago by those who look back to that time with fondness and nostalgia. And it is with grave concern that we see the eyes of the world once again closed to this tragedy. This awful history must not be allowed to repeat itself. . . . At the heart of this conflict is the very real fear of cultural and physical annihilation of the Serbian people living within the present borders of the Croatian state.

Whether or not this fear is rooted in political reality, there is no doubt that the American Serbs sincerely share the anxieties of their co-religionists in the post-Communist independent republics of the former Yugoslavia. The 1991 resolution pleaded for signs of repentance for past Croatian misdeeds from the Croatian government of Franjo Tudjman, a Communist-turned-nationalist:

> If the Germans can admit their genocidal acts, and if the communists can acknowledge the massacre of Poles in the Katyn Forest and their own people in the Soviet Union, and so undergo a cathartic cleansing of old wounds, then the question begs an answer: Why cannot the Croatians acknowledge the genocide against the Serbs, and so begin the process of reconciliation? . . . National repentance is necessary for all crimes committed during that time [1940s]. In the quest for perfection and the Kingdom of God, the saving Grace of repentance can never be ignored or passed over in public reference to such monumental sin. . . . As long as there is not acknowledgement of the truth, there can be no reconciliation.

The assembled SOC clergy and laity concluded their uncompromising insistence on public confession with a practical concrete proposal:

In the interest of such reconciliation, we call on Pope John Paul II to visit Croatia and to join in prayer with Patriarch Pavle at Jasenovac. It is our conviction that a true expression of recognition on the part of the heads of our churches would go far towards freeing the Serbian people from their fears and the Croatian people from their dark past, and would open the path to true and lasting peace.

In an unusually bold gesture, Metropolitan Christopher reiterated this invitation in a personal letter sent to Pope John Paul II on August 13, 1993, while the Roman pontiff was visiting Denver, Colorado. Christopher reminded the pope that the death camp at Jasenovac had recently been bulldozed by Tudjman's Croatian regime "in an effort to erase from history what occurred there." Christopher even went so far as to express his shock at "the silence of the western countries—and yes—even the Vatican—about this barbarism." A polite response two weeks later from the Vatican Secretary of State, Cardinal Angelo Sodano, reminded Metropolitan Christopher that the pope had invited Patriarch Pavle of Serbia to join him and other prominent religious leaders in Assisi, Italy, for the Day of Prayer for Peace on January 9-10, 1993.[160] But the cardinal said nothing about Jasenovac. The Vatican's continued silence on that extremely sensitive issue is at once baffling and galling to Metropolitan Christopher and Serbian Orthodox Christians.

The regularly scheduled SOC *sabor* in September 1993 reacted forcefully to the way the U.S. Holocaust Museum was dedicated on April 22, 1993. President Clinton refused to invite President Milosevic of Serbia to this moving event, but Croatian President Franjo Tudjman attended alongside all the other democratically elected heads of state from Eastern Europe. This was too much for the delegates to the *sabor*, notwithstanding their pronounced dislike for Milosevic as the elected leader of their spiritual motherland. The *sabor* dispatched a letter to President Clinton, Secretary of State Christopher, and all 535 members of the U.S. Congress that read in part:

To have invited the representative of Croatia to the recent dedication of the Holocaust Museum in Washington, D.C., who himself had the Jasenovac Memorial to the 750,000 victims destroyed, is an irony and an affront to the moral conscience of the American people, especially Americans of Serbian descent.

The same letter also requested that the U.S. Congress "pass a joint resolution expressing the sense of Congress" that "a lasting peace and reconciliation" will not be achieved in Croatia and Bosnia-Hercegovina until "the present governments of those lands condemn the genocide of 750,000 Serbs, Jews, and Gypsies on the territories of those republics in World War II."[161] There has been no response to date. Nor should the Serbian Orthodox expect one. The U.S. government has never formally acknowledged any of this century's mass slaughters of Orthodox peoples, whether the Turkish genocide of Armenians in 1915, the Soviet-engineered starvation of Ukrainians in the artificial famine of 1932-33, or the Croatian genocide of Serbs in the 1940s.

Forms of Activism

The SOC hierarchy in North America has zealously witnessed on behalf of freedom and human rights in historic Yugoslavia and the new rump "Yugoslav" state in deeds as well as words.

The Holy Synod of Bishops in Belgrade, to which each of the four (five, since February 1992) diocesan Serbian Orthodox bishops in North America belongs *ex officio,* proclaimed a special Year of Kosovo beginning on Vidovdan 1988 (June 28 on the Julian calendar, or June 15 on the Gregorian) and concluding on Vidovdan 1989, the six-hundredth anniversary of the celebrated Battle of Kosovo. In an unusual step for a conservative liturgical Church, the bishops also decreed that each litany in all worship services during this period should include the following petition, to be chanted by the deacon or priest:

> Again we pray that the Lord our God will hear the cry and petition of His suffering people in Kosovo and for all those who suffer for the sake of righteousness and endure persecution and abuse, and that He will expediently send down His grace and might and protect the innocently persecuted. . . .[162]

The SOC bishops in North America have resorted to even less conventional measures in their public moral witness to government officials and the media in the United States. For example, though not exactly comfortable in the political realm, the bishops themselves have "lobbied" public officials.

In December 1981, Metropolitan Christopher—then bishop of Eastern America—hosted Senator Arlen Specter (R-Pa.) at the diocesan headquarters, with the status of the Serbian Orthodox Church in Yugoslavia heading the agenda.[163] In October 1983 an SOC delegation including three bishops, one priest, and two laymen met in Washington with a group of senators, congressmen, and State Department officials led by the late Congressman Clement J. Zablocki (D-Wis.). The SOC delegation presented a thirty-one-page typescript entitled "The Serbian Orthodox Church in Yugoslavia," a detailed compendium of historical information, testimonial and anecdotal evidence, and documents from the Holy Synod of Bishops pertaining to the persecution of the Church by the Communist authorities and ethnic Albanians. The delegation prefaced this compendium with a list of requests for the assembled government officials. This list would establish the SOC leadership as an unofficial moral/political lobby on behalf of the suffering Church in the old country, and it included the following priorities:

1. That the U.S. Congress send a delegation to Yugoslavia, accompanied by SOC representatives, to investigate the charges;

2. That the SOC be afforded opportunities to testify on this subject before all relevant government bodies;

3. That the U.S. government apply, pending documentation of the charges, its "full and unrelenting power" to persuade the Yugoslav government to stop the anti-Serbian terrorism in Kosovo, return "expropriated and stolen properties" to the Church, and halt "all covert and overt persecution" of believers and "all other outrageous actions against the church." Continued "Most Favored Nation" status and all future financial boons for Yugoslavia would depend on its compliance with these requests.[164]

SOC activism in Washington has been enhanced by the high political profile of Helen Delich Bentley, a Serbian Orthodox laywoman elected to the U.S. Congress in 1984. Congresswoman Bentley (R-Md.) provides the Serbian cause with an outspoken champion and congressional insider.

Although Bentley served as Maryland chairwoman of the 1988 presidential campaign of George Bush and as national chairwoman of an ethnic organization known as "Serbs for Bush," neither honor prevented her from rallying the Serbian-American community against her candidate when a letter from Bush to Congressman Joseph J. DioGuardi was made public. In the letter, then Vice President Bush expressed his support for "the preservation of human and political rights and the autonomy of all nationality groups in Yugoslavia." But he raised the ire of the Serbs by adding, "I remain concerned about ethnic Albanians in Kosovo. The Albanians are a proud and brave people whose rights must be protected."[165] To the SOC Clergy Brotherhood and to Congresswoman Bentley, both of whom wrote letters of vigorous protest to Bush only two weeks before the November election, the Vice President's concern was misplaced and demonstrated ignorance of the political reality in Kosovo, which Bentley described as "the birthplace of Serbian culture, heritage and religion." Bush's comments also were, in Bentley's words, "extremely offensive" to the Serbian-American community.[166] In the last week of the presidential campaign, Bush responded in writing to the letter from the Clergy Brotherhood. Without backing away from his earlier comments about ethnic Albanians, he deftly broadened his advocacy of "human and political rights" in Yugoslavia: "Certainly, the rights of the Serbian minority in Kosovo must be respected and safeguarded."[167]

Perhaps energized by this unprecedented political success, in September 1989 Congresswoman Bentley successfully mobilized the Serbian-American community in what must have seemed to most Americans to be a rather arcane political battle in the U.S. Congress between pro-Serbian and pro-Albanian champions. With the timely assistance of Senator Paul Sarbanes (D-Md.), a member of the Greek Orthodox Archdiocese, she managed to block language in a U.S. Senate bill (S. 1160) that would have condemned the Serbs in the Kosovo conflict. Her clarion call to battle appeared in an open letter to the Serbian-American community, which the official SOC newspaper published in lieu of an editorial in its October 1989 issue.

In July 1990, Bentley, together with the Los Angeles–based American Serbian Heritage Foundation, conducted an educational forum on the Serbian heritage and spearheaded a large-scale lobbying effort in Washington. Three months later, perhaps owing to this campaign or to Congresswoman Bentley's own political skills, the U.S. House of Representatives rejected an amendment to a bill (H.Con.Res. 385) that would have blamed the Serbs alone for the troubles in Kosovo. Similarly, in June 1991 Bentley prevented language in the House foreign-aid authorization bill (H.R. 2508) that would have kept Yugoslavia from receiving "seed money."

Congresswoman Bentley has indeed been a tireless defender of the good name of Serbia and its Orthodox Church in the Congress, even since the eruption of open warfare in Croatia and Bosnia-Hercegovina, for which the world press and most U.S. government officials blame Serbia. More important, as an elected public official and legislator, she has sought an evenhanded U.S. foreign policy toward the former Yugoslavia, based on all the available evidence of violations of freedom and human rights in that region. On September 29, 1992, she arranged a special hearing on Capitol Hill for members of the House subcommittee on human rights with Bishop Atanasije Jevtic, Serbian Orthodox bishop in Hercegovina. The bishop was prepared to testify that dozens of Orthodox churches in his diocese had been razed and that other senseless war crimes and atrocities had been perpetrated against his people by various Croatian and Muslim contingents. Not one member of the press or one U.S. congressman attended the hearing. Bishop Atanasije gamely gave his horrifying testimony to six junior staffers and a scattered audience of Serbian-Americans and others sympathetic to the Serbian side in this bloody conflict.

Having survived a momentary scare in her 1992 campaign for re-election when her Democratic opponent accused her of misusing her congressional office to lobby on behalf of Belgrade, Congresswoman Bentley remains one of the strongest and most respected Republican leaders in her home state of Maryland. In spring 1994 she was contemplating a run for the governor's mansion, which, if successful, would unfortunately remove from the U.S. Congress a powerful moral advocate for justice toward Serbia and the Serbs.

One more form of SOC activism on behalf of freedom and human rights should be noted here. As we have seen, the Serbian émigré community has a fractious history that has precluded the Serbs from mounting a unified public moral witness. The reunification of the two ecclesial jurisdictions in February 1992 healed a festering wound. Ironically, the wars of the Yugoslav secession may be pushing the Serbs in America toward greater unity and cohesion. Although an earlier attempt in March 1989 to organize a political lobby—the Serbian American Voters Alliance, or SAVA, after the patron saint of the Serbs—never got off the ground, another venture launched in January 1992 may prove more durable. "Serb Net, Inc.," or the Serbian American National Information Network, aspires to become a "national umbrella organization of all the recognized Serbian organizations in the U.S.A." that will enable those ethnic organizations to speak "with a united voice on national issues."[168] An ethnic Serbian-American newspaper reported in September 1992 that Metropolitan Christopher of the Serbian Orthodox Midwest Metropolitanate and Bishop Mitrophan of the Serbian Orthodox Diocese of Eastern America had "endorsed" this organization.[169]

UKRAINIAN ORTHODOX CHURCH OF THE U.S.A.

Finding any evidence in the Ukrainian Orthodox Church (UOC) of interest in freedom and human rights in countries other than Ukraine requires a thorough search of the archives and official publications of the UOC, particularly the *Ukrainian Orthodox Word*. Occasional resolutions at the annual conventions of the Ukrainian Orthodox League—a lay organization of the UOC—have touched on such concerns. The 1979 convention, for example, resolved to send a telegram to President Carter "commending him on his interest in human rights and requesting that he continue his efforts for the release of religious and political prisoners."[170] The 1986 convention prayed for "the end of social injustices being perpetrated by the Soviet regime upon innocent people throughout the world."[171] And the Ukrainian Orthodox League has repeatedly voiced its opposition to abortion and its unqualified support for "the restoration of full protection for the unborn child."[172]

The biennial clergy-laity councils, or *sobors,* have only rarely manifested a wider interest in human rights. The 1967 *sobor* was "deeply spiritually moved by the sufferings and torment of other freedom loving nations of the world, who are fighting against the ungodly and hateful communistic aggression," especially "for the defense of Christ's Church and free nations against the advance of

Satan—the hateful Communism."[173] Similarly, the 1977 *sobor* summoned "all the faithful of our Church and . . . all people of good faith to actively participate in defense of the oppressed in the USSR, particularly in Ukraine, in defense of the fighters for the human rights, of public and religious freedom of conscience and for native language and culture."[174] But that is the extent of the extra-Ukrainian public moral witness of the UOC.

Hierarchical Initiatives

The virtually exclusive interest in the human rights of Ukrainians manifested by the UOC hierarchy and biennial *sobors* reflects the position that this jurisdiction has occupied in worldwide Orthodoxy. Together with its two sister jurisdictions with which it has shared a cause—the Ukrainian Greek Orthodox Church in Canada and the Ukrainian Autocephalous Orthodox Church in Western Europe—the UOC represented for decades the only genuinely free expression of Ukrainian Orthodoxy in the world. It was the sole bearer of the faith and culture of a people oppressed, from their standpoint, alternately by Russians, Poles, Soviet Communists, Nazi Germans, and Soviet Communists a second time.

To be sure, the Ukrainian Autocephalous Orthodox Church (UAOC) has resurfaced in Ukraine. An extraordinary synod of Orthodox clergy—both "Ukrainian" and "Russian" by self-appellation —met in Lviv (Ukrainian for Lvov) on October 20, 1989, and elected Bishop Ioann Bodnarchuk, retired "Russian" Orthodox bishop of Zhytomyr—whom the Moscow Patriarchate summarily deposed for this alleged breach of canon law—to lead the new jurisdiction. At least ten Orthodox parishes in the Lviv region had already broken from Moscow and transferred their canonical obedience to the new Church.[175] Then, at its June 1990 *sobor* in Kyyiv, the UAOC elected Metropolitan Mstyslav Skrypnyk to the office of patriarch, although there has never been a "patriarch" of Ukraine! As noted in chapter 2, Patriarch Mstyslav and the UOAC contended vigorously with the Ukrainian Catholics and the Moscow Patriarchate for the spiritual allegiance of Ukrainians during the three years prior to Mstyslav's death in June 1993.

The UAOC's rising popular appeal persuaded the Moscow Patriarchate to bow halfway to a burgeoning Ukrainian nationalism. In October 1990, Moscow finally allowed its exarchate in Kyyiv to call itself the Ukrainian Orthodox Church and accorded Metropolitan Filaret Denisenko of Kyyiv the title of "primate." But the most recent twists in the continuing saga of Filaret, as noted in chapter 2, have had Filaret "deposed" by Moscow, received by the UAOC despite his dubious moral reputation, and precipitating a schism within the nascent UAOC between pro- and anti-Filaret factions, each with its own "patriarch."

Yet there are still occasional signs of hope for the contentious Ukrainians. The Ecumenical Patriarch in Constantinople had already decided, as noted earlier in this chapter, to receive under its jurisdiction the Canadian branch of this "autocephalous" Ukrainian Orthodox community.[176] And prominent leaders in SCOBA jurisdictions such as Fr. Anthony Ugolnik and Bishop Nathaniel Popp have made a point in print of including the UOC of the USA among the canonical or mainstream Orthodox jurisdictions in America.[177] Despite their heretofore twilight existence in world Orthodoxy, the Ukrainian Orthodox, in Ukraine and the diaspora alike, may at last find themselves in a privileged position, squarely in the middle of the mounting ecclesial rivalry between Moscow and Constantinople.

Before these unanticipated events, the late UOC primate, Metropolitan Mstyslav, reminded his flock in his Paschal message in April 1988 that "due to historical circumstances, we, the Orthodox Ukrainians of the free world, are now the only pillars of Ukrainian Orthodoxy, the only rightful heirs of the Kievan Metropolia of Saint Volodymyr, the only defenders of our forefathers' religious legacy."[178] Naturally, the Russian Orthodox Church would dispute this claim to the legacy of the pre-"Ukrainian" and pre-"Russian" St. Volodymyr, or St. Vladimir, as the founder of the Kyyivan Rus state is better known.

In 1968 the UOC hierarchy issued a "Declaration" to an international conference on human rights in Teheran, Iran, that effectively launched the UOC on an internationally recognized, prophetic trajectory concerning freedom and human rights in Ukraine. The UOC bishops sought to focus the attention of the assembly on the "gross violations of the Universal Declaration of Human Rights which adversely affect the lives of millions of our brothers" in the Soviet Union. They demonstrated how specific articles of the United Nations document were routinely violated by the Soviet government and "the government-controlled Russian Orthodox Church." The suppression, for example, of the hierarchy of the Ukrainian Autocephalous Orthodox Church from 1928 to 1936 subverted Article 18, which enunciates a right to freedom of thought, conscience, and religion. Similarly, the bishops declared that "the deprivation of Ukrainians of their own Ukrainian Church, of their own language i[n] ecclesiastical practices is a perfidious violation" of Article 15, which asserts the right to a nationality and a national culture. These human-rights abuses, the bishops concluded, "emanate from the colonial status of the Ukrainian Soviet Socialist Republic, from the rigid subordination of this republic to the central Soviet government in Moscow."[179]

Their unyielding, vitriolic criticism of "Moscow" as the *bête noire* of Ukrainians reveals, however, a "dark side" of the UOC bishops' prophetic role. It is one thing to denounce a hostile government in language that is often eloquent but also exaggerated and sensational. In his Christmas message published in the January 1978 issue of the *Ukrainian Orthodox Word* (the UOC Christmas occurs on January 7, according to the Gregorian calendar), Metropolitan Mstyslav pleaded the Ukrainian cause as follows:

> Today, the Ukrainian mother uniquely and indesirably sheds bitter tears over her children, for insatiable Moscow strives to tear away the soul and lead them into a bear-like condition of parentlessness divested of roots. Purposely, Moscow conditions Ukrainian children to forget the language of their fathers and grandfathers, knowing that those who disdain and forget their native language will become liken to dumb herds, ready material for those who enslave.[180]

Similarly intemperate, though understandable, was the charge by Mstyslav in 1985 that Moscow "bears the biblical mark of Cain for its genocide of our Ukrainian nation and our Martyr-Church."[181]

But the UOC primate crossed the boundary of hyperbole into spiritual fratricide when his impassioned defense of Ukrainian religious identity and freedom led him to demonize other Orthodox Churches. Mstyslav directed his ire against not only the excessively compliant Russian Orthodox Church under Soviet tyranny but also the pre-Communist Russian Church, thereby demonstrating an excellent memory but an unforgiving spirit. His unseasonal Christmas encyclical for 1988/1989 spoke harshly against this sister Orthodox Church, "which from the time of Peter the First," he asserted, "has been well known as a means of enslavement and denationalization of other peoples, especially on the linguistic sector."[182] In the current titanic struggle for spiritual preeminence in worldwide Orthodoxy between the Patriarchates of Constantinople and Moscow, the late Patriarch Mstyslav and the other bishops in every Ukrainian jurisdiction have closed ranks behind the Ecumenical Patriarchate, notwithstanding the latter's refusal, thus far, to accord canonical status to the various branches of the UAOC in Ukraine, Western Europe, and the United States.

This ecclesiastical partisanship, together with a historical antipathy toward all things Russian, apparently led the UOC hierarchy to see a sinister, Communist-directed conspiracy in the Moscow Patriarchate's granting of autocephaly to the Orthodox Church in America in 1970. At a meeting of the UOC bishops in March 1978, Metropolitan Mstyslav, having duly noted the refusal of the ancient Patriarchates of Constantinople, Alexandria, Antioch, and Jerusalem to recognize the autocephaly of the OCA, accused the OCA leadership of single-mindedly aiming at, in the words of a reporter for the *Ukrainian Orthodox Word*, "the liquidation of all ethnic Orthodox Churches in North America, an effort which agrees with Moscow's intention."[183]

Meanwhile, Patriarch Mstyslav and his local successor in the United States, Metropolitan Constantine, forged an alliance of convenience, though perhaps a genuine fraternity as well, with their opposite numbers in the hierarchy of the Ukrainian Catholic Church in the United States. On at least two occasions Mstyslav issued joint appeals with the Uniate primate on matters of common Ukrainian concern, which apparently transcended confessional differences. In November 1982, Mstyslav and Metropolitan Stephen Sulyk co-signed a letter to President Reagan, thanking him for his support for a congressional resolution on "the resurrection of the national churches in Ukraine," and urging the president "to implement this resolution in the name of justice and human rights with all haste."[184] Six years later on the feast of Pentecost, Mstyslav and Cardinal Myroslav Lyubachevskiy issued a "joint statement" in honor of the millennium of Christianity in "Ukraine." Referring, surprisingly, to "our zealous faith," in the singular, the two primates, one Orthodox and one Catholic, lamented the suffering and persecution of the Ukrainian people, particularly the liquidation of the hierarchy of the Ukrainian Autocephalous Orthodox Church, the famine of 1932-33, and the elimination of the Ukrainian Catholic Church on the territory of the Soviet Union. This remarkable ecumenical moral witness concluded with an "appeal to the Christian nations of the world and all people of goodwill to demonstrate their Christian solidarity with our Churches and nation and thus help ensure that the Light of Christ's Truth again [will] illuminate our anewly [sic] freed fatherland Ukraine."[185]

Five Cases

The depth of the UOC bishops' dedication in the pursuit of justice for the Ukrainian nation may be seen in five particular cases.

First, they have reminded the world of the notorious **famine in Ukraine** that Soviet dictator Josef Stalin engineered to subjugate the Ukrainian people, especially the peasants and the middle-class *kulaks*. In July 1983—the fiftieth anniversary of the nadir of this atrocity in which some seven million persons perished—the UOC bishops reminded their flock in an encyclical, "We are called upon to speak loudly of the famine and to remind the entire world of it. For this purpose we must utilize the foreign press, print special publications and sponsor requiem manifestations. We cannot be silent!"[186] The first fruits of this campaign included a well-received scholarly book on the famine by Robert Conquest entitled *Harvest of Despair* and a documentary film with the same title that appeared on television's Public Broadcasting System.

The UOC has frequently invoked the memory of these victims of attempted Soviet genocide. In August 1993, the bishops of the UOC and the UAOC in Western Europe commemorated the sixtieth anniversary of "the Ukrainian Holocaust" in a pastoral letter that denounced "this new Golgotha" as "one perpetrated by the Moscow regime headed by a new Herod, Joseph Stalin." While urging forgiveness toward the Soviets, "as Christ commands us," the bishops also vowed that "we will never forget the sufferings endured by our nation, nor shall we forget whose children we are, our identity, our glorious roots."[187] The UOC clergy conference two months later viewed the famine as somehow redemptive. In a resolution containing language strikingly familiar to that of Jews who regard the modern state of Israel as a phoenix rising out of the ashes of the Nazi Holocaust, the UOC clergy expressed their "gratitude to Almighty God for having accepted our sufferings and prayers, . . . deemed fit that these sacifices were not in vain, [and] . . . blessed Ukraine with statehood and independence and the rebirth of independent Ukrainian Orthodoxy."[188] Despite the faithful prophetic witness of the UOC, the Ukrainian holocaust remains largely unknown or ignored in American social consciousness.

Second, the UOC bishops interceded repeatedly with U.S. officials on behalf of the persecuted Ukrainian historian and dissident **Valentyn Moroz**. In June 1974, the bishops appealed directly to President Richard M. Nixon to secure Moroz's release from prison; in a follow-up letter they promised that all expenses of the dissident's emigration to the United States and his living expenses here "will be covered by our Church."[189] In the second half of 1974, Mstyslav sent similar letters of supplication and/or appreciation to Senator Henry Jackson (D-Wash.), President Gerald P. Ford, Secretary of State Henry Kissinger, Senator Jacob Javits (R-N.Y.), and Kurt Waldheim, the secretary general of the United Nations. The letter to Kissinger, for example, attempted to link the value of the U.S. foreign policy of détente directly to the freedom and human rights of Soviet prisoners such as Moroz.[190]

Third, Metropolitan Mstyslav and the UOC bishops proved to be effective advocates of **Fr. Vasyl Romaniuk**, whom the Ukrainian primate described in a 1976 letter to Patriarch Dimitrios of Constantinople as "the most courageous martyr for Christ" among the Ukrainian Orthodox people. Mstyslav expressed pardonable pride in his ethnic group when he suggested to the Ecumenical Patriarch that during the last fifty years "they have made the greatest sacrifice upon the Altar, in defense of Christ's Truth upon earth." In light of the filial devotion of the Ukrainian Orthodox to the Ecumenical Patriarchate, Mstyslav besought Dimitrios "to take under Your protection and guardianship the Ukrainian Martyrs for Christ," particularly the worthy priest Vasyl Romaniuk.[191] Fr. Vasyl had been arrested in 1972 for "anti-Soviet agitation and propaganda" (Article 62 of the criminal code of the Ukrainian SSR) and sentenced to ten years in a labor camp. In August 1975, Fr. Vasyl appealed to the World Council of Churches for an investigation by a special WCC commission of "violations of elementary human rights in the USSR."[192]

After his release at the end of his sentence, Fr. Vasyl continued to benefit from the vocal support of the UOC leadership until the Gorbachev government allowed him to emigrate to the United States in July 1988. After a brief hiatus in Canada, Fr. Vasyl returned to his native Ukraine, was consecrated to the episcopacy in 1990, and, in what must rank as one of the supreme ironies of the post-Communist era, was elected "patriarch" of Kyyiv in October 1993 by the pro-Filaret faction in the UAOC (the self-described Ukrainian Orthodox Church–Kyyivan Patriarchate, or UOC-KP). The former dissident and survivor of the Soviet gulag now reigns as Patriarch Volodymyr I over, to be sure, half (or perhaps only a third) of a very divided Church.

Fourth, the entire UOC was mobilized to champion the cause of **John Demjanjuk**, a Ukrainian American accused of Nazi war crimes who was extradited to Israel by the U.S. government in February 1986. He was presumed by many in the international media and even by some living eyewitnesses of the Nazi Holocaust to be "Ivan the Terrible," a brute responsible for the deaths of more than 100,000 Jews at the Treblinka death camp in Poland. In May 1986, Metropolitan Mstyslav sent a telegraph to the president of Israel protesting (courteously) his government's acceptance of Demjanjuk despite its awareness of "evidence that Ivan Demjaniuk was not the person whom the Jerusalem mob would like to see on Golgotha." The inflammatory and possibly anti-Semitic language notwithstanding, Metropolitan Mstyslav apparently believed he could persuade the Israeli leader that "the prime architect" of the case against the "pious" Demjanjuk was the old common enemy of Jews and Ukrainians alike —namely, "the political police agencies of the U.S.S.R."[193] The Metropolitan Council of the UOC two months later declared this "shameful attack upon Ivan Damaniuk" an instance of "the widespread action aimed at defaming the good name of the Ukrainian nation by Soviet agents and their servitors in Israel."[194] It is unclear who the latter were supposed to be.

Since Demjanjuk had been a member of the UOC cathedral in

Parma, Ohio, for thirty-four years when he lost his U.S. citizenship, Archbishop Antoniy Scharba of New York and Washington, D.C., the suffragan for the metropolitan, visited the accused war criminal in his prison cell in Israel in September 1986. Back in the United States, Archbishop Antoniy, accompanied by Demjanjuk's son-in-law, Edward Nichnic, began a national tour of the UOC parishes to inform the Ukrainian Orthodox faithful about his trip to Israel, voice his opinion of the controversy, and seek, as the *Ukrainian Orthodox Word* described it, "prayer, support, and financial assistance for the defense of an innocent man."[195] Metropolitan Mstyslav's 1987 Paschal greeting to Ukraine, which was broadcast by the Voice of America, included another impassioned protestation of Demjanjuk's innocence that unfortunately invoked anti-Semitic images:

> And again an innocent person is on trial in Jerusalem—this time a Ukrainian—and faithful member of the Ukrainian Orthodox Church, John Demjanjuk. Again the streets of Jerusalem became turbulent, again the crowd awaits a sentence. Again the cries "crucify him!" resound in Jerusalem. . . .[196]

The annual UOC clergy conference added its voice to this cause in an October 1992 resolution that appealed to the U.S. and Israeli governments "to correct the legal error" of "the unjust sentencing of Ivan Demjanjuk" and "to free the innocent person from further torment." The resolution also urged the faithful to make "generous donations" to help Demjanjuk's family "liquidate the indebtedness brought about as a result of his legal defense."[197]

   In another profound irony for the Ukrainian community, Demjanjuk's conviction by an Israeli court, which sentenced him to death, was overturned by the Supreme Court of Israel on September 19, 1993. That court, persuaded by newly revealed evidence from the former Soviet Union that Demjanjuk had been, all along, a victim of mistaken identity, ordered him freed from jail and deported from Israel. Demjanjuk arrived home three days later. On November 17, the Sixth U.S. Circuit Court of Appeals overturned its 1987 extradition of Demjanjuk, criticizing the U.S. Justice Department for attempting to defraud the court by withholding evidence in favor of Demjanjuk's plea of innocence. There were, however, no celebratory public statements by Demjanjuk himself (who immediately went into seclusion) or his family members or by the UOC leadership, whose loyalty and arduous efforts on his behalf had finally been vindicated. Zealots who refuse to accept the verdict of Israel's highest court and those who now insist that Demjanjuk was guilty of similar crimes at yet *another* death camp will not leave him alone. Some continue to picket his home, while others press for his re-deportation from the United States. Among the latter is the U.S. Justice Department, which in May 1994 appealed to the U.S. Supreme Court the Sixth U.S. Circuit Court's November 1993 decision. The saga of Ivan Demjanjuk continues.

Fifth, the Metropolitan Council of the UOC joined its moral voice to that of a committee of Ukrainian Orthodox religious activists in the homeland who began in early 1989 to demand the restoration of an **autocephalous Ukrainian Orthodox Church**. After receiving a petition from this committee in February 1989, the Metropolitan Council, as reported in the *Ukrainian Orthodox Word,* "acting in the name of the entire Ukrainian Autocephalous Orthodox Church in the United States of America, . . . proclaimed its solidarity with the committee and pledged its members' total support."[198] This committee proved to be the precursor of the Ukrainian Autocephalous Orthodox Church that emerged in Lviv in October 1989. Metropolitan Mstyslav finally returned to his native land in triumph as patriarch on October 20, 1990, and remained there until December 2. One of his most dramatic appearances was before the second Congress of the National Popular Movement for the Restructuring of Ukraine (known in Ukrainian as *Rukh,* the word for "movement") in Kyyiv on October 25, 1990. Mstyslav gave the opening invocation and briefly addressed the delegates, who responded with what the *Ukrainian Orthodox Word* described as "a prolonged standing ovation."[199]

As we have already seen, however, this euphoria eventually gave way to rancor among the Ukrainian Orthodox when Patriarch Mstyslav died in June 1993. Mystyslav's successor in the United States, Metropolitan Constantine Buggan of Chicago and Philadelphia, and his auxiliary, Archbishop Antoniy Scharba, tried in vain to prevent the impending schism between the pro- and anti-Filaret factions of the UAOC. On July 12, 1993, the two American-born bishops issued a fervent appeal to both sides "to conclude an immediate unification, to forget all discord evidenced up this time and to, as befits Christians, forgive one another all manner of wrongs and omissions."[200] But this moral exhortation fell on deaf ears, and a personal UOC mission to Ukraine in October, led by Archbishop Antoniy, also failed to forestall the spiritual scandal of rival claimants to the patriarchal throne in Kyyiv.

Resolutions and Political Action

The biennial *sobors* of the UOC have issued numerous resolutions concerning freedom and human rights in Ukraine. These sentiments, naturally, echo the language of the many statements by the metropolitan and other bishops. The 1988 *sobor,* however, took a decisive turn in a more sophisticated political direction.

Among the many resolutions in 1988 was a rather cryptic condemnation of "the anti-Ukrainian campaign of hatred and degradation which is promoted by some circles in the United States of America and abroad." The *sobor* delegates also railed, as usual, against the Moscow Patriarchate, condemning the sister Church for "its continued enslavement" of the national Ukrainian Orthodox Church, for "depriving said Church of its inalienable (from time immemorial) rights of independent life and self-administration," for "the ruination of its traditions," particularly the use of the Ukrainian language in worship, and for "its efforts to present the Millennium of Baptism of the people of Kievan Rus, a feast exclusively of the Ukrainian nation, as a feast of the Russian Church."[201]

The decidedly new element at the 1988 *sobor* appeared in the twenty-first resolution, which proclaimed the local church of St. Andrew in Washington, D.C., the cathedral of Archbishop Antoniy Scharba.[202] The peripatetic Antony lives in South Bound Brook, New Jersey, but travels frequently to Washington to engage U.S. policymakers on their home turf. The only other Orthodox bishop whose see is the nation's capital — Metropolitan Theodosius of the OCA — resides on Long Island, New York, and actually appears in his diocese mainly on festive occasions. The UOC decision may help increase public awareness of Orthodoxy "inside the Beltway," as Washingtonians are wont to say.

The UOC has, to be sure, been cultivating a direct witness to the movers and shakers in Washington during the past two decades. In

November 1985, the Reagan White House included Metropolitan Mstyslav in a group of only twenty national religious leaders invited to a special briefing on the eve of the president's summit with Mikhail Gorbachev. At that briefing, Mstyslav was able to witness to President Reagan and his staff on behalf of the oppressed nationalities in the Soviet Union.[203] Also, during the presidential election campaign in 1988, Vice President Bush—the Republican candidate—issued a statement congratulating the Ukrainian-American community "on this 1,000th anniversary of Christianity in the history of the Ukrainian nation."[204] Bush, in the throes of a difficult campaign, was, it seems, appealing for political support from a segment of the electorate that he and his campaign staff considered potentially more significant than the Russian-American community. The action signified the arrival of the Ukrainian-American community on the American political scene and, presumably, the growing moral and political influence of the Ukrainian Orthodox Church.

In another unprecedented activity, the Ukrainian Orthodox churches in Chicago have become full partners with their Catholic and Protestant co-nationals in the Ukrainian Congress Committee. This ecumenical organization conducted a fund-raising drive to support non-Communist candidates in the elections to the *rada,* or parliament, of the Ukrainian Socialist Republic in October 1990.[205] Another strictly secular measure of the committee won an endorsement by the *Ukrainian Orthodox Word* in its July-August 1993 issue: a call to the faithful to lobby the U.S. Congress to amend U.S. foreign aid policy so that Ukraine would receive no less than 34 per cent of the dollars appropriated for Russia, or what the committee and *UOW* deemed Ukraine's "fair share."[206]

Finally, the UOC, like other ethnic Churches in the United States, has cultivated potentially useful friendships with American and Ukrainian diplomats. For example, in June 1992 at the Old Executive Office Building next to the White House, Archbishop Antoniy attended the induction of Roman Popadiuk as the first U.S. ambassador to the new Republic of Ukraine. Popadiuk, a Ukrainian Catholic, requested the continuous prayers of Antony and the UOC for his new mission, and the archbishop was glad to oblige. In February 1993, Archbishop Antoniy joined Ukrainian Catholic Metropolitan Stephen Sulyk of Philadelphia and clergy of both communions in blessing the new Ukrainian embassy building, which is located in the Georgetown section of Washington, D.C.

THE PRICE OF PROPHECY

"Parochial" may serve as an apt one-word description of the public moral witness of the Orthodox jurisdictions in the United States on issues of freedom and human rights. Derived from the Latin *parochia*, "parish," this term designates a confined, narrow, provincial perspective. For the most part, the statements, resolutions, and activities emanating from the hierarchies and clergy-laity assemblies of each of the five jurisdictions we have examined represent the collective religious voice of a particular immigrant or "hyphenated-American" community, speaking on behalf of the religious/political freedom and human rights of the co-nationals "back home" in the mother country. Of the three alternative Orthodox identities proffered by Richard John Neuhaus, the Orthodox jurisdictions in the United States have generally projected a distinct, albeit not entirely intended, image of Eastern Churches in exile from the mother Churches overseas.

This predominance of parochial concerns has both positive and negative features. On the credit side, the relentless determination of the several jurisdictions to champion the cause of religious and political freedom in their countries of origin has provided oppressed Orthodox believers there—who would be virtually neglected by the major American print and broadcast media—[207]with intrepid advocates in the most powerful nation on earth. Both Jews and evangelicals in the Soviet Union, for example, have their American "protectors," but who would speak for the Russian and Ukrainian *Orthodox* if not the OCA and the UOC and their sympathetic brethren in the other Orthodox jurisdictions? Similarly, the interests of the Serbian Orthodox in Kosovo or Croatia or Bosnia-Hercegovina, or the Greek Orthodox in Cyprus, or the Romanian Orthodox under Ceauşescu, or the Arab Christians in Lebanon have not figured prominently in the agendas of other religious communities or most human-rights organizations in the United States. In their roles as advocates of these forgotten or neglected peoples, the several Orthodox jurisdictions obviously provide much needed comfort and assurance. They also demonstrate a willingness to pay the price of prophecy for their brothers and sisters in the faith by taking up relatively unknown or even unpopular causes.

On the debit side, however, this parochial public moral witness betrays two dangerous tendencies: one toward phyletism and a corresponding one away from catholicism. Bishop Kallistos Ware, an Anglican convert to Orthodoxy and a professor at Oxford University, once lamented, "Nationalism has been the bane of Orthodoxy for the last ten centuries."[208] The excessive preoccupation with one's own ethnic group, which contrasts sharply with the ecumenical transnational vision that prevailed in the Orthodox empires of Byzantium and even tsarist Russia, was condemned as "phyletism" (from the Greek *phyletismos*—"blood union") by the Synod of Constantinople in 1872 and as "ethnoracism" by Patriarch Joachim of Constantinople in 1904.[209] The fervent support of the Antiochian Archdiocese for the beleaguered Christians in Lebanon and the Palestinians in Israel and the West Bank has a dark obverse side: in glorifying the Arab Christians (and Muslims!), the Antiochians somehow feel compelled to demonize the state of Israel. Similarly, while apotheosizing the oppressed Ukrainians in the former Soviet Union and certain Ukrainian personages in the West such as Ivan Demjanjuk, the UOC resorts facilely to vilification, not only of the Soviet regime as symbolized by the term "Moscow," but also of all things Russian including the entire Russian Orthodox Church, past and present.

The tendency of the Orthodox jurisdictions to narrow their moral compass to their "own" peoples in Eastern Europe and the Middle East also precludes a truly universal vision of human rights more in accord with the traditional Orthodox concern for the religious freedom of all persons irrespective of race or national identity. Such parochialism reduces the "People of God" from the catholic "holy nation" of believers envisioned by St. Peter in the New Testament (I Peter 2:9) to a congeries of nations determined by bloodline alone. This has the inevitable effect of ignoring the often equal and sometimes greater pleas of other peoples, nations, or religious communities for freedom and recognition of their human rights. The moral credibility of the Orthodox Churches must invariably suffer from this skewed prophetic vision.

Hopeful signs of a broader vision appear from time to time. Archbishop Iakovos has been untiring in his personal witness on behalf of the civil rights of all Americans regardless of race, and his example has clearly encouraged the entire Greek Archdiocese in its resolutions on this set of issues. Occasional encyclicals and resolutions—however poorly worded or ideologically motivated—from each of the five spotlighted jurisdictions on abortion, the underprivileged, and the politically and/or religiously oppressed in the United States or in other countries far removed from the historic Orthodox milieu aspire to a universalism consonant with that which is most noble in Orthodox moral tradition. Even those measures by which one jurisdiction recognizes the plight of fellow Orthodox in another country of origin bespeak an inter-Orthodox solidarity that transcends the usual parochialism. A concrete expression of this solidarity was the formation—with the blessing of SCOBA—in March 1992 of International Orthodox Christian Charities to provide relief and long-term assistance to the poor in countries where the local Orthodox Church would welcome such support. Finally, the attempts that Metropolitan Theodosius of the OCA has made to strike "a balance on human rights" consciously eschew political partisanship and religious favoritism in the service of an uncompromisingly universal vision of a free humanity.

If this Theodosian perspective becomes normative, if even the most parochial of the ethnic jurisdictions can expand their moral parameters in this way, the Orthodox community in America may, at last, assert its historic identity in America as *the* Church, pure and simple.

5

Peace and Security: Conventional

The extraordinary spirit of freedom that swept across Eastern Europe in the last few months of 1989 revived several dormant strains of nationalism in the former Soviet bloc. The American news media focused naturally on the most spectacular examples in the three Baltic states, Ukraine, the Moldavian Soviet Socialist Republic (actually the former Romanian provinces of Bessarabia and Bukovina), and the rambunctious regions of Armenia and Azerbaijan in the Caucasus. When the major print media, beginning with the February 5, 1990, issue of *The New Republic,* finally noticed Russian nationalism, crude caricatures and simplistic stereotypes substituted for serious analysis of this complex social phenomenon.[1] Meanwhile, the popular uprising of December 1989 in which Romania threw off its Communist shackles was fueled as much by Romanian nationalism and religious fervor as by sheer desperation over conditions under the despot Nicolae Ceauşescu.[2] More recently, the barbaric violence that has convulsed the nascent successor states of the former Yugoslavia is driven, at least in part, by deadly combinations of religion and nationalism within the Serbian, Croatian, and Muslim communities. The Serbs, of course, are overwhelmingly Orthodox by custom.

From an Orthodox moral perspective, such intense nationalism among predominantly Orthodox peoples in Eastern Europe tends to obscure the fundamental virtues of peace, tolerance, and forgiveness. More often than not, ethnic or nationalistic glorification has been expressed through some form of militarism, further undermining the Orthodox witness on behalf of the Gospel of peace.

Nationalism in Orthodox experience, as noted at the end of the last chapter, tends to glorify ethnic or racial distinctions, while paying lip service to more noble principles of common security and self-determination. The late Russian-American archpriests John Meyendorff and Alexander Schmemann named the romantic type of nationalism that has gripped Europe, Eastern as well as Western, since the French Revolution as the taproot of the particularly divisive forms of nationalism in the Orthodox Balkans.[3] These forms contrast sharply with the ecumenical, trans-national vision of an Orthodox commonwealth that prevailed in Byzantium and even for a while in tsarist Russia. We shall see in this chapter the pervasive role of such extreme nationalism in the proclamations of the Orthodox Churches in the former Soviet Union, Romania, and the United States concerning war and peace in conventional—that is, non-nuclear—contexts.

Compounding the moral problem, various shades of **militarism** seem inextricably yoked to the more virulent expressions of nationalistic pride among the Orthodox. In his classic study of militarism, Alfred Vagts contrasted this phenomenon unfavorably to the "military way." The latter is simply the pragmatic concentration of men and materials to achieve civilian political objectives "with the utmost efficiency, that is, with the least expenditure of blood and treasure." Since the mid-nineteenth century, however, "militarism has connoted a domination of the military man over the civilian, an undue preponderance of military demands, and emphasis on military considerations, spirit, ideals, and scales of value, in the life of states."[4] A less sweeping description of militarism appeared in a document produced by the World Council of Churches in January 1979, "The Programme on Militarism and Armaments Race." Juxtaposed with the usual leftist criticisms of "unjust class and racial structures" was the following indisputable insight: "Many educational systems glorify combat and use of force, exalt patriotism and national chauvinism and military values of hierarchisation and strict conformity."[5]

Several general points should be kept in mind as we examine the militarism of the Orthodox Churches. First, full-blown militarism has surfaced only intermittently in the recent history of the Orthodox Churches in the former Soviet Union, Romania, and the United

States—that is, especially when the host nation was at war or on the brink of war. The statements and activities of the Moscow Patriarchate during the Second World War will serve as a particularly egregious example.

Second, the winds of militarism have usually blown hot or cold depending on the fortunes of the host nation on the battlefield. The most dramatic instance of this tendency in recent years was the *volte-face* reflected in the resolutions of the Greek Orthodox Archdiocese of New York on the Vietnam War between 1966 and 1972.

Third, the official documents of the Russian and Romanian Orthodox Churches in the last decade or so are replete with charges of militarism directed against the enemies—real or imagined—of their governments. Yet while these Communist-dominated Orthodox hierarchies condemned "militarism" and "imperialism" and promoted "peace" and "disarmament," they also reveled in the past military exploits of their nations and glorified the often bellicose foreign policies of their present regimes.

Finally, the Orthodox Churches worldwide do manage sometimes to rise above their nationalistic and militaristic tendencies. The "Message" of the June 1990 *sobor* that elected Aleksii as patriarch of Moscow included the following definitive statement: "Any sign of nationalism contradicts the Divine law and is against human morality. Nationalism is especially inadmissible in the church circles where it leads to tearing the unsewn tunic of Christ."[6] Even more powerful was Patriarch Aleksii II's admission to the Moscow meeting of the Conference on Security and Cooperation in Europe on September 10, 1991, three weeks after the failed coup by Communist hard-liners:

> For a long time our fate was decided through arbitrariness and violence: whole generations grew up with the habit to obey blindly and venerate power. The loss of morality by one man is a great misfortune, so how can we call the ignorance of morality by whole nations?[7]

One of the preconciliar documents prepared in 1986 in anticipation of the long-awaited "Great Synod" of all the autocephalous Orthodox Churches is entitled, albeit awkwardly, "The Contribution of the Orthodox Church to the Realization of Peace, Justice, Freedom, Fraternity and Love among People and to the Suppression of Racial and Other

Discriminations." Imbedded among the paeans to peace, socialist economics, and pluralism that usually found their way into such pan-Orthodox documents in the Communist era is the following moral gem:

> We Orthodox Christians, having grasped the meaning of salvation, feel it our duty to struggle for the relief of sickness, unhappiness and anguish. Enjoying peace, we cannot remain indifferent to its absence from modern society. Having benefited from divine justice, we struggle for more justice in the world and for the abolition of all oppression. Experiencing every day divine clemency, we fight against every form of fanaticism and intolerance between people and peoples. Continually proclaiming the incarnation of God and divinization of man, we defend human rights for all men and all nations. Enjoying the divine gift of freedom thanks to the redeeming work of Christ, we are able to announce more completely its universal value for every person and every people.[8]

This multi-faceted perspective on peace, freedom, and justice proves that ecumenical Orthodoxy can respond, at least incipiently, to the call to provide an integral moral worldview. The document is all the more remarkable in that it emanated from the Orthodox Church of Czechoslovakia, which was at that time thoroughly subservient to the wishes of the Moscow Patriarchate, the Soviet regime, and its own Communist government.

Perhaps the most encouraging sign of burgeoning Orthodox supranationalism was an extraordinary inter-religious conference hosted by the Ecumenical Patriarchate in Istanbul (Constantinople for the Orthodox) in February 1994. Inspired by the Appeal of Conscience Foundation, an educational organization based in New York and headed by Rabbi Arthur Schneier, the event gathered prominent international Jewish, Muslim, and Christian leaders, including Metropolitan Theodosius of the Orthodox Church in America and other Orthodox representatives from Russia, Romania, Georgia, Bulgaria, and the United States. The distinguished conclave produced the "Bosporus Declaration," which proclaimed without equivocation: "We reject any attempt to corrupt the basic tenets of faith by means of false interpretation and false nationalism."[9] Conspicuous by their absence, however, were representatives of the Orthodox and Roman Catholic Churches in the warring states of the former Yugoslavia.

THE MOSCOW PATRIARCHATE

The Moscow Patriarchate secured its international reputation as a mainstay of the Soviet "peace and disarmament" campaign in the revived nuclear debate that took place during the late seventies and the eighties. The introduction of a regular section on the "Peace Movement" in the *Journal of the Moscow Patriarchate* signaled this new preoccupation with the evils of war in the nuclear age.

But the "peace" activism of the Russian Orthodox Church actually dates back to the first conference of the World Peace Council in the Soviet Union in August 1949. At that supposedly irenic gathering, Metropolitan Nikolai Yarushevich of Kiev, the renowned predecessor of Metropolitan Nikodim of Leningrad as head of the Patriarchate's Department of External Church Relations, was hardly a promoter of peace when he denounced the United States as "the rabid fornicatress of resurrected Babylon" that was "trying to seduce the people of the world while pushing them toward war."[10] That same year Patriarch Aleksii I issued his first appeal on behalf of peaceful relations among nations. In 1952, the first inter-religious peace congress of all the registered religious bodies in the Soviet Union met at Trinity–St. Sergius Monastery in Zagorsk near Moscow—the spiritual center of the Patriarchate. The formation of the Soviet Peace Foundation (SPF) in April 1961—only one month after the Holy Synod of the Russian Orthodox Church decided to seek membership in the World Council of Churches—was another milestone in the growing peace conscious-ness of the Patriarchate. The ostensible purpose of the SPF was to render financial assistance to those Soviet social organizations dedi-cated to peace, solidarity, and friendship among nations. The SPF functioned, however, as an arm of the Soviet regime, coercing "vol-untary" donations from the religious communities. The 1945 statute on Church administration legalized such contributions for patriotic purposes. The regime eventually, however, used this law as a pretext for taxing the churches for peace funds, sometimes expropriating huge sums of money for self-serving peace propaganda.

The use of coercion notwithstanding, spokesmen for the Patriar-chate pointed with pride to their generous contributions to the SPF. At the 1969 conference, for example, Metropolitan Aleksii of Tallinn and Estonia—now Patriarch Aleksii II—reviewed the history of donations: Patriarch Aleksii I contributed 20,000 rubles per year in 1967 and 1968; the diocesan administrations donated 903,760 and 876,774, respectively, in those years; and the parishes throughout the country contributed millions of rubles![11] The Russian Orthodox Church had already demonstrated its willingness to support Soviet military aims financially when, during the Second World War, Metropolitan Sergii zealously solicited funds from his flock for what became known as the "Dmitry Donskoi" tank column and the "Aleksandr Nevsky" aircraft squadron. The names are those of two medieval Russian Orthodox prince-saints.

The Soviet government and its front organizations rewarded the loyalty of the Patriarchate in times of peace and war by bestowing medals and honors upon the bishops and other clergy. Soviet religious publications, particularly the *Journal of the Moscow Patriarchate,* often displayed photographs of Orthodox clergy in cassocks bedecked with all manner of military medals and awards from ecumenical "peace" organizations. Patriarch Pimen, for example, received the highest award of the World Peace Council—the Joliot-Curie Gold Medal—in June 1988 for his great contribution as leader of a Church that "has always been on the side of those who fight to prevent war."[12] The honor was granted by the president of the World Peace Council, Romesh Chandra, an Indian Communist and longtime apologist for Soviet aggression throughout the world, including Afghanistan. Professions of faith in "peace" by the Russian Orthodox hierarchy ran the gamut from platitudes to thinly veiled projections of nationalism or ideology. Metropolitan Aleksii of Tallinn and Estonia reminded the patriotic *Rodina* ("Motherland") Society in November 1982, "For us, Soviet people, there is nothing more important than peace! We know from our own bitter experience the hardships, privations, suffering and losses brought on by war."[13] This contention became, of course, a veritable refrain in Soviet propaganda and was usually accompanied by the statistic of 20 million Soviet dead during the Second World War. Patriarch Pimen declared to a peace seminar in Moscow in July 1984 that "force offers no reliable guarantee of security in our time." That is true enough. But the patriarch also spliced together several disparate concepts: "The true guarantee of peace lies in the good will of nations and peaceful political realism of government leaders, their adherence to a policy of detente and disarmament."[14]

During the Soviet era, peace went hand in glove with patriotism for the Russian hierarchs. In March 1979, Patriarch Pimen pronounced "patriotism and peacemaking" an "inalienable part of our Church life."[15] At an ecumenical peace assembly at the Trinity–St. Sergius Monastery in November 1986, Metropolitan Aleksii of Leningrad (the present Patriarch Aleksii II) affirmed everyone's need for a motherland and suggested ominously that people who are alienated from their motherland "have always been held in contempt."[16]

Frequently the patriarch or his bishops blended socialism with their advocacy of peace. Patriarch Pimen issued such an overtly ideological statement to the Soviet Peace Committee in September 1977:

> Lenin's Decree on Peace heralded the great programme for the creation of a just, democratic, and universal peace. This gives us justification to state that socialism and the liberation of man, that socialism and peace, are concepts which cannot be separated one from the other.[17]

Sometimes the best defense was a good offense. During the 1980s, as the United States modernized and augmented its nuclear capability, Soviet churchmen resorted increasingly to shrill condemnations of Western "militarization." In July 1984, for example, Patriarch Pimen scored what he termed "the unabating western propaganda concerning an alleged 'Soviet threat.'" These distortions were "truly insane," since they "belie our country's policy which has always been based on a desire for peaceful coexistence and cooperation with all nations of the world."[18]

In the last two decades the Moscow Patriarchate has celebrated three military events in Russian/Soviet history: the Battle of Kulikovo, the liberation of Bulgaria, and the Great Patriotic War (World War II). In at least one case, a traditional Orthodox moral posture grounded ostensibly in the "justifiable war" perspective seems to have degenerated to militaristic "holy war."

Battle of Kulikovo, 1380

In 1980 the Patriarchate marked the six-hundredth anniversary of the Battle of Kulikovo. The Mongols of the Golden Horde, who had conquered and held Kyyivan Rus and the lands of what is now central

Russia since the mid-thirteenth century, finally met their match in the army of the Muscovite prince Dmitry Donskoi. In 1380, Prince Dmitry, whom the Russian Orthodox Church proclaimed a saint in 1988, defeated the Mongols led by Mamai, their regional governor, at Kulikovo Pole. To be sure, Mamai was replaced by another khan, and Russia had to endure another century of appanage rule by the Mongols. But the victory at Kulikovo marked a definite turning point in the life of the nascent Russian nation and its Orthodox Church.

On the eve of battle, the prince had requested and received the blessing of the monk who would become the patron saint of Russia, Sergius of Radonezh, who also exhorted the army to victory and dispatched two of his fellow monks, Peresvet and Oslyabia, to assist the prince in battle. According to the *vita* of St. Sergius by St. Epiphanius the Wise, the monk declared to the prince: "It suits you, my Lord, to take care of the Christian flock entrusted to you by God. Go against the godless, and with God helping you, you will conquer them and will return to your Fatherland with great honors."[19]

This was a classic example of justifiable war from an Orthodox moral perspective. In a speech in 1981, Metropolitan Aleksii of Tallinn and Estonia thanked the Russian warriors for defending "the happiness, freedom and independence of our great country" — moral goods that may serve as a just cause for military action.[20] Metropolitan Yuvenaly of Krutitsy and Kolomna boasted in 1980 that "it was our Church that inspired our ancestors to fight the conquerors of the Russian land." Kulikovo "saved European nations from invasion and enslavement."[21] Patriarch Pimen used similarly ambiguous, possibly xenophobic language when he rejoiced that the Russian troops "saved the states of Europe, having shielded them from the terrible invasion of the aliens." That Pimen referred to repeated invasions "by alien forces" in the six centuries since Kulikovo suggests, however, that the problem may be semantic rather than substantive. The patriarch also added an unquestionably Orthodox cause. The Church inspired the nation to cast off the Mongol yoke, he asserted, because the Golden Horde had desecrated the shrines, devastated the land of Russia, and "threatened the very life of the Moscow state."[22] The role of the Church, particularly St. Sergius, in the Battle of Kulikovo met the justifiable-war requirement of a sufficient cause: defense of the people of God. In 1980 neither Pimen nor any other hierarch commented on the dubious role of monks as warriors. More recently, however, Metropolitan Ioann of St. Petersburg and Ladoga explicitly commended St. Sergius for this gesture. Though "in violation of all customs and regulations," Ioann admitted, the saint furnished thereby "a visible image of the Russian Church's participation in the struggle for the freedom of the Motherland."[23]

Liberation of Bulgaria, 1877

The protests in January 1990 by thousands of Bulgarians against the decision of the post-Communist government to grant religious and political rights to the Turkish minority surprised most Westerners.[24] But the brutal oppression in the bygone era when Turkey controlled their land still lingers in the memory of Bulgarians, especially the Bulgarian Orthodox Christians, who constitute the vast majority of that nation. Turkish cries of suppression of national identity thus ring hollow among many Bulgarians. They note, for example, that a little more than a century ago, Bulgarians were required by their Turkish Muslim overlords to wear fezzes as an outward sign of their national submission to Turkey.[25]

The modern Bulgarian nation-state dates from 1877, when a Russian army fought and won another of imperial Russia's many wars against the Ottoman Turkish Empire. After six months of difficult military operations and some 200,000 casualties, the Russian and allied Romanian forces, together with a corps of Bulgarian volunteers, finally dislodged the Turkish forces garrisoned in Plevna. A few additional victories in Asia Minor and throughout the Balkans, culminating in the advance of the allied forces toward Constantinople, led to an armistice in January 1878. The decisive role of these Russian forces and, in particular, the special contributions of the Russian Orthodox and Bulgarian Orthodox Churches were repeatedly commemorated in the *Journal of the Moscow Patriarchate* in 1977 and 1978.

Russia's motives for declaring war against Turkey in April 1877 were mixed, of course, and included the projection of imperial power to secure the ancient capital city of Byzantium, the advancement of Slavophilism, rivalry among the "great powers" in the Balkans, and perhaps revenge against Russia's perennial enemy, who had been saved from defeat in the recent Crimean War only by the intervention of

Britain and France. But the Patriarchate's centennial commemorations of this military venture dwelt only upon the ostensibly noble reasons for fighting the Turks.

Archimandrite Kirill, dean of the Bulgarian Orthodox parish in Moscow, described the Russians who entered his country in 1877 as fraternal liberators who sought neither conquest nor vengeance but wished to establish peace.[26] In various speeches in October 1977, Patriarch Pimen of Moscow referred to the Bulgarian campaign as a "sacred cause," and spoke of "that great and selfless feat of the Russian people," "the immortal feat" of those soldiers who "paid with their lives for the freedom and independence" of the Bulgarian motherland. Pimen also commended the Bulgarian nation, whose courageous volunteers "did not bow their heads before the oppressors and never stopped fighting for their freedom and independence."[27]

Patriarch Maksim of Bulgaria returned the compliments in a speech delivered at the cathedral of St. Aleksandr Nevsky in Sofia in October 1977. (This church was named after the great Russian saint in gratitude for the Russian victory against the Turks in 1877.) Maksim lauded "fraternal Russia" for responding "not merely compassionately but sacrificially to the call of the Slavonic Orthodox Bulgarian people, its coreligionist." The Russians shouldered "the burden of the sacred war of liberation," providing the proper political authority, as required by the Orthodox justifiable-war ethic. Further, the Russians' intent in launching the military campaign was properly spiritual and just: they "rose to the defence of the profaned Bulgarians, their tribesmen and coreligionists, inspired by the awareness that in defending their profaned brothers' rights, honour and faith they were defending their own rights, honour and faith." Finally, the cause was clearly justifiable insofar as the Russian forces responded to the plea of an Orthodox people to undo centuries of religious and political bondage. Maksim described those conditions as follows:

> For five long centuries did Bulgaria direct its agonized gaze through the impenetrable gloom of the heavy yoke towards the heroism of liberation. Dreadful were those five hundred years in whose depths merged the poignant song of Tsar Shishman's soldiers, sorrowful moans of people in captivity, bitter tears of hapless mothers, the burning blood of the wretched children, the profaned sacred church

objects, the locked doors of our national schools, the degraded rights of human dignity and the manifestations of national consciousness brutally suppressed. A grievous situation which is appropriately remindful of the biblical words: . . . *lamentation and weeping, and great mourning* (Mt. 2:18).[28]

The contributions of the Russian Orthodox Church to this cause were many and varied. Patriarch Pimen, though hesitant, to be sure, to separate the Church from the entire Russian people, noted that the officers and men of the Russian army were Church members; that before each battle Orthodox clergy blessed the combat banners and exhorted the troops; that the Holy Synod donated sizable sums of money to the Red Cross to care for wounded and infirm Russian and Bulgarian soldiers; that the Orthodox convents sent hundreds of nurses to staff the military hospitals; and that the Holy Synod required each diocesan bishop to solicit donations to the cause from the parishes.[29] Another source indicated that in May 1876 the nuns of a convent in Samara sewed and embroidered a military standard that depicted a black cross on a piece of heavy silk with white, blue, and red edgings—the Russian national colors. The citizens of Samara gave this standard to the Bulgarian insurgents, who carried it into battle after battle against the Turks.[30]

An article in the Patriarchate's *Journal* listed approvingly the military exploits of the Bulgarian Orthodox clergy: "At times priests ran military detachments, exhorted the people to rebellion, took part in the work of collecting funds, buying arms and military supplies, and were in the fore at fierce battles."[31] At least two hundred clergy and an unspecified number of monks and nuns rendered this kind of military support, despite the Orthodox canonical prohibitions.[32]

Great Patriotic War, 1941-45

The militant atheism and extreme hostility displayed toward the Church by the Soviet regime since its inception disqualified the Soviet state as worthy of military defense by Russian Orthodox Christians. Despite this lack of a proper spiritual ethos, as required by the Orthodox justifiable-war ethic, the Moscow Patriarchate acted as if the Soviet regime were a morally legitimate government and the Soviet state a legitimate heir of the ancient Christian Russian empire. The following remark of Patriarch Pimen typifies this nationalistic attitude:

> Not a century has passed without a war. Aggressors have invaded our land from the west and east, north and south. And every time the tocsin sounded from the holy cloisters and churches summoning the people to the defence of the Motherland.[33]

Every five years since 1975, the *Journal of the Moscow Patriarchate* has featured dozens of documents and articles commemorating the victory of the Soviet Union in the Second World War, dubbed by the Soviets the "Great Patriotic War." Russian Orthodox Church leaders recall with pride the contributions of the Church to that war effort. We shall look at three aspects of the Moscow Patriarchate's position on that war: its attempt to establish a *justifiable cause,* its *wartime activities,* and its *post-war reflections*.

1. *Justifiable Cause.* Since the beginning of the Great Patriotic War, the Patriarchate's hierarchy has endeavored to establish the justice of the Soviet resort to arms and of the active participation of the Church in the national war effort.

On June 22, 1941, the day after Hitler invaded the Soviet Union, Metropolitan Sergii of Moscow sent an encyclical to all the parishes in which he tried to rally the entire Church to defend the motherland by invoking past invasions of *Orthodox* Russia:

> The blood of peaceful civilians is being shed on our native soil. The times of Batu Khan, the Teutonic Knights, Carl of Sweden and Napoleon are being repeated again. The wretched descendants of the enemies of Orthodox Christianity are trying again to bring our people to their knees before untruth and brute force, to make them sacrifice their Motherland's goodness and integrity, the testaments of love for their country made in blood. . . . Our Orthodox Church has always shared the fate of our people. She has shared their trials and rejoiced in their achievements. She will not abandon her people now either. She blesses with a heavenly blessing the forthcoming national feat.[34]

At a prayer service four days later, Sergii issued another rousing call to arms:

Our Motherland is in danger, and she is calling us: everyone into the ranks, everyone to the defence of the homeland, its historical shrines, its independence from foreign envlavement. Shame on anyone, whoever he be, who remains indifferent to this call.[35]

Events had, it seems, defined the Church's position. A year into the war, Sergii reminded the Holy Synod that "the fascists had attacked our country, they were plundering it, leading our compatriots into captivity, tortured and robbed them, and so on." National self-defense was at stake: "Common decency could not allow us to take any other stand than the one taken, i.e., unconditional negation of everything that bore the seal of fascism, the seal of hostility towards our country."[36] And yet not everyone deemed the external threat greater than the internal one. The late Russian Orthodox dissident Boris Talantov testified that the Orthodox faithful received with tremendous misgivings the initial appeal of Metropolitan Sergii to support the Red Army: "All believers in Russia regarded the Second World War as the wrath of God for the immense lawlessness, impiety, and persecution of Christians which occurred in Russia from the beginning of the October Revolution."[37]

The current generation of bishops has echoed the Sergianist position, sometimes with equal eloquence, sometimes more shrilly. At an inter-religious gathering at the Trinity–St. Sergius Monastery in Zagorsk (now Sergiyev-Posad) in April 1985, Patriarch Pimen, ignoring the manifest evil of Stalin's reign in his own country—indeed, virtually anointing the Soviet state and the Red Army as just warriors —condemned Nazism and the German invasion of the Soviet Union in absolute terms:

For never before in world history had evil bared its essence so openly as in Nazism, never before had it pitted so haughtily its misanthropic ideas against the humane principles of human intercourse, never before had claims to world domination drawn on such mighty military strength. And it is above all to our Motherland's credit that this force was crushed, that the peoples of Europe and the rest of the world were liberated from fascist slavery. It is with gratitude to God that we recall at this time the glorious victory of our nation over a powerful and ruthless enemy. This victory was not only proof of the military superiority of one of the belligerents over the other. This was the victory of a just cause over evil. The victory of creation over destruction. For us, for our common inter-religious ministry for peace the victory we are recalling here today serves as an inspiring symbol of the destruction of any evil design aimed at ruining the life created by God.[38]

Metropolitan Aleksii of Tallinn and Estonia painted a similar picture of good and evil in a sermon in September 1984, commemorating the Soviet "liberation" of the Baltic republic of Estonia from Nazi occupation:

Our nation won the war because we were fighting a just cause, because truly victorious strength lies not in the destructive might of arms, but in the power of the human spirit, in patriotism, in the righteousness of the Divine Economy: it lies in the unity of all peace-loving nations and people. With the hands of its hero-soldiers, the Soviet nation hoisted on the Nazi Reichstag the banner of victory. The avenging sword of justice fell on the heads of those who had unleashed the frightful tragedy of World War II, not only in retribution for what had been done, but in order to put an end once and for all to the evil and save mankind from the corrupt man-hating ideology of fascism.[39]

In assigning guilt for the outbreak of that war, Metropolitan Aleksii chose not to mention the 1939 Molotov–Von Ribbentrop Pact by which Hitler's Germany and Stalin's Soviet Union agreed to "divide" Poland between them. In 1990, however, Soviet historians and political leaders began to admit publicly the imperialistic role of their own country in the invasion of Poland and the subjugation of the three Baltic republics, including Estonia.

Besides whitewashing their own government's guilt, some of the Patriarchate's spokesmen have demonized the enemy. In Nuremberg, Germany, in 1987, Metropolitan Aleksii of Kalinin and Kashin, a much-decorated veteran of the Great Patriotic War, chronicled the "acts of blasphemy" perpetrated by the "savage foe"—the "fascist invaders" who launched the "perfidious attack" on the Soviet Union. From there it was only another step to the complete dehumanization of the German military: "The Nazi henchmen lost all traces of humanity and compassion, behaving like savage beasts and extermi-nating with diabolical hatred defenceless civilians on temporarily occupied Soviet territory."[40] This remark was a subdued version of a shocking comment by Metropolitan Nikolai of Kiev to Stalin on the occasion of the twenty-fifth anniversary of the October Revolution: "I request you . . . to accept from me and from the believers of the Ukraine warm and prayerful wishes for the Almighty to give you health for long years in our dear Motherland and for the earlier liberation of our land under your direction from the German vermin."[41] It would have been difficult, perhaps impossible, for Russian Orthodox leaders who so regarded the Germans to maintain in their advocacy of the war effort a proper spiritual intent, as required by the Orthodox justifiable-war ethic.

Other leaders of the Patriarchate boldly proffered the inverse of this demonization of the enemy of the Soviet state. If the Germans were, or had become, so evil and even somewhat less than human, then the mission to defeat them on the battlefield was nothing less than a "holy war"! Metropolitan Aleksii of Leningrad, the future Patriarch Aleksii I, consecrated his flock for holy battle in July 1941:

> But war is a holy thing for those who are forced to fight—in defence of righteousness and their country. Those who take up arms in such cases perform a feat of righteousness, and, suffering hardship, wounds and death for their kin and country, follow in the footsteps of the martyrs to win unwaning and eternal crowns. For this reason the Church blesses these feats and everything each Russian does in defence of his country.[42]

Aleksii misapplied the biblical image of the "crown of righteousness" that awaits one who has "fought the good fight" (II Tim. 4:6-8) —traditionally reserved for martyrs in Christian parlance—to literal soldiers, who had fought, moreover, on behalf of an atheistic and virulently anti-Christian government. One month later, Aleksii demonstrated the extent to which he was willing to turn Orthodox moral and spiritual values on their heads. The individual Russian, he asserted, "does not merely view the cause of national defense as a duty, albeit a holy duty; it is an irresistible prompting of the heart, an outburst of love which he is unable to stop and which he must exhaust to the end."[43] The loss of emotional control described by the bishop, far from being an ennobling or holy experience, conforms more closely to the ascetical interpretation of the "passions" (*pathē* in Greek) of the soul—untoward disturbances of the spiritual equilibrium and rational self-control of the Christian.

In a retrospective article in 1980, the monk Innokentiy from Odessa Theological Seminary actually used the term "holy war" to describe the campaign of "our glorious warriors" against the "cruel enemy."[44] Further, in July 1984, Metropolitan Filaret of Minsk and Byelorussia (now Belarus) coined an oxymoron: "Byelorussia took the first blow of the enemy whose perfidious attack aroused in the Orthodox a wave of holy anger and strengthened their insuperable will for Victory."[45] Orthodox moral and spiritual tradition has never blessed the passion of anger for anyone, much less an entire nation overcome by such an alien "crusader" spirit.

2. *Wartime Activities.* During the course of the Great Patriotic War, the hierarchy of the Moscow Patriarchate pulled out all the stops in supporting Stalin's national war effort. Metropolitans Sergii and Nikolai sent special appeals to the Orthodox Christians in enemy lands or enemy-occupied lands, urging them either to renounce their alliances with the Nazis or to resist the Nazi invaders.[46] As for any Russian Orthodox priest who collaborated with the Germans or refused to suffer with the Russian people under German occupation: Sergii warned these "traitors" that they would be called before the bar of justice of both Church and country.[47] Patriarch Pimen later hinted ominously at Sergii's prosecutorial role regarding conscientious objectors:

> It was with great pain that His Holiness Patriarch Sergei of blessed memory sent messages to those of our brothers by blood and faith who failed to discharge their duty during that hour of trial, exposing and exhorting them, as we still do today.[48]

"Exposing" draft resisters to the wrath of the civil Communist authorities reduced the wartime Patriarchate to a tool of the Soviet regime.

Perhaps the most dramatic service rendered by the Church was the active participation by Orthodox clergy in combat as "partisans" or in supportive roles. Metropolitan Sergii commended "your local partisans" as "an example and an inspiration" to his wartime flock and encouraged noncombatants to "supply the partisans with bread and everything they need in their danger-filled life."[49] More recently,

Metropolitan Filaret of Minsk and Byelorussia boasted that "many clerics by word and personal example inspired the people to defend their native land and actively supported the partisan movement."[50] In 1975, to commemorate the thirtieth anniversary of victory in the Great Patriotic War, an instructor at the Leningrad Theological Academy published in the *Journal of the Moscow Patriarchate* the names of war veterans who subsequently served the Church as bishops, priests, deacons, and docents, as well as the names of seminarians who later served in the Soviet Army. These persons had performed "their sacred duty to their country, in the war." And the surviving veterans "were given places of honor" at the celebration in Leningrad, many of them proudly wearing military decorations on their clerical robes.[51]

Indeed, on five-year anniversaries of the victory the pages of the *Journal of the Moscow Patriarchate* are filled with such photographs and with memoirs by and testimonials to the clergy combat veterans, notwithstanding the canonical strictures against violence by clergy or future clergy.[52] In a 1985 article Metropolitan Aleksii of Kalinin and Kashin recounted his exploits as the deputy commander of a platoon and as a sergeant-major.[53] Deacon Mikhail Tultsev served the "resistance" in Tartu, Estonia, as a military intelligence agent, keeping the partisans informed about German troop movements in the area around Lake Chudskoe.[54] Archpriest Anatoly Novikov related that he was decorated as a private with the "For Combat Merit" medal for fighting on the Karelian Front.[55] Archdeacon Ksenofont Roshchupkin dramatically retold the story of his military prowess—how he single-handedly manned a 76mm anti-tank gun in one firefight, "knocked out two of their machineguns," buried the "enemy spotters . . . under the rubble," disabled three tanks, and so on.[56]

3. *Post-War Reflections.* The Moscow Patriarchate reserved special blessings for those who fell in battle in the uniform of the Red Army. Upon his accession to the Patriarchal throne in April 1945, one month before the conclusion of the war in Europe, Aleksii I concluded his first sermon as patriarch with a bold reference to the war dead: "You and I have prayed together for our dear soldiers and for those who fell in battle for their country and are now in the Kingdom of Heaven, crowned with a wreath of glory for their deeds."[57]

When Nazi Germany finally surrendered, Patriarch Aleksii rejoiced that this was the "joyful day of the Lord—the day on which God passed righteous judgment on these vicious enemies of mankind." Consequently, "Orthodox Russia" (!) now stood "before the Lord of Hosts in prayer, thanking the very Source of victory and peace for His heavenly help in time of war, for the joy of victory and for the gift of peace to the world." In this spirit of prayerful thanksgiving, Aleksii congratulated the victorious Soviet war machine, "their great supreme leader" (Stalin), "and "all true sons of our country who stand behind their leader and his victorious army." He also pledged never to cease praying for "our valiant soldiers and those of our near and dear ones who laid down their temporal lives for our happiness."[58]

Religious themes also have been assimilated to these civil concerns. There is no greater Russian Orthodox symbol than the empty tomb of Christ on Pascha (Easter). Metropolitan Pitirim of Volokolamsk, who heads the publishing department of the Patriarchate, resorted to what has become a homiletic convention in a sermon on Victory in Europe Day in May 1983:

> May Victory Day always be our earthly, human Easter, because this is the day of deliverance from the great evil which befell our sacred land, and to which here too, on the fields round Volokolamsk, as everywhere else in this country, courageous resistance was put up. It was a stand for Truth, the fight against Evil, and therefore I boldly say that Victory Day is our civil Easter.[59]

Contemporary Cases

The current generation of bishops enlarged the scope of the Patriarchate's support of Soviet military and diplomatic ventures. William Fletcher and other specialists on the Soviet Union have chronicled the role of the Moscow Patriarchate in promoting Soviet foreign policy, whatever its objectives.[60] A few examples should suffice here to illustrate the Patriarchate's peculiar application of the Orthodox teaching on peace, national security, and justifiable war.

Patriarch Pimen furnished a laundry-list of special causes at the first "world conference" of "peace-loving" Soviet religious leaders in June 1977. The world, Pimen announced, had arrived at a crossroads and faced a choice between the way of life and the way of death. This "way of life" as Pimen envisioned it was skewed toward the political left. Besides implementation of the principles of peaceful coexistence and détente in international relations, the way of life included:

> the defeat of fascist regimes in Greece, Spain and Portugal, the establishment of peace in South-East Asia and the re-unification of Vietnam, the liberation from colonial regimes of Mozambique, Angola and the Cape Verde Islands, successes in the struggle for liberation of the peoples of Zimbabwe and Namibia, the growing part played by the United Nations Organization in the fight against militarism and for disarmament, and the UN Declaration on a New International Economic Order.[61]

The "Appeal" of the assembled Soviet religious leaders filled out the leftist agenda by (1) insisting that the "racist minority regimes" in South Africa, Namibia, and Zimbabwe "be removed from power"; (2) scoring the "gross and continued violation of democratic freedom in South Korea" (with no mention of the truly grievous abuses of human rights in Communist North Korea); (3) encouraging the "progressive" religious forces in Latin America in their "struggle" to have "the exploitative neo-colonialist system dismantled"; (4) urging all governments to "give full support and assistance" to Cuba, Puerto Rico, and Panama in their anti-colonial (read anti-U.S.) struggles; and (5) demanding the "withdrawal of Israeli troops from all areas occupied by war" and condemning "the continuous Israeli attacks" against the southern borders of Lebanon.[62]

The "support" rendered by the Patriarchate to its favorite causes was not necessarily "peaceful" or non-violent. With amazing candor, Metropolitan David of the Georgian Orthodox Church—an autocephalous sister Church of a new republic located in the Caucasus region of the former Soviet Union—boasted in 1988: "In recent years the Orthodox Churches in the Soviet Union, like the churches in other countries, have been providing material assistance to the South African freedom fighters. This is only natural."[63] Perhaps it was not so "natural," since some of these "freedom fighters" routinely resorted to terrorism—which sometimes included such barbarous practices as "necklacing" their fellow black Africans deemed insufficiently opposed to the South African regime.

Hardly any military conflict or foreign-policy issue escaped comment by the Moscow Patriarchate in the Soviet era. Even the establishment of a centralized military command by the U.S. armed forces on the island of Diego Garcia in the Indian Ocean drew the moral ire of the Patriarchate. Soviet and Indian religious leaders at a meeting in October 1984 condemned this American action as "an encroachment on the national interests and independence of the states in the area" and resolved "to continue the struggle for the demilitarization of the Indian Ocean, for the liquidation of all foreign [read U.S.] military bases in the area and for the realization of the UN declaration on turning the Indian Ocean into a zone of peace."[64] This resolution was not without precedent. In April 1977, the Working Committee of the Christian Peace Conference — undoubtedly encouraged by the Moscow Patriarchate — reaffirmed "the need to keep the Indian Ocean a zone of peace, free from military, naval or air bases" and noted the construction of a "nuclear air-naval base" on Diego Garcia for use by "imperialist powers."[65]

Ecumenical Activities. The Moscow Patriarchate was for decades a prime mover of the moral statements of international ecumenical organizations such as the Christian Peace Conference. Metropolitan Nikodim of Leningrad served as president of the CPC from October 1971 until June 1978, just three months before his death. After that a strong Muscovite influence continued in the person of Metropolitan Filaret of Kiev and Galich, who, prior to his 1992 break with the Moscow Patriarchate, served as chairman of the CPC's "Continuation Committee. This is one of the three key leadership positions, alongside that of the president, now Bishop Karoly Toth of Hungary, and the general secretary, now Lubomir Mirejovsky of Czechoslovakia. In virtually every resolution concerning conventional military conflicts, the CPC has vigorously attacked the United States or its perceived allies, such as Israel and the Republic of (South) Korea, or extolled the virtues of the former Soviet Union or its client states.

The CPC has unstintingly endorsed leftist or Communist factions in the revolutionary struggles and civil wars of Third World nations. In January 1976, for example, when Angola was in the throes of a post-colonial civil war, Metropolitan Nikodim and Bishop Karoly Toth declared that the MPLA — a Marxist-Leninist faction that eventually emerged victorious — was "the only force in Angola which opposed the exploitation of the country by foreign powers and spearheaded the redistribution of wealth and power."[66] A statement produced at a meeting of the Working Committee of the CPC in Kiev in March 1981 (at which Aleksii S. Buevsky and Archimandrite Sergii Fomin represented the Moscow Patriarchate) advocated "the just struggle of the people of El Salvador and its people's organizations—the Farabundo Marti National Liberation Front and the Democratic Revolutionary Front."[67] Similarly, the fifth All-Christian Peace Assembly in Prague in June 1978 proclaimed the Palestine Liberation Organization "the sole and real representative" of the Palestinians and reaffirmed the support of the CPC for the MPLA government in Angola and several other violent Marxist revolutionary movements: "the PAIGC government in Guinea-Bissau, the FRELIMO government in Mozambique, and . . . the liberation movements SWAPO (Namibia), ANC (South Africa), as well as the Patriotic Front (Zimbabwe) and POLISARIO (Democratic Arab Republic of Sahara)."[68]

This political partisanship is frequently aggravated by the use of shrill ideological rhetoric in the name of "peace and justice." In December 1982, for example, the CPC claimed that "the 'rape of Lebanon' by Israel" was an "atrocity . . . matched only by the extermination programmes of Hitler and Pol Pot."[69] An "enlarged" meeting of the presidential board of the CPC in December 1982 condemned the "US policy of domination, exploitation and aggression" in Central America. The delegates scored the "crudely imperialistic policy of the Reagan Administration's military intervention in the area": it rendered that government "guilty of violently and unjustly threatening the sovereignty of countries in this area." The CPC statement also included the following seemingly prophetic criticism: "The Christian faith is misused by those who, in the name of God, seek only to perpetuate an ungodly system of oppression and murder."[70] But of course the delegates leveled that charge not at their own mostly Soviet-bloc governments but at the United States.

The United States is indeed the *bête noire* of the CPC. A communiqué from a meeting of the CPC's International Secretariate held in Minsk in September 1986 accused the United States of exercising "state terrorism" against the peoples of Libya and Nicaragua.[71] It is an "obvious fact," the CPC said in an earlier document, that in Latin America "the US is always on the side of the most reactionary forces and governments." Further, "US imperialism has exposed itself as the major enemy" of the Latin American peoples.[72]

The Soviet-dominated CPC was not alone among religious bodies in its blatant anti-Americanism. Despite a much larger and more diversified ecumenical membership, the World Council of Churches has maintained essentially the same party line, in large measure because of the imposing presence of the delegations from the former Soviet Union (particularly the Moscow Patriarchate) and its erstwhile satellite states. The most dramatic, controversial episode occurred at the 1983 Vancouver Assembly. While refusing to cite the Soviet Union as a foreign aggressor in Afghanistan, the delegates dealt at length with the "military intervention" of the United States in Central America. "The current United States administration," the statement read, seeks "to destabilize the Nicaraguan government, renew international support for Guatemala's violent military regimes, resist the forces of historic changes in El Salvador [i.e., the Communist rebels], and militarize Honduras in order to insure a base from which to contain the aspirations of the Central American peoples." While denouncing U.S. foreign policy toward Central America, the WCC Assembly lauded the "life-affirming achievements of the Nicaraguan people and its leadership since 1979"—the year of the Sandinista revolution.[73] Attempts by fair-minded moderates to delete explicit references to the United States or to include criticism of Soviet activities in the region failed in vote after vote.

The WCC Central Committee (the authoritative agency between the Assemblies) added fuel to the fire at its regular session in Geneva in January 1987. A statement on Nicaragua blamed the United States and its economic embargo against the Sandinista regime, "the war imposed by the White House through the counter-revolution and the misinformation campaigns and pressures," for the social and economic hardships in that country. Further, the WCC leaders charged the United States with threatening the sovereignty of Nicaragua, violating its territorial integrity, challenging the right of the Nicaraguan people to self-determination, thwarting "their efforts to shape their own destiny," and imposing "pain and suffering" on them.[74] Nothing was said about the gross violations of fundamental liberties and the persecution of the Miskito Indians by the Sandinista regime, which the Nicaraguan people finally were able to vote out of office in February 1990. Among the representatives of the Moscow

Patriarchate at the meeting that produced this one-sided statement were several of the illuminati of Russian Orthodox ecumenism: Metropolitan Filaret of Minsk and Byelorussia, Metropolitan Kirill of Smolensk and Vyazma, Archpriest Vitaly Borovoi, Aleksii S. Buevsky, and Nina Bobrova.

Two recent conventional wars, those in Vietnam and Afghanistan, also received special attention from the Moscow Patriarchate.

Vietnam War. From the beginning of the full-fledged American military involvement in southeast Asia in 1965, and long after the withdrawal of U.S. forces, the Moscow Patriarchate echoed prevailing Soviet policy concerning Vietnam. It sided openly with the Viet Cong, the Communist guerrilla forces in the Republic of South Vietnam, and with their parent organization, the army of North Vietnam. As early as February 1965, Patriarch Aleksii I reacted to news of the alleged bombings and shelling of cities and villages in North Vietnam by condemning the United States. "These arbitrary and inhumane actions," he protested, "no matter how the U.S. government tries to justify them, are in direct contradiction not only with the elemental norms of international law, but also with Christian morality. . . ."[75] The patriarch charged the United States with violating the 1954 Geneva Accords and recklessly endangering the peace of the whole world.

A year later Patriarch Aleksii I expanded his argument. The United States, he declared, had "entered on the path of flaunting justice, preventing by force the Vietnamese people from deciding their own internal affairs." He rejoiced at the courageous witness of those American Christians who had begun to protest the U.S. involvement in Vietnam. And he appealed to the U.S. government to abide by the 1954 Geneva Accords and a United Nations declaration on the self-determination of states. That would lead, he suggested, "to rapid cessation of military activity in South Vietnam, of bombardment of North Vietnam, and to the proper withdrawal of foreign troops from that country."[76] These foreign troops presumably did not include the Soviet advisors in Hanoi or traveling with the Viet Cong.

Two collective proclamations also merit mention. An inter-religious "peace conference" at Trinity–St. Sergius Monastery in Zagorsk issued an appeal on July 4, 1969:

We demand to stop [*sic*] the US and their allies [*sic*] aggression against Vietnam. We voice our solidarity with the heroic people, with the Provisional Revolutionary Government of the Republic of South Vietnam [i.e., the Viet Cong]. We welcome the realistic and just program for peaceful settlement of the conflict advanced by the Provisional Revolutionary Government at the Paris talks, and we urge the US government to hearken to these proposals, and thereby hasten a peace settlement in Vietnam.[77]

Two years later, in 1971, a national *sobor* of the entire Russian Orthodox Church was allowed to meet—from May 30 until June 2 —for only the second time since the Communist takeover in 1917. It, too, added its collective voice on the Vietnam conflict. While electing Metropolitan Pimen of Krutitsy and Kolomna as Aleksii's successor, the delegates adopted a special resolution that appealed to Christians throughout the world "to struggle for," among other objectives, "the stopping of American armed intervention in the internal affairs of the countries of southeast Asia."[78] (By that time, U.S. forces had launched their "incursion" into Cambodia in pursuit of the North Vietnamese enemy and were actively combating the North Vietnamese regulars and the native Communist Pathet Lao in Laos.) The Church said nothing about the armed intervention of Communist Vietnamese forces in Cambodia and Laos.

The unyielding loyalty of the Moscow Patriarchate to Soviet policy toward its client state in southeast Asia was demonstrated again in February 1979. By then the U.S. presence in the region was a distant memory. When the People's Republic of China invaded the Socialist (i.e., Communist) Republic of Vietnam, Patriarch Pimen immediately issued a statement in support of Vietnam. The Vietnamese, he said, had "just recently repelled prolonged and cruel foreign intervention by their heroic and selfless struggle." Now the Chinese—perceived by the Soviet government at that time as dangerous, unpredictable rivals—had compelled the Vietnamese once again "to take up arms to uphold their independence, territorial integrity and national dignity."[79] A few weeks later, the Patriarchate, through the efforts of Metropolitan Filaret of Kiev and Galich, helped to engineer the so-called International Emergency Conference in Support of Vietnam, held in Helsinki under the aegis of President Urho Kekkonen of Finland. According to a report in the *Journal of the Moscow Patriarchate,* the delegates "arrived at the unanimous conclusion that China's aggression be cut short and peace be restored in Vietnam."[80]

Representatives of the Patriarchate also scored major victories on the Vietnam War issue in the WCC and CPC. As early as 1967 the WCC Central Committee chose sides, predictably taking an anti-U.S. position. In August of that year, the Central Committee reaffirmed a statement made by its executive committee in February that called on the United States to stop the bombing in North Vietnam, summoned North Vietnam to "indicate by word and deed its readiness to move toward negotiations," and insisted that South Vietnam allow the Viet Cong insurgents to be represented at those negotiations. But this relatively moderate policy statement was skewed by the Central Committee's need to assign blame:

> That is why we consider, that from our point of view, the origin of the Vietnam tragedy is the entirely unjustified military intervention of the USA in the internal life of the Vietnamese people. The withdrawal of the American troops from the territory, without any condition, is absolutely necessary, and the Vietnam problem must be settled on the basis of the Geneva Agreements.[81]

Among the seven signatories of this statement were five Russian Orthodox: Metropolitan Nikodim of Leningrad, Metropolitan Filaret of Kiev and Galich, Bishop Vladimir of Kirov and Slobodskoy, Archpriest L. Voronov, and Professor Nicholas Zabolotsky.

From the beginning of the escalation of the U.S. military intervention there, the Christian Peace Conference was clearly in the Communist camp. In November 1965 the president of the organization, Josef L. Hromádka, sent a letter of protest on behalf of the CPC to President Lyndon B. Johnson that condemned U.S. "aggression" against the Vietnamese people.[82] Metropolitan Nikodim in his presidential message to a meeting of the Working Committee in Kenya in April 1977 rejoiced over the "victories won by the peoples of Vietnam, Laos, Kampuchea, Guinea-Bissau, Mozambique, Angola, and other countries."[83]

When the People's Republic of China replaced the United States as the Soviet adversary in Vietnam, the CPC turned its ire on the Communist Chinese. In a statement issued from Prague in February 1979, the CPC leadership (including Metropolitan Filaret of Kiev) declared that they were "deeply shocked by the irresponsible and shameless attack on Vietnam by China."[84] A year later, the CPC declared that the Chinese leaders had "aligned themselves with the forces of reaction and imperialism here as well as elsewhere"—the most serious charge that Communists can lodge against other Communists.[85]

Afghanistan War. An Agence France-Presse photograph in the December 12, 1989, *New York Times* depicted Metropolitan Pitirim listening attentively to a wheelchair-bound veteran of the Soviet war against Afghanistan.[86] The occasion was the tenth anniversary of the Soviet invasion, and Pitirim had come to Friendship Park in Moscow to conduct a memorial service for the estimated 14,000 Soviet soldiers killed in that war. By then Mikhail Gorbachev had completed the Soviet military withdrawal from Afghanistan, and the Church—personified in this photograph—had reverted to the missions for which it is best suited: pastoral care, reconciliation, and healing of those who are broken by sin.

The role of the Moscow Patriarchate in the Soviet imbroglio in Afghanistan was not always benign. However, Patriarch Pimen and the rest of the hierarchy were not as forthright on this issue as on the others discussed above. Perhaps their reticence was due to a sense of foreboding about world opinion concerning this particular Soviet gambit. If so, the controversy over Afghanistan that erupted within the previously compliant World Council of Churches at its Vancouver Assembly in 1983 served to validate the Patriarchate's low profile.

In a statement issued in March 1980, Patriarch Pimen and the seven other bishops in the Holy Synod supported the official Soviet version of the events that led to the Soviet invasion in December 1979. The "revolutionary events in Afghanistan"—particularly the socio-economic changes in a socialist direction enacted by the Islamic republic—"aroused severe opposition on the part of the feudal lords of Afghanistan, whose attempts to turn back the historic development by force of arms have been generously backed by a number of conservative regimes of imperialistic states." In light of the Soviet-Afghan "Agreement on Friendship, Good-Neighborly Relations, and Cooperation" (a family pact between Moscow and the puppet regime it had installed in Kabul), the besieged government of Afghanistan had turned to the Soviet Union "to ward off the aggression from outside."

The position of the Patriarchate on the Soviet military action was, however, couched in unusually defensive, even nuanced terms:

> We, churchmen, understand and accept the reasons which prompted the Soviet Government to take such a step and we by no means recognize as justifiable the use of the Afghan events by the USA and other countries to forcefully intensify tension in the relations between East and West, between the USSR and some non-European countries.[87]

This was hardly the fervent patriotic bombast that characterized most of the statements on peace and security by the Patriarchate. A subsequent article in the *Journal of the Moscow Patriarchate* referred in passing to the "selfless, friendly efforts" of the Soviet Union in support of "the people's democratic revolution" in April 1978. But even here the reference to Afghanistan was bracketed by complaints about unfair treatment of the Soviet venture in the Western mass media and vague "intrigues against Afghanistan."[88]

The Moscow Patriarchate also maintained this unusually subdued position in the Christian Peace Conference. A special statement by the CPC leadership (including Metropolitan Filaret of Kiev and Galich) in January 1980 extolled the "achievements" of the April 1978 revolution that brought to power a Communist regime of "progressive forces" in Afghanistan. But this "humanistic" and "democratic" government, the CPC leaders warned, was being destabilized by "the military and political activities of the USA," as well as those of China and Pakistan.[89] A surprisingly muted comment in December 1982 mentioned no names: "The cessation of all subversive foreign intervention in the region should also make possible the withdrawal of the foreign forces now in Afghanistan."[90]

The most decisive action by the Moscow Patriarchate regarding the Soviet war in Afghanistan was the intervention of the Church's delegation to the 1983 Vancouver Assembly of the World Council of Churches. The critical analyses of the WCC by Ernest W. Lefever and J. A. Emerson Vermaat have chronicled the debates within the WCC on this thorny issue.[91] But the vacillation of Metropolitan Kirill (then Archbishop of Leningrad) deserves special mention here.

Early in 1980, the Central Committee of the WCC linked the Soviet actions in Afghanistan to other "threats to peace." Archbishop Kirill had argued that the Soviet government merely responded to a cry for help from the Afghan government, but he finally allowed a compromise statement. That compromise ranked the Soviet invasion ahead of six other "threats to peace" but interpreted the Soviet military decision as a response to the decision of NATO in December 1979 — the month of the invasion — to deploy new intermediate-range nuclear missiles in Western Europe.[92]

By the time the Vancouver Assembly of the WCC debated the issue, Kirill, sufficiently chastised by his colleagues in the Patriarchate, was prepared to add his voice to the rest of the Patriarchate's delegation in its endeavors to keep the heat off the Soviet Union. The WCC's final resolution on Afghanistan, in contrast even to the position of the United Nations General Assembly, refused to demand the immediate, unconditional withdrawal of Soviet troops from Afghanistan. Instead the WCC urged this withdrawal only "in the context of an overall political settlement" between the two nations.[93]

Prior to the surprisingly close vote on the wording of this resolution, Metropolitan Kirill intervened to caution the Assembly against any language that "would be politically misused" as propaganda. He also warned that any amendments rendering the resolution critical of the Soviet Union would challenge the Patriarchate's "loyalty to the ecumenical movement" — a thinly veiled threat that the Moscow Patriarchate might have to withdraw from the WCC.[94]

On this sensitive issue of conventional war, the Soviet invasion of Afghanistan, the Moscow Patriarchate appeared almost stymied from the beginning. Perhaps Patriarch Pimen and his fellow bishops were finally constrained somewhat by a prophetic conscience.

More recently, Patriarch Aleksii II manifested a stronger moral conscience during a trip to Budapest in March 1994. He personally apologized to the government and people of Hungary for the Soviet regime's brutal suppression of that country's anti-Communist revolution in 1956. Aleksii denounced the Soviet leaders as "the executioners of evil deeds" and admitted that their action "casts a shadow on my people."[95] The patriarch's conciliatory gesture, we may hope, promises a long overdue reassessment of the tragic Soviet military role in the world.

THE ROMANIAN ORTHODOX CHURCH

Despite the occasional utterances of patriarchs and other bishops on topical issues of war and peace, the Romanian Orthodox Patriarchate, like its counterpart in Moscow, commenced its well-oiled campaign for peace and disarmament only in the early 1980s. The last 1981 issue of the *Romanian Orthodox Church News* credited the Communist dictator Nicolae Ceauşescu with taking the initiative to establish a new Romanian peace movement. The "Appeal for Disarmament and Peace" was launched in November 1981 by the Democratic and Socialist Unity Front, described in *ROCN* as "the most representative forum in our country — comprising all the mass and public organizations, as well as the religious bodies." This appeal called upon all nations to work together "for the immediate implementation of the urgent objectives of security, détente and international cooperation."[96] Explicit condemnation of the U.S. government's "neutron bomb" (see chapter 6) twice in this short document indicates perhaps the chief reason for the Church's sudden involvement in the peace crusade.

Patriarch Justin did manage to propose a reasonable definition of peace during the "peace assembly" held in Bucharest in conjunction with the "Appeal." It is worth quoting at length for its balance and its similarity to the classic Western liberal democratic conception of natural rights and justice.

Many a time peace is considered as an absence of wars. But in its essence peace has a positive character. It is a natural attribute of the life of peoples in understanding, in respect for each others [sic] natural rights and property, and as equal parts of the human community, of the world. Thus peace is rooted in justice, and if one or another side of justice is trespassed upon, then peace in the world is troubled.

The basic natural rights of each people are freedom, independence and sovereignty. They are closely related to national dignity and so no nation would give them up willingly, as no man would give up willingly his human dignity. By infringing upon these rights, and by suppressing the perfect equality among peoples, conflicts, and misunderstandings and reasons for wars are brought about. On the contrary, the freedom, independence and sovereignty of all peoples strengthen the feeling of equality and create, in their way towards progress, the conditions for passing from peace to friendship, and from friendship to love.[97]

The Kantian quality of that statement was, however, mitigated by Justin's simplistic reduction of the alternatives confronting nations to "the good and the evil, life and death, peace and war." Men have "no right," he insisted further, "to choose evil, death or war." Not only war—the deadly clash of men in battle—but "arming in itself is evil; it is the main cause of the present economic crises in the world."[98]

The patriarch also resorted to the platitudes and nostrums that often punctuate public proclamations on peace. In June 1984, at another inter-religious "peace assembly" in Bucharest, Patriarch Justin declared, "Peace is not a simple silence of arms, but their abolition." He proposed "a permanent education which should eradicate from the minds of the people any warlike thoughts and plans." Continuing in the utopian vein, he virtually pleaded, "All conflicts of ideas should be solved by ideas, by appealing to reason and not by resorting to force" (by which he meant, presumably, violent or military force).[99] Peacemaking had, therefore, become an essential mission of the Church. "Nothing could be more beautiful, better and wiser," Justin announced in March 1985, "than the voice of the one who preaches peace."[100]

And yet there was room in this anti-militaristic pursuit of peace to acknowledge the value of national security. At the June 1984 peace assembly, a committee chaired by the priest-monk Nifon Mihăiță (then Patriarchal counselor for foreign affairs and now bishop) concluded, "Security, which is essential to peace, has always been one of the most profound and legitimate strivings of mankind."[101] Further, the July-September 1984 issue of *Romanian Orthodox Church News* included an article by Metropolitan Nestor Vornicescu of Oltenia that summarized succinctly the "just cause" requirement of the classic Western just-war tradition:

Christianity which is a religion of peace, cannot accept war as a natural event in the life of the peoples. As a matter of fact war is in favour of the great and powerful countries and causes moral and physical misery to the masses of people. War cannot be defended on any religious grounds or considerations. An exception to this are the wars for the defence of the homeland and of the national freedom, sovereignty and independence.[102]

In one of the first indications of the public moral posture of the Church in the post-Ceauşescu era, the National Assembly of the Patriarchate pledged support in March 1991 for all "peoples who reject dictatorship and forced occupation of their territory," with special reference to the Baltic States and also to Kuwait, newly freed from its Iraqi invaders.[103] Thus for the first time since World War II, the Patriarchate was on the same side as the United States in a war.

Peace Romanian-Style

The Romanian Orthodox bishops have been, on the whole, even more diligent than their Russian brothers in perceiving peace through the prism of patriotism. Metropolitan Nicolae Corneanu of Banat must certainly regret his obsequious praise of Nicolae Ceauşescu as "justly considered 'the man of peace.'"[104] But even if one discounts these Ceauşescuisms as obviously politically motivated, the genuine nationalism that permeates the statements of the Patriarchate is still overwhelming.

There is, for example, a tendency to identify Church and nation in the pursuit of peace. Bishop Nifon observed as a priest-monk in 1983 that in the best Orthodox tradition the Romanian Orthodox Church "always supported the Romanian faithful in their most noble actions, and made the defence of life one of its main concerns throughout the centuries." And yet the Church has known that "peace is a prerequisite of the material and spiritual development of the people its serves."[105] Metropolitan Nestor of Oltenia went further in a message published three years later: "Our Christian conscience is to the same extent our patriotic conscience. . . ." This accounts, apparently, for the "direct participation" of the Church "in support of all the initiatives, proposals and actions of our country for the defence of peace and for the preservation of life."[106]

An even more self-serving rewriting of Romanian history presents the Romanian people as inherently peace-loving and always just. Even before the violent popular uprising that toppled Ceauşescu in December 1989, Romania's history since the mid-nineteenth century, like that of its Balkan neighbors, had been marred by frequent palace revolts, internal conflagrations, and violence on a massive scale. And yet Bishop Nifon could insist that "the call for peace is characteristic of the Romanian people who have known the suffering and destruction caused by wars and devastating invasions."[107] In 1983 Patriarch Justin blessed Romania's heritage of peace with justice: "It never waged any aggression war [sic] and threatened nobody by force. But it did defend its country and faith in case of need."[108]

At the Bucharest peace assembly the following year, Patriarch Justin gave an expanded imprimatur to Romania's alleged adherence to the classic just-war tradition:

> Our people has never allowed itself to be tempted by expansionist thoughts, it has never coveted territories that did not belong to it; it has never carried out any conquest wars. The whole chain of struggles which our forefathers were forced to carry were limited to the defence of their own land; to defending "their property," namely the territory inherited from our forefathers, grandfathers and great-grandfathers. The Romanians have endeavoured to defend their national being; and strove to preserve their entire cultural heritage. They fought bravely for their life and material and spiritual goods.[109]

Justin surpassed this in a telegram he sent to Ceauşescu during that same peace assembly: "Romania is the brilliant image of a country striving for the triumph of peace and cooperation, for ensuring life to all peoples in the world, and for setting up international ethics."[110]

This kind of ludicrous hyperbole reached its zenith at the March 30, 1989, meeting of the Holy Synod of the Patriarchate. The bishops wrote to Ceauşescu:

> We also wholly approve of the ardent activity which you, as the greatest and most brilliant hero of peace and tireless fighter for understanding and peaceful collaboration, wage for the victory of mankind's progress, and for complete equality in law, respect for national independence and sovereignty, and for the development of the principles of non-interference in internal affairs, i.e. those principles which Romania consistently and determinedly applies to its relations with all the states of the world.[111]

Such claims seem cynical at best. This "brilliant hero of peace" and his government conducted sinister, round-the-clock international intrigue. They were involved hip-deep in the international arms trade, furnished substantial funding to terrorist organizations, and unleashed the dreaded Securitate at home and abroad against Romanian nationals who had fallen into disfavor.

Denunciations of Enemies

The Patriarchate's record of intemperate, ideological pronouncements on peace did not begin in the 1980s. Three earlier cases of conventional warfare drew a response from Patriarch Justinian.

In July 1950 Justinian rushed a telegram to the Security Council of the United Nations to protest its decision to resist by military force the invasion of South Korea by Communist North Korea. Justinian ignored the actual aggression by the North Koreans and offered instead the following partisan observations:

> Filled with bitterness and deeply pained in our hearts by the echo of the sufferings of the aged, of the women and of the innocent children of Korea, which was transformed into the most torturing hell by the merciless bombardments of the American Air Force, which ruins the villages and the cities with their hospitals and schools, defenseless children and of the dying old people are heard, — the faithful members and the clergy of the Romanian Orthodox Church, through me and through the Holy Synod, are raising their voices for the defense of justice and they all protest against the savageries and against the atrocities committed by the American Army in Korea.[112]

Even this was tame compared to subsequent documents. In January 1951, Justinian issued an "Appeal" to the Romanian nation, which was published in all the major newspapers in the country. The patriarch charged wildly that the American armed forces in Korea were decapitating children and burying other children alive. He pledged the "brotherly help" of the Romanian nation to the heroic, suffering North Koreans against the "American murderers."[113] Another anti-American diatribe was offered by Metropolitan Sebastian Rusan, who represented the Romanian Orthodox Church at a "peace conference" in May 1952 hosted by the Moscow Patriarchate at Trinity–St. Sergius Monastery in Zagorsk. Sebastian accused the "American imperialists" of employing "the bacteriological weapon in the war with Korea."[114]

Fifteen years later, Patriarch Justinian turned his attention to the U.S. involvement in Vietnam. The Patriarchate's official journal, *Biserica Ortodoxa Română*, reported in its first issue for 1967 that the patriarch had expressed a "growing anxiety" over "the American imperialist intervention in Vietnam."[115]

A year later, Justinian was forced by events to turn his moral wrath against Romania's fellow signatories to the Warsaw Pact. In the wake of the invasion of Czechoslovakia by the Soviets and four Warsaw Pact allies in August 1968, the Grand National Assembly in Bucharest, in keeping with Nicolae Ceauşescu's new "independent" foreign policy, denounced Moscow's resort to military force. The national religious leaders naturally followed suit, with Patriarch Justinian signing an extraordinary inter-religious pastoral message on behalf of the Orthodox. That message criticized the invasion as "a violation of certain fundamental principles of the relations between nations," including national independence and self-determination. The "five Socialist countries" that occupied "the neighboring friendly Republic of Czechoslovakia" were also deemed guilty of "hampering the free development of the life of the Czech people which in no way threatens any other country."[116] On this issue, Patriarch Justinian clearly distanced himself from his Soviet counterpart, Patriarch Aleksii I. The Russian Church leader predictably defended the Soviet invasion as a merciful act in response to "the destructive actions of anti-socialist forces," an act that "averted great shedding of blood and, perhaps, international armed conflict."[117]

The prophetic value of Patriarch Justinian's position on the Soviet invasion of Czechoslovakia was mitigated by the need he perceived to adjust his thinking to the currents of Romanian foreign policy. In August 1968 those currents ran sharply against the Soviet elder brother. Earlier in the life of the Communist regime in Romania, its hostility was directed chiefly toward the West, particularly the United States, and the ecumenical posture of the Romanian Orthodox Church reflected this. At the beginning of his reign, Patriarch Justinian together with his clergy dutifully denounced the Vatican and the nascent World Council of Churches. For example, in a pastoral letter that he ordered all parish priests to read in church on March 5, 1950, Justinian contended that "part of western Christendom, including the Vatican and the World Council of Churches, has placed itself in the ranks of those preparing for war."[118]

After the Soviet attitude toward these Western institutions changed dramatically in 1961, Justinian and the Romanian Orthodox Church became ardent ecumenists and wholehearted supporters of the WCC's leftist proclivities, which emerged full-blown at the Uppsala Assembly in 1968. In an article first published in April 1967, the patriarch revealed this *volte-face:*

> The World Council of Churches therefore supports the action for the liberation of nations and individuals from any bondage and is the defender of the freedom of any nation and individual in so far as they do not use their freedom in order to deprive other nations and individuals from their own freedom.[119]

But in the matter of Czechoslovakia in 1968 Justinian did prove that he could still in some cases proclaim moral truth.

From Moldavia to Moldova

The demise of the Communist regime did not, unfortunately, usher in a new era of moral responsibility in foreign affairs on the part of the Patriarchate of Romania. Patriarch Teoctist and the Holy Synod appear to have exploited an ethnic civil war in the Republic of Moldova (the succesor state to the former Moldavian Soviet Socialist Republic) and generated an embarrassing, morally enervating conflict between the Romanian and Russian Orthodox Churches.

When the Republic of Moldova declared its independence on August 27, 1991, only a week after the failed coup attempt against Mikhail Gorbachev in Moscow, the prospect of reunification with Romania raised hopes in Bucharest but caused considerable anxiety among the Russian- and Ukrainian-speaking minorities in this historic Romanian province between the Prut and Dniester Rivers known as Bessarabia. A rebellion by neo-Soviet ethnic Russians and Ukrainians against the newly independent Republic of Moldova erupted in the sliver of territory east of the Dniester River. This led, by the end of 1991, to the birth of yet another secessionist state—the so-called Transnistrian Republic, or Dniester Republic. The rebellion turned violent in May 1992, as Moldovan armed forces clashed with the 14th Russian Army and irregular military elements in "Dniester."

We have seen in chapter 4 how the 1992 clergy-laity congress of the Romanian Orthodox Episcopate of America reacted to this civil war. The Patriarchates in Moscow and Bucharest also pursued their parochial self-interest in this affair. In June, Metropolitan Vladimir Cântărianu of Chişinău (Kishinev in Russian) exhorted Russian President Boris Yeltsin to halt the violence, and in October Vladimir persuaded the Moscow Patriarchate to grant administrative autonomy to the Church in Moldova, as it had already done for its branches in Ukraine and Belarus. But Patriarch Aleksii II and the Russian Church were obviously determined to keep this Church in their rapidly disintegrating ecclesial realm and to prevent the Moldovians from reverting to the jurisdiction of the Patriarchate of Romania. On December 20, 1992, the Romanian Holy Synod reactivated its metropolitan see of Bessarabia (dormant since Stalin annexed the region in 1944) and named Bishop Petru Păduraru of Bălţi—one of Metropolitan Vladimir's assistant bishops—as *locum tenens,* pending the election of a ruling bishop. The official decree asserted that Bishop Petru and his "delegation" of twelve priests "express the will of the faithful and clergy over the Prut River" in their desire to be received by the Patriarchate of Romania.[120]

The Moscow Patriarchate was not amused. Bishop Petru had already been suspended by the Russian Holy Synod for his disagreeable revanchist activities. Now the decision of the sister Church in Bucharest created a furor in Moscow. Patriarch Aleksii sent a message of vigorous protest to Patriarch Teoctist, in which Aleksii objected to Bucharest's "anticanonical actions" and warned of a "severance of relations between the two Churches."[121] According to the Moscow-based democratic newspaper *Nezavisimaya Gazeta,* a large portion of the parishes in Moldova shifted allegiance from Vladimir to Petru, leaving only the trans-Dniester region firmly in the hands of the Moscow Patriarchate. But Moldovan president Mircea Snegur, who is in no hurry to yield control over his republic to Bucharest, publicly attacked the Patriarchate of Romania for accelerating the political dismemberment of his fledgling state.[122]

Tensions between the two Patriarchates continued unabated through spring 1994. What began as an ethnic civil war in a forgotten corner of Eastern Europe has, tragically, expanded into an ecclesial civil war between the two largest Orthodox Churches in the world. And both sides seem determined to exacerbate the dispute.

THE ORTHODOX IN AMERICA

The five representative Orthodox jurisdictions in the United States have produced a wide array of resolutions, encyclicals, and other official pronouncements on issues of conventional war and national security. We shall look at some of these statements dealing with opposition to violence and war and the commemoration of military events, then give special attention to the public moral witness of the Churches on the Vietnam War, the Persian Gulf War, and the civil war still raging in the former Yugoslavia.

Statements of *opposition to violence* often seem rather obvious and unremarkable. A resolution of the 1986 clergy-laity congress of the Greek Orthodox Archdiocese "condemns international terrorism in all its forms" and "expresses its sympathy to the victims of terrorism, and its indignation to the governments which support this terrorism or cover it up."[123] The 1988 convention of the Ukrainian Orthodox League said it "deplores the use of terrorism in whatever form and for whatever purpose throughout the world."[124] The 1975 convention of the Antiochian Orthodox Archdiocese in its condemnation of violence called attention to one type that the delegates deemed characteristic of their archenemy Israel: "We, as Orthodox Christians, deplore all forms of violence, whether by individuals, private groups, or governments, but we consider the premeditated act of technological terror by a government as the most deplorable of all. . . ."[125]

The 1975 All-American Council of the Orthodox Church in America passed a resolution that reflected the Orthodox moral mainstream, though its wording was too general to have much of an impact on either Church or society:

> The overwhelming trend in our society to glorify violence and to use violence for gaining power, pleasure and profit is to be forthrightly rejected. Violence in any form — physical and psychological — has no place in human life and can never be the source of human freedom and dignity. All "ideologies of violence" are evil and destructive of human life and community, and any particular acts of violence which may be undertaken as the least of evils must never be glorified. They must rather be repented of and suppressed as quietly as possible through the spiritual and moral cultivation of

personal and social peace and well-being through individual and corporate self-control and self-sacrifice.[126]

The caveat against glorifying "any particular acts of violence which may be undertaken as the least of evils" accepted a proportionalist "lesser evil" approach to moral decision-making—an increasingly popular, though hardly authentic, mode of Orthodox moral decision-making. Further, this statement did not endorse absolute pacifism. The added requirement of repentance for certain violent acts that "may" be undertaken placed the OCA firmly on the side of those contemporary moralists who, though not rejecting *a priori* all military actions, demand an overriding justification for violence in all permissible cases.

The *commemoration of the military past* of their national homelands is a second theme in this area for the Orthodox Churches in the United States. For instance, in 1989 the Serbian Orthodox Church engaged in a year-long celebration of the 600th anniversary of the Battle of Kosovo—the decisive defeat by the Muslim Turks that marked the end of the medieval Serbian Orthodox empire in the Balkans. The Eastern Diocese of the SOC resolved in February 1989 to "*welcome* the decision of our Mother Church to organize the 600th Anniversary celebration of the Battle of Kosovo at the Monastery of Gracanica on the Field of Kosovo to memorialize the Holy Martyr, Prince Lazar, and the immortal heroes who gave their lives for the defense of *the Holy Cross and Golden Freedom.*"[127] The second italicized phrase quickly became a rallying slogan for Serbs, especially in times of foreign threats or aggression. But the exaltation of popular suffering and national defeat epitomized in the commemoration of Kosovo also has served ironically as a counterweight to the bellicose nationalism and "holy war" tradition that run throughout Serbian history, particularly the revolutionary national independence movement in the nineteenth century.

Clerical and lay leaders of the Ukrainian Orthodox Church of the U.S.A. similarly invoke Ukraine's glorious military past. An encyclical of the Council of Bishops in December 1986, referring to the 1654-67 war against Poland led by the Cossack chieftain Bohdan Khmelnytsky, observed that "the Church blessed the warriors for freedom" and greeted the Cossack as "the national liberator upon his arrival in

Kiev."[128] To cite only one additional example, the 1967 *sobor* of the UOC commemorated another seminal event in military history—the Ukrainian national revolution that began in 1917. The delegates extolled the "immortal glory gained in the combat for freedom and independence of Ukraine."[129]

The Greek Orthodox in America have not neglected the military exploits of the Hellenes. Archbishop Iakovos has liberally infused his encyclicals with invocations of modern Greek heroism. His "Ochi Day" encyclical in 1962, for example, proclaimed "a sacred obligation to glorify God, by piously offering our prayers in behalf of our brothers, who made the supreme sacrifice on the fields of battle" in the national resistance to Benito Mussolini's Fascist military occupation of Greece in 1940.[130] The archbishop's Ochi Day encyclical in 1972 blended religious and ethnic images by situating this event in the Greeks' "three-thousand year history of holy struggle: defensive struggles against force. Struggles of freedom from oppression. Struggles of the spirit against ignorance. Struggles of human ideals against international tyranny." The sacrifice in 1946 of "the thousands of our brothers who fell on the battlefield, or in detention camps, from enemy and communist fire" but who ultimately vanquished the tyrants cried out, Iakovos said, for memorials from those who had reaped the fruits of liberty.[131]

The other decisive military event in modern Greek history—the Greek Revolution, which began on March 25, 1821, in conjunction with the Orthodox feast of the Annunciation—has figured even more prominently in Archbishop Iakovos's glorification of Greek heroism. His encyclical for March 25, 1968, attributed the victorious uprising in 1821 to "the total involvement of the people," who had been "persuaded that the time had come for faith and morals and the soul of man to be resurrected."[132] In an encyclical to the clergy, teachers, and parish councils of the Greek Orthodox Archdiocese three years later, the archbishop tried to situate this event in post-Byzantine Greek history:

> The vision of Eternal Greece, protagonist in the arena of eternal values, which was kept alive in the souls and hearts of our forefathers during the 400 years of slavery, and which the gallant fighters of 1821 together with the philhellenes who fought with them always kept before them, was a constant fountain of inner power.[133]

Contemporary military conflicts, particularly those involving U.S. forces, are a third theme in the American Orthodox public moral witness on war, violence, and nationalism. There are endorsements of American efforts to keep the peace or to reestablish it when violated by aggressors. For example, the *sabors* of the Serbian Orthodox Church in 1980 and 1984 produced virtually identical resolutions that reflected the patriotism of the American and Canadian delegates: "We express our loyalty to our homelands, the United States of America and Canada, by supporting their efforts in maintaining peace in the world and in defending all human rights which are jeopardized by totalitarian regimes, and especially by godless international communism."[134] In its November 1989 annual assembly, the Midwest Diocese added an explicit reference to military defense: "We deeply believe that only a moral and militarily strong America will be able to fulfill her historical mission and to respond to the difficult tasks set before her."[135] Similarly, in April 1985, Metropolitan Mstyslav of the Ukrainian Orthodox Church gave a plenary endorsement to President Reagan's "policy of active opposition to the aggressive imperialistic policy of the USSR," especially his efforts "to quell the spread of Communism on the American continent" and his moral support of those nations "enslaved by communist imperialism."[136]

Occasionally a resolution attempts to approach contemporary violence and conventional wars more even-handedly. The delegates to the 1980 clergy-laity congress of the Greek Orthodox Archdiocese, for example, rededicated themselves "to the cause of peace" and condemned

> all armed aggression including the invasion and continued occupation of Cyprus by Turkish armies; the invasion of Vietnam by one of its neighbors, the invasion of Afghanistan by Russia and the use of chemical warfare in said invasion; the presence and active participation of Cuban troops in African political turmoil.[137]

Perhaps the most balanced, nuanced document on this subject appeared at the OCA's 1983 All-American Council. A "Resolution on Justice and Peace" acknowledged that the Church prays for "all civil authorities" but qualified this seeming political advocacy by noting that "our ultimate battle can never be a political one. . . . Since justice and peace cannot be achieved by force, their spiritual dimensions are our only hope." The council reserved special criticism, however, for the activities of the World Council of Churches' 1983 Vancouver Assembly. The OCA delegates prophetically scored the WCC's "one-sided and unfair" selection of and manner of addressing "situations where justice is betrayed and peace is threatened." The "flagrant omission" of the violent persecution of believers and the suppression of human rights in the Communist world "indicates that the statements made by the World Council of Churches are determined by political expediency" and hence "deprived of their moral significance."[138]

This balanced approach contrasts sharply with the policy statements and resolutions of the Governing Board (since late 1990 called the General Board) of the National Council of Churches, in which four of the five Orthodox jurisdictions examined in this study participate regularly. As K. L. Billingsley has demonstrated, the NCC almost invariably takes a "liberal," or even "leftist," position on contemporary cases of conventional war, particularly when the military forces of the United States or of countries to which it gives aid are involved.[139] Criticisms of official U.S. policies abound, and sometimes the statements of NCC officials reflect a rush to judgment even before the smoke of battle has cleared.

An egregious example was NCC General Secretary Claire Randall's 1983 telegram on behalf of the NCC to President Reagan decrying "the injection of our U.S. military forces" into the Caribbean island of Grenada as a violation of that nation's sovereignty, a contravention of international law and of the United Nations Charter, and "a dangerous precedent." She also urged the "prompt withdrawal of U.S. forces from Grenada."[140] The telegram was dated October 25—the *first* day of this military operation during which there was a media blackout and hence no details available to the public. This venture ultimately proved to be not only highly successful in achieving its stated aims but also extremely popular both in the United States and in Grenada itself.

In a notorious resolution adopted on May 17, 1990, the NCC Governing Board declared war on the memory of Christopher Columbus. Rather than celebrate the 500th anniversary of his first landing in the Western Hemisphere, U.S. Christians were urged by the NCC, with Fr. Leonid Kishkovsky of the OCA presiding, to repent for "the subsequent invasion, genocide, slavery, 'ecocide,' and exploitation of the wealth of the land." Resolutions of this sort call into question the continued participation of the usually more conservative Orthodox delegations in this ecumenical body.

Vietnam War

The public moral witness of the Orthodox Churches in America on the most controversial and divisive military venture in recent American history was itself controversial and divisive.

Most surprising perhaps is the high correlation of the positions of the Churches with changing popular sentiment concerning the war. Between the escalation of the U.S. military involvement in the Vietnam conflict in 1965 and the withdrawal of all remaining U.S. forces from that war-torn country in 1973, the consensus in the United States shifted dramatically from fervent support of the war effort to determined opposition. The public positions of the Orthodox Churches did likewise.

In the initial stages of the U.S. military action, Archbishop Iakovos occasionally referred to the U.S. role in glowing terms. His Annunciation encyclical in 1965 praised the sacrifices "being made today by the youth of this great American nation in far-away South Viet-Nam." Their cause was just, because they were defending a people whose freedom was being "trodden underfoot" (the archbishop did not name the offender).[141] An encyclical to the clergy in September 1966 declared that the "War in Vietnam against the unjust and unjustified intervention of the strong at the expense of the weak" must, like other wars against evil, "be won in the name of Christ and for the sake of man."[142] Similarly, at its *sobor* in October 1967, the Ukrainian Orthodox Church passed the following succinct resolution: "The Sobor prays to the All Merciful Lord to grant victory to the heroic people of South Vietnam and hails the United States of America and her allies for their help in the struggle against communist imperialism."[143]

But in August 1970, when the tide of public opinion had begun to turn against the expansion of the war in Southeast Asia, Metropolitan Philip of the Antiochian Orthodox Archdiocese said: "We have already had two barbaric wars during the first half of this century and we continue to wage a senseless war in Viet Nam."[144]

The clearest example of the shifting moral ground within the various jurisdictions is the resolutions on the Vietnam War produced by the four clergy-laity congresses of the Greek Orthodox Archdiocese from 1966 to 1972. The 1966 congress promised unqualified moral and civic-minded support for a nation in what was then perceived to be "a time of need." In its resolution on "World Peace," the congress acknowledged "the suffering and oppression of our fellowmen" and said it therefore

> wholly supports America's commitment to the pursuit of peace in Viet Nam. We deplore, however, such hypocritical acts of pacifism as draft-card burning and the evasion of military service, for we affirm that freedom is not and has never been totally free. The preservation of our cherished rights and liberties requires the solemn obligation and duties of citizenship among which the Church recognizes as most important, the service to and defense of country in time of need.[145]

This denunciation of explicit anti-military actions in the public arena, though typical of the mainstream attitude in 1966, may now appear misguided. In addition, the attempt to equate those variously motivated actions with "pacifism" reflected, in retrospect, at least a poor choice of words and was perhaps an unfair impugning of the motives of conscientious objectors.

Two years later, in 1968, the clergy-laity congress, held in Athens, Greece—far from the political and social turmoil raging in the United States, especially at the Democratic National Convention in Chicago —passed a noticeably subdued resolution that lamented the tragic inhumanity of war. The delegates implored President Lyndon B. Johnson "to keep seeking a solution that is just and equitable," while assuring him that "we stand solidly behind him in his agony to preserve these ideals which comprise the essence of humanity." The congress also appealed to Hanoi, Peking, and Moscow "to take seriously the pursuit of peace and to find the way in Paris to end the holocaust."[146] The tone of this resolution was at once somber and plaintive. But a separate statement on "civil disobedience" repeated the harsh criticism voiced two years earlier of anti-military demonstrators.[147]

By 1970 the Greek Orthodox clergy-laity congress had achieved a new measure of equilibrium on the subject of Vietnam. Noting the "carnage" and "demonic destruction" of the last half century, the congress decided "to commend every effort and every movement to terminate war and hostility in every area, whether it be Southeast Asia, the Middle East or anywhere else." Conspicuously absent, however, were any suspicions about anti-military demonstrators, any explicit support for the U.S. military effort in Vietnam, and any criticism—implicit or explicit—of Communists for the oppression and suffering they caused in that part of the world. The most pressing need was no longer the "service to and defense of country in time of need," but rather the cooperative pursuit of an "equitable" end to the war at the Paris peace talks.[148]

The reversal was complete at the 1972 clergy-laity congress. The resolution on "peace" was sobering:

> The wars of the 20th century, history's most destructive, affirm that war destroys, kills, wastes, and embitters. It provides no cures. It produces no victors. Vietnam offers the latest testimony to these tragic facts. Already too many have died and suffered. Too much has been wasted. Too often we have heard false reports of a termination.
>
> We urge ceaseless activity towards the goal of peace in Vietnam, especially by the leaders of all nations involved on both sides. Also, we appeal to all world leaders to work towards this end.
>
> We who have been called the "sons of God" when we pursue the avenues that make peace, pledge ourselves to labor in all possible ways to bring peace in Vietnam. No time can be too soon for the conclusion of this tragic war.[149]

Gone was the spirit of optimism, purpose, and patriotism that marked the initial foray of the Greek Orthodox congresses into the public debate on Vietnam. Now, six years later, a bitter taste of failure and betrayal, both moral and social, was all that remained among the assembled representatives of Greek Orthodoxy in America. "Peace" in Vietnam was all that seemed to matter, but no political conditions were stipulated for the establishment of this peace. These delegates would have had much to dispute with their predecessors at the 1966 congress and possibly that of 1968, even as delegates to future clergy-laity congresses may find cause to regret the style and substance of the 1972 statement on "peace."

The metamorphosis of the Greek Orthodox Archdiocese's moral position on the Vietnam War mirrored that of the National Council of Churches. The record of the NCC on this most controversial of U.S. wars began inconspicuously enough with a "Resolution on Vietnam" by the Governing Board (February 25, 1965) that recognized "the concern of the United States for the freedom and independence of all peoples" and acknowledged "our responsibility to the people of South Vietnam who have been depending upon our aid." Nine years later, after all U.S. military forces had been withdrawn in keeping with President Nixon's "Vietnamization" policy, the NCC Governing Board issued a "Resolution on Ending Further Involvement in Indochina War" (February 27, 1974). This resolution urged that the Nixon administration "cease military assistance to the Republic of Vietnam so long as that nation fails to comply with the provisions of the Paris Peace Agreements" of 1973 and did not afford its citizens freedoms of speech, assembly, and religion. No such standards of liberal democracy were applied to North Vietnam or its Viet Cong guerrilla force in the south. Meanwhile, the NCC still blamed the United States for its indirect "support of continued warfare in Indochina."

The various Orthodox members of the NCC were, for the most part, swept up in this changing tide of opinion. One shining moment, however, remains as a testimony to the prophetic courage of at least four Orthodox representatives. After the NCC had reached its turning point on this issue, the Governing Board's "Resolution on the Cambodia-Vietnam Situation" (June 21, 1970) explicitly endorsed two amendments to a bill in the U.S. Senate "designed to end US military participation in the war in Cambodia and Vietnam." Voting against this particular paragraph in the NCC resolution and requesting that their names be recorded in opposition were thirteen delegates including Fr. Robert G. Stephanopoulos, Fr. Demetrios J. Constantelos, and William K. Condrell of the Greek Orthodox Archdiocese and Constantine H. Kallaur of the OCA. Unfortunately, this is the only NCC resolution on an issue of war and peace in which Orthodox dissent is on the record.

Persian Gulf War

The Persian Gulf War in 1990-91 furnished the Orthodox Churches with a rare opportunity to apply their justifiable-war ethic to U.S. defense policy with confidence and relative ease. This case study in international conflict began on August 2, 1990, when Iraqi armed forces invaded Arab emirate of Kuwait and proceeded to subjugate the people ruthlessly, pillage the capital city, and set fire to oil wells. The United States joined this military conflict on January 16, 1991, after—arguably, to be sure—pursuing all reasonable peaceful alternatives and marshalling the good offices of the United Nations Security Council. The incredibly brief ground war—the 100 hours from February 24 until Saddam Hussein's Iraqi government sued for peace on February 28—caused a remarkably low number of American and allied military casualties and of civilian casualties in Kuwait and Iraq.

Unlike the Orthodox positions on the Vietnam War, the public moral witness of the several Orthodox jurisdictions in America was virtually uniform in opposition to U.S. policy throughout the duration of the Persian Gulf conflict.[150]

In its September 14, 1990, "message," the NCC Executive Coordinating Committee sounded the alert to its member communions. Though the message "condemned Iraq's invasion and occupation of Kuwait," it also raised "serious questions about the decision of the U.S. government to send troops to the Gulf region and about the growing magnitude of the U.S. presence." Two months later, in its November 15, 1990, "Message and Resolution on the Gulf and Middle East Crisis," the NCC's General Board, with Fr. Leonid Kishkovsky of the OCA presiding, warned that as a result of the Bush administration's "reckless rhetoric and imprudent behavior," the United States might "initiate war." The NCC specifically called for "an immediate halt to the buildup and the withdrawal of U.S. troops from the Gulf region except those which might be required and explicitly recommended by the Security Council of the United Nations in accordance with the relevant provisions of the United Nations Charter."

When on November 30 the U.N. Security Council set a January 15, 1991, deadline for the withdrawal of all Iraqi forces from Kuwait, the NCC expanded its opposition: it was now against *any* use of military force for *any* reason by the United States, the U.N., or any combination of Western powers. A November 29, 1990, letter to President Bush produced under NCC auspices and signed by fifteen church leaders—including Archbishop Iakovos of the Greek Archdiocese, Metropolitan Philip of the Antiochian Archdiocese, and Fr. Leonid Kishkovsky (as NCC president and presumably not representing the OCA)—expressed the crypto-pacifist view that "war as a means of settling international disputes is in conflict with the teaching of our faith." This letter, which preceded by one day the expected resounding affirmation of U.S. policy by the U.N. Security Council, also tried to shift the burden of decision for entering the Iraq-Kuwait war to the U.S. Congress, which, the church leaders complained, had not "debated adequately the options before our nation."

However, when the Congress endorsed President Bush's position after a memorable two-day debate in January on the eve of the U.N. deadline for Iraqi withdrawal, the same church leaders turned in desperation one more time to President Bush himself. In an "urgent letter" sent to the president by fax on the very day of the January 15 U.N. deadline, the NCC pleaded with him to "give peace another chance" and not to "lead our nation into this abyss." The letter took on an apocalyptic tone: "Once begun, it is unlikely that this battle can be contained in either scope, intensity, or time"; and, referring to anticipated casualties among "aggressors and victims alike," "this sacrifice is out of proportion to *any conceivable gain* which might be achieved through military action" (italics added). The Orthodox signatories to this letter were Metropolitan Theodosius of the OCA, Metropolitan Philip, Metropolitan Christopher of the Serbian Orthodox Church in the U.S.A. and Canada, and Fr. Miltiades B. Efthimiou, representing Archbishop Iakovos. The name of Fr. Leonid Kishkovsky also appeared on the document in his capacity as NCC president.

Meanwhile the Orthodox had contributed a few documents of their own along the same lines. Two days before the November 30, 1990, U.N. Security Council resolution, the Standing Conference of Canonical Orthodox Bishops in the Americas (SCOBA) issued a statement that effectively placed the moral weight of the Orthodox Churches behind "continued firm application of the [economic] sanctions against Iraq"—one of the policy alternatives then confronting the U.N. This statement also objected to "the irresponsible political demagoguery and inflammatory rhetoric"—without naming the source or sources—that the bishops deemed an obstacle to "a permanent solution" to the crisis. Like their NCC colleagues, the SCOBA bishops were pessimistic about the future course of the conflict if the United States should resort to a military solution. Any military action, they feared, would leave "no hope" for the millions of persons in the region. "It is through negotiations," they declared, "and not through troop deployments that a lasting and just peace will be found."[151]

In an editorial in the December issue of *The Word,* Metropolitan Philip railed against "this Western jingoistic policy in the Middle East," resorted to the simplistic anti-war slogan "Blood is more precious than oil," and engaged in political fortune-telling: "The United States must realize that it will undoubtedly win the battle, but ultimately lose the war." The Antiochian primate did not miss the opportunity to point a finger at Israel: "Why does our military might not protect the little Palestinian children who are being cut down daily by Israeli bullets?"[152]

On January 17, 1991, the second day of aerial bombardment of Iraqi military targets in Kuwait and Iraq, Metropolitan Theodosius sent a pastoral letter to his OCA flock that signaled a shift toward moderation. Though he referred anachronistically to "the breakdown of peace" as if it had occurred with the U.S. intervention on January 16, 1991, instead of with the Iraqi aggression the previous August, Metropolitan Theodosius approached the escalation of the conflict soberly and with an equanimity rare among his colleagues at that juncture. He urged his flock to pray for their relatives and friends in the U.S. armed forces who were "honorably fulfilling their sacred duty," and expressed hope that the terrible suffering and carnage of the war would be "transformed into a saving and redemptive act, establishing the foundation for a better world order and a permanent peace for the peoples of this region."[153]

The NCC, however, was undaunted. On the same day that Metropolitan Theodosius dispatched his encyclical, Fr. Leonid Kishkovsky and NCC general secretary James A. Hamilton issued a joint statement that pronounced bitter judgment on the two-day-old military counteroffensive against Iraq: "Operation Desert Storm may be a success for advanced military technology, but the resort to war reflects a failure for the human spirit."

The NCC reached its nadir on this issue in its February 12, 1991, "Call to the Churches," which was signed both by American religious leaders and by some seventy delegates to the Assembly of the World Council of Churches, then meeting in Canberra, Australia. Among the American signatories were Metropolitan Philip, Fr. Miltiades B. Efthimiou, and, as NCC president, Fr. Leonid Kishkovsky. Archbishop Makary of the Moscow Patriarchate's parishes in North America also signed the document in New York. Conspicuous by his absence from the list was Metropolitan Theodosius. As the anticipated commencement of the allied ground offensive drew near, the signatories declared confidently, "War would bring nothing but loss to us all." The statement included a litany of suffering people that among other things (1) implicitly equated the indiscriminate targeting of civilians in Israel by the Iraqis to the highly discriminate bombing practices of the multinational alliance against Iraq, (2) raised the irrelevant point of the racial composition—"a disproportionate number" of "people of color"—of the all-volunteer American armed forces, and (3) tried to link the Israeli-Palestinian conflict to the Iraqi invasion of Kuwait that precipitated the allied intervention. The statement also called for a ceasefire and "a fresh effort to find a diplomatic solution," which probably would have served Saddam Hussein's interests more than those of the suffering people for whose sake, the NCC said, it "opposed this war on moral grounds." Further, the signatories pledged their support not only to American conscientious objectors but also "to those who cannot obey military orders that conflict with the church's teaching on the sacredness of human life" —an open invitation to deserters from the line of duty. Finally, this statement reflected a hubristic certitude that the NCC's views, and not the policy of the U.S. government, conformed to the will of God: "The word of the gospel cannot be reconciled with what is now happening in the Gulf. It is on Jesus' call to be peacemakers that we are united and will take our stand."

After the decisive victory of the U.S.-led alliance, the NCC and the Orthodox leaders who spoke publicly on this issue continued to cast the event in the worst possible moral light, with no admission of any errors of prudential or moral judgment on their part. On February 28, the day of the ceasefire, Fr. Leonid Kishkovsky and James Hamilton issued a hasty lament for the pain and suffering of "this terrible tragedy," accepting as fact the outlandish Iraqi allegation that "Iraqi victims are now counted in the hundreds of thousands." Lest any Americans lose sight of what they saw as the dire outcome of the recently concluded war, Fr. Leonid and new NCC general secretary Joan Brown Campbell issued a March 28, 1991, "letter of pastoral concern" to the NCC member communions that hammered home this theme during the Lenten season. The war "could have been avoided," they insisted; because it was not, "ancient enemies are again set against one another—now with renewed vengeance." In the wake of an overwhelming chastisement of Hussein's Iraq, they asserted that "little has been resolved and the level of conflict has not diminished." The NCC leaders impugned President Bush's motives: "In recent times our American leaders have frequently sought to distract public concern for domestic needs by responding to a perceived external threat to our national security." They also referred simplistically to the "obsessive appetite for oil." Perhaps the most egregious comment was this: "The earth has been scorched and waters fouled as Iraq was driven from Kuwait." This made the calculated ecological damage wrought by the Iraqis in Kuwait and the Persian Gulf sound like a by-product of the allied counteroffensive.

If such statements produced under NCC auspices—whether with or without the overt collaboration of Orthodox members—may be dismissed as the products of a highly politicized organization, faithful Orthodox Americans must take seriously the utterances of their own hierarchies. Thus it is particularly painful to review the March 7, 1991, statement of the Holy Synod of Bishops of the OCA on the Persian Gulf War.[154]

Crafted under the tutelage of Fr. Leonid Kishkovsky in his capacity as "ecumenical officer," this statement was clearly intended as a sober, even-handed, "moderate" alternative to the NCC's increasing radicalism. For example, the bishops stressed their pastoral role: "[W]e embrace in our pastoral care both those who argued that the war against Iraq was just and necessary, and those who argued that the war and the suffering it brought to civilian populations was not proportional to the Iraqi aggression, and that means short of war to resist and reverse the invasion of Iraq had not been fully tested and given time to work."

But this pastoral vision was undercut by the OCA bishops' astonishing disavowal of the justifiable-war ethic. "We are moved, furthermore," they proclaimed, "to point out that the 'just war theory' does not reflect our theological tradition. . . . If the assertion that a war is just makes it appear that war is theologically justified, that there can be a 'theology of war,' then we believe such an assertion is erroneous and morally misleading." What was erroneous and morally misleading was the bishops' flight from their own mainstream moral tradition on war and peace. If they had opted for the absolute pacifist ethic, this rejection of the justifiable-war ethic (leaving aside any quibbling about their use of the terms "just" and "theory") might have made sense. But they freely admitted in the same paragraph "that a lesser evil must sometimes be chosen to resist a greater evil."

The OCA bishops apparently wish to allow for military action on occasion, but without blessing it or calling it "just." If they persist in this sophistry, they will paint themselves into a moral corner as *neither* just warriors nor pacifists.

CIVIL WAR IN YUGOSLAVIA

Although it may seem perverse to search for a positive effect of the tragic civil war in the former Yugoslavia, one glimmer of light does indeed shine in the darkness that has overcome that historically troubled region: Orthodox spokesmen in Europe and the United States have closed ranks behind the embattled Serbs, while maintaining an unequivocal prophetic witness on behalf of justice for all the warring factions. We shall examine how the Orthodox have managed this delicate moral balancing act. But first a little background is necessary to illustrate the complexities of this civil war and the predicament of the Serbs as an Orthodox nation embroiled in an ungodly religio-ethnic armed conflict.

The civil war in the former Yugoslavia began in earnest in June 1991, when Croatia and Slovenia seceded from the Communist multiethnic federation. The Slovenes drew only a token and short-lived military opposition from the federal government in Belgrade, but ethnically heterogeneous Croatia was a different matter. Approximately one-eighth of Croatia's pre-civil-war population of 4.5 million was Serbian, living mostly in densely settled ethnic pockets in the Krajina region and along the eastern border with Serbian-controlled Vojvodina. The prospect of living in an independent Republic of Croatia cut off from the rest of the Serbian community in Yugoslavia was horrifying to the majority of Croatia's Serbs. Their collective memory of anti-Serb atrocities committed with great zeal by the Croatian "Ustasha" Fascists during the Second World War was still palpable. The pro-Ustasha and anti-Serb activities of the Croatian government of Franjo Tudjman—a longtime Communist and anti-Semite, but now a born-again nationalist—only magnified Serbian fears of another attempted genocide. Sporadic violence had occurred in the Krajina even before the June 1991 secession. But a full-scale armed rebellion by Serbian militia erupted in autumn 1991 in eastern Slavonia, with most of the fighting in the cities of Vukovar and Osijek. The Serbian rebels were supported by the Socialist government of the rabid nationalist and ex-Communist Slobodan Milosevic in Belgrade. Their cause was fueled, no doubt, by the international recognition granted to the Republic of Croatia in January 1992. Spearheading that recognition was Germany, the historic *bête noire* of the Orthodox nations in the Balkans.

A similar pattern of events describes the advent of the civil war in Bosnia-Hercegovina. In March 1992, this so-called republic seceded from what remained of Yugoslavia. It quickly achieved international recognition as a sovereign state on April 7, 1992, with the United States and Germany leading the way. Bosnia-Hercegovina was a Yugoslavia-in-miniature, a religio-ethnic patchwork: 44 per cent Muslim, 33 per cent Serb (at least nominally Orthodox Christian, mostly agrarian, occupying some 60 per cent of Bosnian territory), and 17 per cent Croat (at least nominally Roman Catholic, concentrated in the southwest corner of the region). The Muslims, whom the new "republic" and the Western media prefer to label "Bosnians," do not constitute an ethnic group or a nation, properly speaking; they are mostly Serbs or Croats whose ancestors converted to Islam during the five centuries of Ottoman Turkish domination of the Balkans.

The majority of Serbs in Bosnia had refused to participate in the national referendum on secession conducted in March 1992 by the central government in Sarajevo. That government was headed by President Alija Izetbegovic, a Muslim whose 1970 work *The Islamic Declaration* called for a fundamentalist Muslim state in Bosnia. When Izetbegovic's government seceded from Yugoslavia anyway, the Bosnian Serbs launched an armed rebellion on many fronts throughout the new "republic." No doubt they were encouraged by the Milosevic regime in Belgrade and by dreams of a Greater Serbia linking the Serb-populated regions throughout the former Yugoslavia. Again history was, ostensibly, the driving force of resistance by the Bosnian Serbs. During the Second World War, Bosnia was one of the principal anti-Serbian "killing fields," and specially designated Muslim SS units assisted their Croatian Ustasha overlords in rounding up and murdering Serbs by the hundreds of thousands.

The question of causation has, however, been reduced and distorted in the Western media and among the Western European and U.S governments to one of "Serbian aggression" across internationally recognized borders. Many prominent political and religious leaders refuse to consider the armed conflict a civil war and lay most of the blame for starting the war and for the atrocious destruction and carnage—at least 200,000 deaths—at the feet of "the Serbs." Media coverage of the Bosnian phase of this civil war has generally demonized the Serbs, sanctified the Muslims as the primary victims, and ignored the Croats—until atrocities committed by Croatian militia in Bosnia or by Croatian regulars from across the Bosnian-Croatian border became too obvious to be ignored any longer. (To cite one example: the senseless destruction of the 500-year-old bridge in Mostar—a venerable historical landmark—by Croatian artillery was duly reported in the West, but without evoking the chorus of outrage that greeted the Serbs' shelling of the medieval fortress of Dubrovnik beginning in October 1991.) Many of the loudest demands to "protect" the Bosnians and to "punish" the Serbs have come from political and religious leaders who either know little about the complex history of the region or are pressing their own agendas.

Some Ecumenical Evenhandedness

To be sure, some ecumenical spokesmen have tried to steer a more moderate course between Serb-bashing and a whitewash of Serbian atrocities. For example, the Vatican nuncio to Bosnia, Archbishop Francesco Monterisi, acknowledged in a candid February 1994 interview: "There are the Serbs who attack Sarajevo but also Moslems who attack Croatian villages of central Bosnia and finally the Croatian artillery that shoots at the Moslem-held eastern zone of Mostar." When Pope John Paul II called for "disarming the aggressor," Archbishop Monterisi explained, he meant the aggressors on all three sides.[155] The National Council of Churches has repeatedly urged the U.S. government to exercise prudence and restraint in responding to the Bosnian tragedy. A May 14, 1993, "Message of Church Leaders" orchestrated by the NCC specifically advised President Clinton and U.S. Secretary of State Warren Christopher "to assume a greater share of the burden" already carried by the United Nations Protection Force (UNPROFOR). This meant "the commitment by the United States of a significant contingent of peace-keeping forces to the UNPROFOR effort," but assuredly *not* the use of airstrikes or the lifting of the arms embargo throughout the former Yugoslavia.[156]

The World Council of Churches also has strained to be evenhanded, in part, no doubt, because of the historic role of the Serbian Orthodox Patriarchate in its deliberations. The WCC Central Committee issued a statement from its January 1994 meeting in Johannesburg, South Africa, that noted the lack of "objectivity" in much of the media coverage of "the tragic conflict"; expressed concern that the economic sanctions applied by the UN against Serbia and Montenegro alone "have caused widespread suffering to the civilian populations, whilst the flow of arms through the region continues unabated"; and rejected as counterproductive any additional armed intervention from outside Bosnia. "The situation is too complex," the WCC Central Committee concluded, "and the aggressors too numerous, for simple solutions to be sought bringing military force to bear on one or another side." At the same time, the Committee condemned "the manipulation of religious symbols and religious feelings for war aims"; called for protection of the human rights of everyone, including every minority group in the region; denounced "ethnic-cleansing" of territory by any nation or ethnic group against any other; and exhorted all Christians in the former Yugoslavia "to resist every attempt to use religious sentiment and loyalty in the service of aggressive nationalism."[157]

Patriarch Aleksii II of Moscow has extended his moral support to the embattled Serbs without, however, compromising his renewed post-Communist commitment to international peace and justice. On May 12, 1993, for example, Aleksii and the Holy Synod of the Moscow Patriarchate issued a statement that echoed the tone of the moderate ecumenical leaders. The statement admitted up front that the Russian Orthodox faithful "take to heart the sufferings of the Serbian people," since "[o]ur common Orthodox faith and the Slav blood, the closeness of our historical destinies cement our single-mindedness." But the Russians also "take the sufferings of any people as our own." Thus the Russian Church was grieved at the attempts to present the political conflict in the former Yugoslavia as "an inter-confessional and inter-religious one" and to "use religious feelings of people to aggravate military tension." Turning to the question of appropriate policy measures, Patriarch Aleksii and the Holy Synod appealed to all parties to the armed conflict "to put an immediate end to military action and work for a peaceful solution of current issues through mutual concessions." The Russian bishops, like the WCC Central Committee, categorically rejected any additional armed interventions, as well as the "unilateral economic blockade of any one party" to the conflict. Finally, they prudently urged the international community to avoid a "prejudiced approach to any side in the conflict," lest it result in "the creation of a morbid climate in the Balkans and thus hamper true reconciliation."[158]

Similarly, Patriarch Bartholomaios I of Constantinople has thrown the considerable weight of the premier see of world Orthodoxy behind the Serbian cause. In an interview with the Paris daily *Le Monde* published on April 20, 1994, the Ecumenical Patriarch categorically denied the existence of a political "axis" linking the Orthodox Churches based in Belgrade, Athens, and Moscow, and he upheld the honor of Patriarch Pavle as a spiritual leader who has not hesitated to distance himself and his Church from the regime in Belgrade. But, Bartholomaios also insisted,

Serbia should not be held solely responsible for the war in former Yugoslavia. Responsibility is shared by the Western powers who, for economic and political reasons, and religious reasons too, were too quick to recognise the independence of certain countries, thus promoting the break-up of Yugoslavia. Those western governments now accept that their eagerness was a mistake.[159]

The Untold Tale

If these evenhanded statements of non-Serbian Orthodox and non-Orthodox ecumenical leaders have failed to resonate with the media and governments in the West, perhaps it should come as no surprise that the efforts of the indefatigable Patriarch Pavle and the other Serbian Orthodox leaders to achieve a just peace in their homelands have been shamelessly under-reported and often ignored in the West. This frustrates and deeply pains Serbian-Americans and many of their fellow Orthodox Christians in the United States, and it surely accounts, in part, for the forcefulness of the collective Orthodox public moral witness concerning the civil war in the former Yugoslavia.

Few Americans, religious or otherwise, know that on May 27, 1992, the Holy Synod of the Serbian Orthodox Patriarchate in Belgrade issued a detailed memorandum that condemned *all* atrocities against civilians, whether Croat, Muslim, or Serbian; called for a new government to replace Slobodan Milosevic's neo-Communist regime in Belgrade; and appealed to the international community to investigate some half-dozen concentration camps in Croatia where Serbs were reportedly subject to human-rights abuses.[160] Fully two years later, those camps—and eighteen others cited by the Serbian Orthodox bishops in the United States on August 6, 1993—remain unexposed.[161]

Few Americans are aware of the eyewitness accounts of Bishop Atanasije Jevtic of Mostar, Hercegovina—now in forced exile—who tried in vain to testify on Capitol Hill in October 1992 that Croatian militia had destroyed fifteen Serbian Orthodox churches in his diocese. As we saw in chapter 4, a hearing arranged for him by Congresswoman Helen Delich Bentley in a conference room of the U.S. House of Representatives drew only six junior staffers barely out of college.

Few Americans know that Patriarch Pavle visited the United States in October 1992 on a good-will mission as spokesman for some ten million Serbian Orthodox faithful—a sizable constituency by any journalistic standard. This gentle, soft-spoken, deeply spiritual man, who like the elder Zossima in Dostoevsky's novel *The Brothers Karamazov* preaches repentance and forgiveness at every opportunity, has also led public protest marches in the streets of Belgrade against the Milosevic regime and its brutal execution of the war effort. But Pavle was apparently too moderate and reasonable to attract the attention of those in the American media who prefer the now familiar stereotype of the rowdy, rapacious Serb. Only a handful of journalists—none from the major news publications and broadcast media—showed up at a press conference in the National Press Building in Washington, D.C. Leaders of no other church or European religious community would be treated with such disdain.

Although the Western media have turned a collective deaf ear to this voice of Serbian Orthodox moderation in Belgrade, the Serbian bishops continue to cry aloud in the wilderness. In November 1993, a special assembly of bishops, evidently distressed by their inability to change international opinion, sounded a more apocalyptic note:

> For us and for our people, these are epic times and the hour of crucifixion on Golgotha. We are witnesses and participants in the suffering of an entire Christian nation, condemned by the domestic and foreign powers of this world. . . .
>
> How can the Serbs as an Orthodox Christian and European people, and especially how can their Church, acquiesce to the humiliation and extortion of the world powers and of one-sided propaganda and renounce their *holy land* of Kosovo and Metohija, where in the span of a hundred kilometers our people have 1,300 churches and monasteries, of which ten are at the pinnacle of the world's spiritual and cultural inheritance? How can the Serbian people renounce Zitomislic or Prebilovac in Hercegovina, monastery Tavna, Ozren, and the old church in Sarajevo in Bosnia, monasteries Pakra and Orahovica in Slavonia, Jasenovac and Glina in Krajina, or monasteries Krka, Krupa and Dragovic in Dalmatia? How can we, under pressure from the world powers, leave our cradles and graves, the holy places of our birth, our death, and our national resurrection? Are we really to become the trash heap of the world, the windblown Balkan stomping grounds of unscrupulous politicians, pacified on a reservation to which they have driven us? But we believe in God's eternal justice: His word is the last word both in history and in the world to come.[162]

The bishops specifically lamented those women, children, and elderly who were languishing in prison camps, exile, hospitals, and poor houses, often without adequate food and medicine because of "the sanctions imposed by the world powers."

In their November 1993 statement the bishops also provided a qualified justification for the conduct of Serbs who had taken up arms in the civil war: they were fighting "in defense of their homes and religious and national shrines." But the bishops hastened to point a critical finger at them also: "Certainly the Serbian people is not without its faults and sins, which they have demonstrated during this unfortunate time, most often in self-defense but also in attacks of madness by individuals and groups. We once again condemn their conduct and their evil deeds, as we have in the past. We call all such to repentance." In a beautifully phrased pastoral appeal, the bishops asked their own people

> to persevere in patience and Christ-like forgiveness, in generosity towards all people, but also to be critical—first of all of themselves, and then of their leaders and of the world's officials. Seek your civil and national rights, but in order to protect your freedom both internal and external, always according to the terms of Christian bravery: "It is better to lose one's head than to sin against your soul."[163]

When on April 10, 1994, NATO (actually U.S.) warplanes attacked Serbian armed forces near the besieged Bosnian city of Gorazde—the first time in history that a NATO contingent had engaged in combat —the war of words came to an abrupt and violent end for the Serbs and their Orthodox Church. Now the Western powers had shed Serbian blood in a cause that Orthodox Church leaders in Europe and the United States deemed tragically misguided at best.

A United Religious Front

Rising above their usual parochial proclivities, the Orthodox Churches in America have developed an unprecedented concord on this civil war. The ethnic preoccupations of the Serbian Orthodox Church as discussed in chapter 4 would lead us to expect the SOC to take a strong pro-Serbian stance. And indeed it has, but not without a measure of prophecy that lends moral balance. In their August 6, 1992, statement, for example, the SOC bishops expressed a firm and prayerful "desire for peace for all the suffering people throughout the tragic lands of the former Yugoslavia," while reserving their most fervent plea for their own people: "We call upon the United Nations, the United States, the Red Cross, and all other concerned bodies, to vigorously pursue human rights and justice for the suffering Serbian Orthodox people" throughout the former Yugoslavia.[164]

More recently, however, the SOC, echoing the mother Church in Serbia, has resorted to more apocalyptic, sometimes hyperbolic rhetoric. The September 1993 *sabor* sent a letter to President Clinton, Secretary of State Christopher, and each member of the U.S. Congress requesting an end to the economic sanctions against Serbia and Montenegro, which the delegates pronounced "unjust, a form of aggresssion and genocidal . . . [causing] an isolation of the whole nation, mostly affecting the children and the elderly, which is unparalleled in history."[165] Another letter to the White House expressed the outrage of Metropolitan Christopher and three other bishops at the April 10, 1994, bombing of Serbian armed forces by NATO warplanes. Ironically, the date marked the fifty-third anniversary of the establishment of the Croatian Ustasha regime that perpetrated such unprecedented horrors agains the Serbian nation and Church. The four bishops concluded their letter with the prayer that President Clinton would be granted the divine wisdom to act more charitably toward the Serbian people, "whose history, life, culture, and now very existence have been so callously ignored and threatened with extinction."[166]

The other Orthodox jurisdictions and organizations in the United States have issued less sobering statements on the civil war, but they all appear to have responded in advance to the clarion call of Bishop Maximos of the Greek Orthodox Diocese of Pittsburgh in October 1993: "The hour has come for Orthodoxy to show a united front not so much from a political point of view, but from a religious point of view."[167] The April 27, 1993, meeting of SCOBA generated a message to President Clinton, advising him to "avoid any use of military intervention" by the United States lest it lead to "a general conflagration in the Balkans." On May 17, SCOBA released another statement, an evenhanded denunciation of "all war crimes and the rapes committed by all three sides, Croatians, Bosnia Muslims, and Serbs."[168]

The bishops drafted and approved two more pronouncements at SCOBA's May 10, 1994, meeting.[169] A "Statement on the Civil War in Former Yugoslavia" reiterates their unequivocal condemnation of all carnage, crimes, and suffering in this war and calls for a "negotiated settlement" of the conflict, "taking into account the legitimate needs and aspirations of all the people involved." The statement also expresses "brotherly appreciation" of the bishops of the Serbian Orthodox Church for their unflagging pursuit of justice for all parties and their "practical humanitarian action." But this SCOBA statement delves more deeply than its predecessors into the political complexities of the case:

> This tragic conflict has roots which defy simplistic analysis. These include, we believe: the historical conditioning of the peoples of the area towards mutual mistrust by events as recent as the unresolved fascist crimes of World War II; the cynical manipulation of these fears and of nationalistic feelings by political leaders among all groups in an attempt to remain in power; the premature recognition of new states by the world powers without the support of all the inhabitants of those states and without other guarantees of basic human rights; and, as the Serbian Orthodox Church has repeatedly asserted, by the breakdown of basic moral conscience brought about by decades of atheistic rule.

The implicit criticism of the Western democracies, particularly the governments of the United States and Germany, under the rubric "world powers" marks a dramatic political turn by SCOBA: solidarity with the Serbian Orthodox people in a generally just cause now trumps public moral support for current U.S. foreign policy.

This shift in conventional allegiance is even clearer in SCOBA's 1994 statement on "the inhumane sanctions" imposed on Serbia and Montenegro by the U.N. Security Council since November 16, 1992. The bishops list the "disastrous and unavoidable results" of this economic embargo on "the innocent native inhabitants" of the region. They also contend that "similar stringent sanctions against Haiti and Iraq are immoral and inhumane for the same reasons." SCOBA prefers to view this issue of "foreign policy and politics . . . from the moral perspective first and foremost."

The Holy Synod of Bishops of the Orthodox Church in America issued an exemplary, albeit more subdued, statement on the civil war in Yugoslavia on May 26, 1993. The OCA bishops offered pastoral sympathy to all the suffering victims, while "referring to God's judgment" all who have committed atrocities, whether Serbs, Croats, or Muslims. They singled out for special denunciation "any form of 'ethnic cleansing'; the use of intimidation, torture, rape, and other unspeakable measures; the arbitrary targeting of innocent non-combatants, women, children, and the elderly; the creation of prison camps; and every other violation of basic rights." The OCA bishops also professed their solidarity with Patriarch Pavle and the Serbian Orthodox faithful in their opposition to the violence and bloodshed, specifically "the courageous stand" taken by Pavle together with Msgr. Vinko Puljic (the Roman Catholic Archbishop of Sarajevo) and Rais ul Ulama Jakub Selimoski (the Muslim leader of Bosnia-Hercegovina) at a November 1992 ecumenical meeting in Zurich, Switzerland, arranged by the Appeal of Conscience Foundation.[170]

The new pan-Orthodox humanitarian organization, International Orthodox Christian Charities (IOCC), also rushed to the rescue of the many thousands of suffering Serbs virtually abandoned by the Western democracies. Working through Belgrade, the IOCC has, since January 1993, channeled over $3 million in food and medical assistance through the Serbian Orthodox Patriarchate to the half-million displaced persons in areas of the former Yugoslavia under Serbian control. IOCC relief is able to pass through Serbian military lines, but it is not earmarked for Serbs alone. For example, a regular shipment of food is directed to a soup kitchen in Belgrade administered by the Muslim mufti. The WCC has designated the IOCC its "lead agency" for humanitarian aid operations in those sections of Bosnia accessible only from Serbia, and additional projects are envisioned between the IOCC and UNICEF and the World Food Program.[171] The IOCC and its thousands of supporters in the United States, including all the SCOBA bishops and jurisdictions, believe it is better to light the way in Yugoslavia through charity than merely to curse the darkness of the economic embargo against Serbia.

Pennsylvania Prelates Speak

The most detailed, cogent, forceful, and prophetic statement on the civil war to date, however, came from the four Orthodox bishops in western Pennsylvania on April 2, 1993. Their statement was a response to a declaration in February by Pittsburgh-area Roman Catholic, Protestant, Jewish, and Muslim leaders that purported to list "the full catalogue of atrocities carried out against the people of Bosnia" and called on the U.S. government to defend the Bosnians, as well as the Albanian majority in Kosovo.[172] Although this intemperate, grossly inaccurate, and politically prejudicial statement refrained from mentioning the Serbs by name, it was clear whom the ecumenical leaders had chosen to designate as the enemy of humanity in the former Yugoslavia. The Orthodox bishops in the area—Archbishop Kyrill Ionchev of the OCA, Bishop Maximos of the Greek Archdiocese, Bishop Mitrophan of the Serbian Eastern Diocese, and Bishop Nicholas Smisko of the Carpatho-Russian Diocese under the Ecumenical Patriarchate—decided to pick up this gauntlet.[173]

Claiming privileged communications from "reputable sources" in the former Yugoslavia and "objective information" from British and other monitors of events there, the four bishops express their disdain at the outset for "all those who are politically held hostage by the biased and one-sided reports presented by the American press." After that shot across the bow of the Serb-bashers in their midst, the bishops then steer a fine prophetic course, both condemning wartime atrocities by all sides —especially the "ethnic-cleansing," carnage, rapes, and suffering of innocent civilians—and defending a people and their Church against what they term "a propaganda effort to demonize the Serbs and incite American hatred and war-mongering against the Serbs."

The four Pennsylvania bishops address six key points.

1. *Alleged Serbian aggression.* The bishops confidently assert that neither in Bosnia nor in Croatia is the armed conflict the result of an international invasion; it is, rather, an ethnic civil war. The Serbian minorities in those new "republics"—who have lived on these lands for centuries—demand "the same right of self-determination that their ethnic neighbors are exercising with the blessing of the international community." The bishops thus cast their lot with their colleagues in the Serbian Orthodox Patriarchate who perceive a *justifiable cause* of Serbian involvement in the civil war in both Croatia and Bosnia in accordance with Orthodox moral tradition—namely, self-defense of the People of God.

2. *Memory of the genocide.* Invoking the Croatian Ustasha and Muslim SS atrocities during the Second World War, the four bishops instruct their ecumenical colleagues: "The power of these memories cannot be ignored when the future of the area is being decided." To many Americans and Western Europeans, the frequent invocation of this horrible collective memory may be little more than—to evoke a

distinctly American image from our own post–Civil War era—
"waving the bloody shirt." But the Orthodox bishops remind their
ecumenical counterparts that the "ethnic-cleansing" visited upon
Serbs in the Nazi era was "on a scale and with a brutality matched
only a few times in history, most notably against the Jews by the Nazis
and the Armenians by the Turks." To be sure, this tragic history does
not justify atrocities of any kind or revenge for any reason by Orthodox
Serbs, but it must be factored into any serious analysis of causation
and resolution of the civil war in the region.

3. *Croatian misdeeds.* Viewing the issue of justifiable cause from yet
another angle, the four bishops specify the reasons for Serbian unease
in the new Republic of Croatia, including discriminatory hiring practices, overt desecration and destruction of Serbian Orthodox churches,
the "ethnic-cleansing" of some 200 Serbian villages in the Slavonia
region, the revival of Ustasha symbols by the Tudjman government,
and continued stonewalling by the current Croatian regime on the
attempted genocide of the Serbs during the Second World War.

4. *Islamic fundamentalism.* Citing Alija Izetbegovic's dream of a
Muslim state in Bosnia (though inaccurately identifying an excerpt
from his 1970 work *Islamic Declaration* with a quotation of it in a 1992
issue of the *London Daily Telegraph*), the four Orthodox bishops warn
that Christians and other non-Muslims have ample cause to fear being
relegated to "second-class status" in a fundamentalist Muslim Bosnian
state. (If Izetbegovic's more recent disavowals of plans to establish an
Islamic state are sincere, this concern may be misplaced. But expecting
Bosnian Serbs to trust Izetbegovic's commitment to a secular multiethnic Bosnia—especially in the wake of the current civil war—may
be like asking them to buy a pig in a poke.)

5. *Artificial territorial boundaries.* The bishops insist that the present
boundaries of the Croatian and Bosnian states "are artificial and do not
reflect the realities of ethnicity or history." Rather, the territories of these
internal Yugoslav "republics" were gerrymandered by the Communist
central government of Josip Broz Tito to weaken the Serbian minority
and thus dampen its potential threat to the Communist regime. Further,
there is no "Bosnian" ethnicity or nation per se—the term is merely a
toponym—and the Croatian minority in Bosnia "is well on its way
towards uniting with Zagreb in a 'Greater Croatia,' with surprisingly
little outcry from the international community, which is so quick to

condemn the Serbian desire for self-determination." In short, the present borders are not set in concrete, and a just resolution of the civil war will require some adjustments, notwithstanding the international recognition of the republics of Croatia and Bosnia "as is."

6. *Right of self-determination.* Returning to this theme adduced earlier, the bishops insist that the Serbian minorities in Croatia and Bosnia have asked for nothing more than the Croats and Bosnian Muslims demanded when they seceded from Yugoslavia. The bishops see the issue, then, as one of simple fairness and political consistency. The Serbs' intent is to establish their own sovereignty (whether independent of or in union with Serbia proper is their choice) in "territories where Serbs are the clear majority." The four Orthodox bishops have thus grounded their argument in a secular version of what we identified in chapter 1 as the *spiritual intent* required for a war to be deemed justifiable according to Orthodox moral tradition. In light of the atrocious conduct of the Serbian factions in the civil war, Orthodox spokesmen on both sides of the Atlantic would have been better advised to stick with the traditional Orthodox standard for proper intent: continually regarding one's enemy as an errant child of God to be resisted instead of viciously punished or "ethnically cleansed" can serve as a powerful spiritual deterrent to war crimes.

Also missing from the Pennsylvania bishops' analysis of the civil war is any discussion of the moral legitimacy of the political leadership of the Serbian communities in Croatia, Bosnia, or Serbia proper. It is doubtful, at best, whether Slobodan Milosevic in Belgrade and Radovan Karadzic in Bosnia, despite their tacit support for the Serbian Orthodox Church, provide a *proper political ethos,* or warrant the loyalty of Serbs willing to risk their lives in mortal combat.

The four Pennsylvania bishops also propose several prudential prescriptions to resolve the conflict justly:

1. "Redrawn borders" in closer conformity to the actual ethnic composition of the region.

2. "Guarantees of full cultural and civil rights" for all minority groups in each successor state.

3. "Reparations and safe passage for anyone who wishes to resettle in other areas after new borders are drawn."

4. International inspection of all detention camps in the region, including those run by the Bosnian and Croatian governments.

5. An "even-handed war crimes tribunal" that would not try Serbs alone.

6. No "use of force by outside third parties with the aim of imposing a political solution."

7. Lifting of the UN sanctions against Serbia in favor of negotiations.

Some of these proposals may resonate well with the views of Western governments. Unfortunately, number six is already moot in view of the April 10, 1994, NATO bombing of Serbian artillery.

The four Orthodox bishops punctuate their extraordinary statement with an aggressive defense of Orthodox honor and dignity: "We protest the implicit or explicit characterization of the Serbian people and Orthodox Christian faith as backward, barbaric, uncivilized, or anti-Western. Such characterizations are racist, inflammatory, and inherently false, and betray a communistic and anti-Orthodox bias." The bizarre red-baiting aside, this unusually strident declaration, and indeed the entire document, serves notice to America that a sleeping moral giant has finally awakened.

The civil war in the former Yugoslavia, especially the popular mistreatment of the Serbs and their cause, has galvanized the four million Orthodox Christians in this country like no other single issue in the recent past. The Orthodox in America have closed ranks behind their co-religionists in their national struggle for communal survival. Neither lacking in self-criticism nor Pollyannish in their pursuit of a just peace in war-torn lands of the former Yugoslavia, the American Orthodox leaders and the Serbian, Moscow, and Ecumenical Patriarchates have nevertheless decided to stand together against world opinion, even if it is reinforced by the international military might of NATO and the United Nations.

But it is not yet, for the Orthodox, their finest prophetic hour. That will come when, God willing, a permanent ceasefire descends upon the benighted lands of the former Yugoslavia and the task of rebuilding these countries begins. The Orthodox will be called upon to demonstrate both forgiveness and repentance for the wartime atrocities inflicted upon and committed by the Serbian people. Whether the Orthodox Churches rise to the occasion and witness as forcefully and prophetically then as they have done so far will be the greatest test of their moral character.

THE PRICE OF PROPHECY

The contradictory resolutions of the Greek Orthodox Archdiocese on the Vietnam War illustrate one of the twin dangers of the contemporary Orthodox public moral witness on issues of conventional war and national security: the slide into moral relativism, or at least moral insignificance. These resolutions suggest a disturbing zeal on the part of the delegates to adjust Orthodox moral teaching to current political sentiment. What was the position of the Greek Orthodox Archdiocese on the Vietnam War? The answer depends, unfortunately, on who represented the archdiocese at any given time. Such a slippery situation hardly conforms to the self-understanding of the Orthodox Church as the universal, essentially unchanging Church of Jesus Christ. Further, the flip-flops of the Greek Archdiocese and the conflicting views of other Orthodox hierarchs in America beg the question as to whether such changing Church pronouncements have any enduring moral value or even social relevance.

The more recent record of pronouncements on U.S. involvement in the Persian Gulf War only aggravates this problem. The self-conscious aspiration of American Orthodox bishops and other Christian leaders to genuine prophecy notwithstanding, the mostly NCC-inspired statements will probably be remembered only for their numerous empirical errors, hysterical predictions, political flavor, and wrong-headed moral judgments. Never before had so many prominent Orthodox and other religious leaders wasted their potential influence on U.S. government officials by consistently warning of terrible consequences that fortunately never came to pass. If this sorry episode fails to convince the leaders of the several Orthodox member-jurisdictions that the NCC's effect on them is corrosive, perhaps nothing will.

The other danger in the Orthodox public moral witness on issues of conventional war and national security is the tendency of the Orthodox communities to form political and moral liaisons with their governments.

A creeping militarism is evidenced by Russian and Romanian bishops and priests bedecked with military combat medals on their cassocks, the routine violation of the historic canons that attempt to separate the clergy from all forms of violence past or present, the celebration of the military exploits and combat heroism of Orthodox clergy in the former Soviet Union, and the intemperate language of hierarchs who demonize national or ethnic "enemies," revealing thereby a distorted spiritual intent in their advocacy of military actions.

Moreover, the advocacy of "peace" by the several national Orthodox leaderships is, despite its fervor, often of questionable provenance. Proclamations of support for peace appear to be innocuous platitudes when, with a few notable exceptions, they are really curious alloys of "peace" and some corrosive impurity such as patriotism, socialism, or the foreign-policy agenda of a particular government. The intervention of the Russian Orthodox Church in the superpower rivalry between the Soviet Union and Communist China, particularly the local Chinese-Vietnamese war that followed U.S. withdrawal from the region, was hardly mandated by the Orthodox justifiable-war ethic. This gratuitous public moral witness, together with the earlier, shriller anti-U.S. pronouncements, betrayed the real political goal of the Patriarchate's involvement in the wars in Southeast Asia.

The glorification of past military exploits poses a third disturbing problem. To be sure, this practice may represent a reasonable moral position based on understandable pride in a common national or ethnic heritage. But this pride too often partakes of an extreme nationalism. The glorification of events in the predominantly Orthodox Christian history of Russia or Romania papers over the discontinuities with the anti-Christian regimes of the past seven or four decades, respectively, and perhaps even the current post-Communist societies. In particular, it serves to obscure the qualitative differences in the political, cultural, and moral character of successive regimes. The Soviet Union was by no stretch of the imagination "Holy Russia." Nor was Communist Romania, especially under the late Nicolae Ceauşescu, a legitimate heir to the pre–World War II Romanian Orthodox nation-state. Even the secular, pluralistic United States may not meet the traditional Orthodox standard of a society with a proper spiritual ethos—one of the criteria of the Orthodox justifiable-war ethic. And yet Orthodox leaders in each of these countries have often provided unqualified, uncritical, and unprophetic public support for the military activities of their nations.

This nationalism reaches extreme proportions when it drives Orthodox leaders into the "holy war" camp, which has no grounding in the Orthodox moral tradition concerning war and peace. Sometimes the rhetoric of the bishops and church councils is racist or xenophobic, as epitomized by the anti-German sentiment of Metropolitan Nikolai of Kiev during the Second World War. Sometimes Orthodox leaders, even in the United States, get carried away by an excessively mystical identification of the People of God with the pagan pre-Christian or post-Christian nation of their ancestry. Sometimes this distracting, debilitating nationalism results in mere silliness, such as the tendency of some Romanian Orthodox clergy to paint an obviously distorted, self-serving picture of Romania's collective innocence in all the military engagements in its national history.

There are laudable instances of genuine prophecy in this tangle of peace and propaganda. Patriarch Justinian and the Romanian Orthodox Church officially condemned the Soviet invasion of Czechoslovakia in 1968. The 1983 OCA All-American Council criticized the World Council of Churches for its ideologically unbalanced record on conventional wars. The Greek Orthodox clergy-laity congresses from 1966 to 1972 testify, despite the self-contradictory product of their deliberations, to a genuine soul-searching on the issue of U.S. military involvement in Vietnam. Similarly, the pattern of opposition to all U.S. policy initiatives in the Persian Gulf War reflects a self-consciously "prophetic" stance of American Orthodox spokesmen — even if events eventually proved them wrong on almost every count. Finally, the unprecedented pan-Orthodox support for the dignity of the Serbian people and their Church in the midst of a return to ethnic barbarism in post-Communist Yugoslavia demonstrates the perennial applicability of St. Augustine's insight: *"O felix culpa"* — O happy fault: because of sin, grace abounds all the more!

But these isolated prophetic moments do not, unfortunately, indicate that the Orthodox Churches in the former Soviet Union, Romania, and the United States are generally willing to pay the full price of prophecy in their public moral witness on issues of conventional war and national security. It remains to be seen whether the united Orthodox front on the civil war in the former Yugoslavia represents a coincidence of moral courage or a genuine turning point.

6

Peace and Security: Nuclear

President George Bush surprised the world on September 27, 1991, ordering massive unilateral reductions in U.S. strategic (i.e., intercontinental) and tactical (i.e., battlefield-level) nuclear arms. For a start, U.S. strategic bombers were immediately taken off alert status and their nuclear weapons placed in storage. The president announced that the entire arsenal of tactical nuclear warheads would be withdrawn from Europe and elsewhere and subsequently destroyed; that all nuclear warheads would be removed from U.S. naval vessels; and that the numbers of long-range missiles in silos and on submarines would be reduced ahead of the schedules established by the first Strategic Arms Reduction Treaty (START I).[1]

This American initiative spurred a quick response from Moscow. Eight days later, on October 5, Mikhail Gorbachev announced a matching downgrading of the alert status of the Soviet strategic bomber force; removal and destruction or stockpiling of all tactical nuclear warheads; removal and partial destruction of all nuclear-tipped antiaircraft missiles; a freeze on the number and location of compact mobile Intercontinental Ballistic Missiles (ICBMs); removal of 503 ICBMs from alert status and the elimination of 1,000 more strategic weapons than the number required by the START I treaty; a personnel cut of 700,000 in the Soviet armed forces; and the suspension of nuclear tests for one year.[2]

These developments, which would have seemed impossible just a few years before, seemed to move the world a giant step in the direction of international peace and security. But the virtue of prudence—a cautious exercise of good judgment, especially to anticipate

277

the likely consequences of one's decisions—must not be forgotten. Tens of thousands of strategic nuclear weapons still remain in silos, submarines, and bomber-aircraft controlled by the United States and by four of the successor states to the former Soviet Union: Russia, Ukraine, Belarus (formerly known as Byelorussia), and Kazakhstan. Despite an announcement in Moscow on May 30, 1994, that Russian missiles were no longer trained on targets in the West, and a similar announcement the next day by the Pentagon that U.S. and British land- and sea-based nuclear missiles had been retargeted, these new computer programs are just as easily reversible.[3] Washington and Moscow—and now Kyyiv—have said they intend to disarm most, if not all, of their tactical nuclear warheads, but thousands of these weapons of mass destruction are still deployed on land and sea and in the air in Europe.

Particularly unsettling in this regard is the statement of official Russian military doctrine released in November 1993. The revised doctrine revokes the old Soviet pledge of "no first use" of nuclear weapons: Russia may now use such weapons defensively against a nuclear attack or even against a conventional-weapons attack by a non-nuclear state allied to a nuclear power.[4] Despite early pledges of mutual cooperation by Russia and Ukraine and the Ukrainian parliament's belated ratification of START I, Moscow and Kyyiv have not yet divided the nuclear-armed Black Sea naval fleet, and the final disposition of Soviet nuclear warheads in Ukraine hangs in the balance. As long as (1) these deadly devices remain poised for battle, (2) other nations are also capable of producing them, and (3), as FBI director Louis J. Freeh warned the U.S. Senate on May 25, 1994, organized crime in Russia might be able to steal such weapons from their national arsenal and sell them to deadly anti-U.S. terrorists, the moral issues pertaining to nuclear defense must still concern us.[5]

DETERRENCE AND DEFENSE

A fundamental issue in the nuclear era is whether this era is unique. Does the use of nuclear energy in weapons of mass destruction represent a quantum leap in the evolution of modern warfare that could threaten the very existence of human life on the planet?

Virtually all advocates of nuclear deterrence would agree that its primary objective is to prevent a nuclear exchange that could trigger a nuclear holocaust. Prevention of nuclear violence is the salient characteristic of all strategies of "deterrence"; it is also a universal prudential and moral duty that should engage religious leaders as much as defense strategists and policymakers. What has been at issue is the best *means* to achieve this common end of preventing nuclear violence.

If nuclear "deterrence" entails, as Robert J. Art says it does, "the threat of retaliation" in order "to prevent an adversary from doing something that one does not want him to do and that he might otherwise be tempted to do,"[6] a nation need only acquire a *sufficient* military arsenal at the strategic, or intercontinental, level. Sufficiency of strategic power, both nuclear and non-nuclear, would be that which, as Michael Howard observes, does not promise to one's own side the chimera of nuclear "victory" but rather guarantees the capacity to deny the adversary any chance for a *meaningful* victory: "to set on victory for our opponent a price that he cannot possibly afford to pay."[7] One might call this the price of imprudence.

The necessary positive complement of this negative quality of deterrence may be furnished by "reassurance." Howard argues that the object of reassurance is "to persuade one's own people, and those of one's allies, that the benefits of military action, or preparation for it, will outweigh the costs."[8] The strategic alternative that offers the most realistic hope of meeting this combined negative-positive goal is likely to emerge as the dominant nuclear-defense strategy in each generation. Whether that dominant strategy is also the most *moral* choice is another question, one that the Churches, more than any other segment of society, are obligated to address.

Two "schools" of deterrence have offered conflicting answers to the question whether the invention of nuclear weapons has essentially changed the recourse to and conduct of war. Bernard Brodie and William Borden set the standards for subsequent generations of nuclear-defense theorists in their signal works on this subject, both published in 1946. Brodie boldly declared that he was "not for the moment concerned about who will *win* the next war in which atomic bombs are used. Thus far the chief purpose of our military establishment has been to win wars. From now on its chief purpose must be to avert them. It can have almost no other useful purpose."[9] Borden argued that the new weapon was an avenue to "a return to eighteenth century warfare and the classical principles of Karl Von Clausewitz, because once again the key to victory lies in defeating hostile military forces."[10]

More recently, Charles-Philippe David pursued the trajectories emanating from these opposing premises and derived a useful typology.[11] What he called the "apocalyptic approach" had eight underlying convictions:

1. Nuclear weapons represent, à la Brodie, a radical revolution in the historical evolution of warfare.

2. Any use of nuclear weapons, however "limited," probably would escalate to a "general war."

3. There is no point in planning for supposedly limited nuclear wars or restricting targeting to military objectives, which cannot, in any event, be isolated from population centers.

4. No technologically feasible defense against nuclear attack is possible.

5. Superiority in numbers of nuclear weapons is irrelevant.

6. The Soviets share this view of nuclear war as unthinkable and mutually devastating.

7. Soviet/Warsaw Pact aggression against nations of the North Atlantic Treaty Organization (NATO) in Europe may be deterred by conventional forces and the uncertainty of a possible nuclear response.

8. Only through the deterrence of "assured destruction" and arms-control agreements may nuclear war be prevented.

What David labeled the "conventional approach" had also eight underlying principles, the mirror opposites of the "apocalyptic" convictions:

1. Nuclear weapons represent, à la Borden, merely another step in the continuing development of military technology, one that provides an opportunity for reviving the classic features of warfare against military targets (known as "counterforce" targeting).

2. The use of nuclear weapons in combat may be subject to rational restraint.

3. The superpowers ought to plan for "limited" nuclear wars.

4. The population, industrial base, and military force of a nation may be safeguarded through strategic defensive measures.

5. A goal of nuclear superiority is not only feasible but also politically significant.

6. The Soviets have never subscribed to the concept of "mutual assured destruction" (or MAD), believing instead that they can initiate and win a nuclear war.

7. Soviet/Warsaw Pact aggression against NATO-Europe may be deterred by the perception of the enemy that the West certainly will use its tactical nuclear arsenal in keeping with concrete contingency plans.

8. Nuclear conflict is conceivable, so the United States ought therefore to develop strategic policies that will contribute to victory over the Soviets in any nuclear exchange.

We shall call these two classic approaches to nuclear deterrence the *apocalyptic* and *continuity* schools, to avoid confusion with the established use of "conventional" to mean non-nuclear warfare. Neither school has ever promised much of a future. If the continuity theorists appear preoccupied with a callous calculus of human carnage—"collateral damage" in the technical jargon—in pursuit of military objectives, the apocalypticists seem prepared to sacrifice too readily the moral goods of human freedom and dignity on the altar of sheer survival.

In response to this kind of moral and poltical unease, President Ronald Reagan introduced what has developed into a third "school" of deterrence, which may be called the *fortress* approach. In March 1983, he announced a new defensive orientation later dubbed the "Strategic Defense Initiative" by the administration and "Star Wars" by the press. Because of the massive cuts in the U.S. defense budget following the end of the Cold War, SDI research and development— to say nothing of the testing, production, and deployment of any functional systems—now suffers from severe underfunding. Under siege in the U.S. Congress, the *fortress* approach to nuclear deterrence may never have a fighting chance to emerge as a practical alternative to the *apocalyptic* and *continuity* schools.

THE PEACE-AND-DISARMAMENT CAMPAIGN

In his report to an inter-religious conference on "nuclear catastrophe" held in Moscow in June 1982, Metropolitan Filaret of Minsk reminded the delegates that the Soviet Union had "launched in the postwar period a total of more than 130 peace proposals aimed at curbing the arms race, creating a climate of trust and détente, and at averting the threat of nuclear war." The Soviet "Peace Programme" was a continual "source of inspiration for all peace champions," Filaret said.[12]

This boast was remarkable in that it revealed the true source of the extraordinary energy expended by the Moscow Patriarchate—and its loyal ally, the Romanian Orthodox Patriarchate—in the "peace and disarmament" campaign. These two Orthodox Churches took their cues from the foreign policies of their governments. Each Soviet or Romanian Communist "initiative" routinely received the full support of the country's Orthodox Church, and the Orthodox hierarchies reflexively denounced any U.S. initiative. Thus the public moral witness of both Patriarchates on issues of nuclear defense has—until the present—been consistently reactive rather than proactive.

Evolution of a Movement

The Moscow Patriarchate launched its anti-nuclear crusade in March 1950 with its support of the Stockholm Appeal to Ban Atomic Weapons. This document, which garnered half a million signatories, originated with the World Peace Congress, a Soviet front organization and precursor of the World Peace Council. The Soviets had successfully detonated their first atomic bomb half a year earlier, but they still lacked the quantity of warheads and the effective means of delivery they needed to offer any serious threat to the United States, which at that time had a virtual monopoly in nuclear power.

The Russian Orthodox Church hosted its first inter-religious conference in May 1952 at Trinity–St. Sergius Monastery in Zagorsk. This event was actually convened by Patriarch Georg VI of the Armenian Orthodox Church in the Soviet Union. Patriarch Aleksii I of Moscow subsequently invited the leaders of all the religious communities in the Soviet Union—Christian, Buddhist, Muslim, and Jewish. Among the seventy-four delegates were distinguished foreigners such as Patriarch Justinian of Romania and Archimandrite Maksim, the future patriarch of the Bulgarian Orthodox Church. The ideological flavor of this conference was evident in the claim made by

Metropolitan Nikolai of Krutitsy and Kolomna, who chaired the pre-
paratory commission, that the threat of a global war was due to the
desire of the ruling circles of the capitalist states "to subjugate to
themselves and to their way of life all nations, the whole world."13

The second inter-religious conference was convened by Patriarch
Aleksii I, also at the Trinity–St. Sergius Monastery, in July 1969. This
time 175 representatives of religious communities in the Soviet Union
attended as well as prominent religious personages from forty-four
countries.

By June 1977 the Patriarchate's peace-and-disarmament movement
had achieved international stature. Patriarch Pimen invited representatives from 107 countries to a conference in Moscow called "Religious Workers for Lasting Peace, Disarmament and Just Relations
Among Nations." The participants entrusted the implementation of
their pronouncement to a "Working Presidium" chaired by
Metropolitan Yuvenaly of Krutitsy and Kolomna. In May 1978, that
body issued an appeal to a special session on disarmament of the
United Nations General Assembly. The Working Presidium recommended that all states recognize disarmament as their "pre-eminent
task"; that "the production of nuclear armaments be stopped
completely by all states"; that "the development and production of
new types and systems of mass-destructive weapons" and "nuclear
tests of any type" be "prohibited"; that the proliferation of nuclear
weapons be prevented and all nations sign the Non-Proliferation
Treaty; that the stockpiles of all "nuclear, atomic and thermonuclear
weapons" be "destroyed"; and that "nuclear-free zones" be declared
"in certain areas of the world."14 By then the Soviet Union had not
only caught up with but surpassed the U.S. nuclear arsenal. This
agenda (except for the unrealistic call for the destruction of all nuclear
weapons), if enacted, would have locked into place a decisive Soviet
advantage over the United States in numbers and types of nuclear
warheads.

In March 1979, the Moscow Patriarchate achieved a significant
international ecumenical milestone with the "Choose Life" statement
issued jointly by the churches in the Soviet Union and the National
Council of Churches of the United States. Bilateral contacts between
the Patriarchate and the NCC began during the first years of the Cold
War. The first fraternal exchanges of delegations occurred in 1956,

and reciprocal visits were repeated in 1962-63 and 1974-75. The "Choose Life" statement committed both ecclesial entities to an apocalyptic position on the nuclear-arms race. The delegations declared "with one voice—NO! in the Name of God—NO!" to the arms race. Citing St. Paul's declaration of war in Ephesians 6:12 against demonic "principalities" and "powers," the two delegations "confessed that seeking our security through arms is in fact a false and idolatrous hope and that true security can be found only in [a] relationship of trust."

The "Choose Life" statement pledged support for several nuclear-defense policies, including the second series of Strategic Arms Limitation Talks (SALT II—the U.S. Senate refused to ratify the treaty after the Soviet invasion of Afghanistan in December 1979). The statement also called for a "full and general prohibition" against testing, development, deployment, and stockpiling of additional nuclear or chemical arms. Participants from the Moscow Patriarchate included Metropolitan Yuvenaly, Archbishop Kirill of Vyborg, who was rector of the Leningrad Theological Academy (he is currently Metropolitan Kirill of Smolensk), Archpriest Vitaly Borovoi, Aleksii Buevsky, secretary of the Department of External Church Relations, and Aleksii Osipov of the Moscow Theological Academy.[15]

The CPC and the WCC

Two ecumenical organizations, the Christian Peace Conference and the World Council of Churches, were apparently quite receptive to the Patriarchate's party line on nuclear weapons. For example, the CPC's Fifth All-Christian Peace Assembly in Prague in June 1978 issued a resolution on security and another on disarmament. The resolution on security posited the principle of "equal security for all nations"; deemed national and international security "inseparable" and hence supported a Soviet proposal to conclude a world treaty renouncing the use of force by all countries; proposed a moratorium on the production and stockpiling of nuclear weapons, especially the "neutron bomb," which at that time only the United States had developed; supported the Warsaw Pact's proposal of a treaty renouncing "first use" of nuclear weapons in combat—a policy that would have been, at that time, contrary to NATO's strategy of nuclear deterrence; and urged the creation of nuclear-free zones and the successful conclusion of the SALT II talks.[16]

Subsequent actions by the CPC continued to support Soviet policy. In March 1981, for example, Metropolitan Filaret of Kiev signed a letter from the CPC Working Committee to Leonid Brezhnev that expressed the committee's "high opinion" of the Soviet leader's "frankness" and desire to achieve peaceful agreements with the West, while scoring the United States for "the tough line" it was pursuing in its negotiations with the Soviet Union.[17] Two years later, the "enlarged presidential board" of the CPC appealed to world leaders "to freeze all nuclear arsenals and stocks of delivery systems at their present level"—the position of the Soviet Union and various "peace" organizations in the United States and Western Europe, in direct opposition to the position of the Reagan administration. The CPC also requested that the United States "abandon its limited nuclear war strategy which is an affront to human dignity."[18] By July 1985 the CPC had joined the chorus of those who vehemently opposed what they called "the militarization of outer space"—a reference to the Reagan administration's Strategic Defense Initiative.[19] Thus the CPC, with crucial input from the Moscow Patriarchate, was on record opposing every major initiative by the United States to modernize its nuclear arsenal or enhance its deterrent capability against the quantitatively superior Soviet arsenal.

The Moscow Patriarchate disproportionately influenced the highly selective "anti-nuclear" perspective of the World Council of Churches. It was probably no coincidence that as early as March 1962, one year after the Moscow Patriarchate and other Soviet-bloc Orthodox Churches joined the WCC, the WCC Executive Committee urged the leading nations of the world to discontinue or refrain from testing nuclear weapons and to agree on a reliable regime of verification. The *Journal of the Moscow Patriarchate* lauded the WCC in 1986 for the "extremely active and creative" participation of its representatives in the 1973 World Congress of Peace Forces in Moscow, the 1977 World Conference in Moscow, and other peace-and-disarmament gatherings.[20]

The WCC could easily return the compliment to the Patriarchate. In August 1980, for example, the WCC Central Committee issued a one-sided pronouncement on the increase in Soviet-American tension "heightened by the NATO decision to base new missiles possessing counterforce qualities and exceptional accuracy." This referred to the U.S. decision to deploy 108 Pershing and 464 cruise missiles in Western Europe to counteract the previous deployment of hundreds of intermediate-range Soviet SS-20 missiles. In an earlier draft, this reference to "the NATO decision" was balanced somewhat by an observation that both the United States and the Soviet Union "seem to be ready to apply a nuclear warfighting strategy."[21] But the WCC Central Committee abandoned even this modest nonpartisanship and substituted language suggesting that only the United States and NATO were devising strategies for "limited nuclear war." The change in text was due to the persuasive skills of the Moscow Patriarchate's Aleksii Buevsky.[22]

Another milestone in the Moscow Patriarchate's peace-and-disarmament campaign was the 1982 World Conference called "Religious Workers for Saving the Sacred Gift of Life from Nuclear Catastrophe." This Moscow conference drew 590 inter-religious delegates from some ninety countries, who, according to the *Journal of the Moscow Patriarchate,* summarily "condemned the doctrine of a limited nuclear war and other similar plans as madness, as bordering on possession by the Devil."[23] In his address, Patriarch Pimen did not hesitate to reduce the complexities of this theory of nuclear deterrence (which we have labeled the *continuity* school) to simplistic slogans. Having asked whether a local nuclear war could be "confined to some fixed regional limits," he answered with a confident statement of the *apocalyptic* point of view:

> Of course, it cannot. Because even those regions of the world which escape direct nuclear strikes, would all the same be affected by radioactive fallout, by global disruptions of economic links, by irreversible ecological changes, by the consequences of genetic changes, by some unpredictable seismic phenomena and so on.[24]

Having virtually consecrated one of the conflicting theories of nuclear deterrence, the patriarch went on to caricature U.S. nuclear-defense policy. He criticized as irresponsible the "mounting chorus of voices in support of the doctrine of a nuclear first strike," as if American policymakers were scheming to score, out of nowhere, a massive knockout blow against the Soviets.[25] The U.S./NATO policy in force at that time simply reserved the right to resort to tactical nuclear weapons in response to a large-scale Soviet/Warsaw Pact invasion of Western Europe: if that meant U.S./NATO might be the first side to use nuclear weapons, then so be it.

New Fronts in the 1980s

In 1983 the Moscow Patriarchate opened several new fronts in its campaign for nuclear disarmament—by, that is, the United States and NATO. Patriarch Pimen dispatched an intemperate open letter to President Reagan in March that responded to the U.S. president's famous description of the Soviet Union as "an evil empire." Pimen railed against Reagan's "sinful" belligerence and his hostility against the Soviets, questioning his profession of Christian values, before concluding with a pitch for "a freeze of nuclear weapons before it is too late."[26]

A month later, representatives of the Patriarchate and Pax Christi International—a pacifist Roman Catholic organization—met in Antwerp, Belgium, for their fifth round of "conversations." Patriarch Pimen's apocalypticism was on display: "One irresponsible decision or an accidental mistake may result in the destruction of all God's creation in a nuclear conflagration."[27]

A fortnight later, a delegation from the Russian Orthodox Church traveled to Uppsala, Sweden, for the Christian World Conference on Life and Peace. The representatives included Metropolitan Aleksii of Tallinn and Estonia, Metropolitan Filaret of Minsk and Byelorussia, Archpriest Vitaly Borovoi, Aleksii Buevsky, and a newcomer, Bishop Sergii of Solnechnogorsk. "Most" of the conference participants (but apparently not all, surprisingly) concluded that "the possession of nuclear weapons is inconsistent with our faith in God." All agreed on the concept of "common security" as an alternative to the classic pursuit by nations of collective security, or "security through strength."[28] This new (albeit neo-Kantian) internationalist notion, increasingly popular among the European left, would have nations explicitly forgo military superiority in favor of checks and balances presumably enforced by a supra-national entity. Patriarch Pimen had already in 1982 lodged his objections to "the false understanding of national security" based on "narrow national interests" and "the force of arms" instead of "the common interests and security of the whole of mankind."[29]

Hiroshima, Japan, provided the setting in August for yet another peace-and-disarmament venture by the Moscow Patriarchate. The 1983 World Conference Against Atomic and Hydrogen Bombs was an occasion for a considerable amount of U.S.-bashing. While commemorating the victims of the atomic bombing of Hiroshima and Nagasaki by the United States during the Second World War, Patriarch Pimen could not resist taking a swipe at "reactionary circles in the USA and in a number of West European countries" intent on devising "ever new systems and types of weapons of mass destruction."[30]

Finally, in March 1983, the Patriarchate convened in Moscow the first annual international inter-religious "Roundtable Conference" of theologians and scientific experts on nuclear war. The topic that year was the so-called nuclear-arms freeze, which the delegates saw as the "foremost step on the road to detente." They examined this policy proposal from every conceivable angle. Among the Orthodox participants, for example, Metropolitan Antonie of Transylvania spoke about the related moral and economic aspects of a freeze. Aleksii Buevsky of the Moscow Patriarchate emphasized the feasibility of a freeze in light of the wide support for it throughout the world. Archpriest Nikolai Shivarov, rector of the Orthodox Theological Academy in Sofia, Bulgaria, explored the prospects of the conversion from military-oriented to civilian-oriented economic production that a nuclear-arms freeze presumably would permit.[31]

Each subsequent Roundtable Conference also focused on one theme—at variance with the stated policy of the U.S. government. The 1984 conference dwelled on what Metropolitan Filaret of Minsk termed the "catastrophic consequences for all mankind of the militarization of outer space"—that is, President Reagan's SDI.[32] (This component of the Moscow Patriarchate's peace-and-disarmament campaign will be examined later.)

The 1985 Roundtable Conference introduced the latest pseudo-scientific *cause célèbre:* "nuclear winter." The delegates heard one speaker after another cite as scientific fact the speculations of scientists such as Carl Sagan of Cornell University concerning the atmospheric and ecological damage to be expected from the detonation of as few as 500 nuclear warheads out of the roughly 40,000 to 50,000 in the combined arsenals of the United States and the Soviet Union. Not one dissenting or merely skeptical scientist or theologian spoke at this conference.[33]

The 1986 Roundtable Conference forged new links between the nuclear-arms race and the problems of hunger and poverty. Its unsophisticated "zero-sum" approach to deterrence and economics posited a direct relation between military spending by nations and the impoverishment of parts of the world. One of the working groups at this conference also urged the establishment of "a new moral order," indeed a "moral revolution — one that helps people to shed outdated, self-centered, narrowly nationalistic views" in favor of "the vision of humanity as a single worldwide family" whose unity would be expressed through "mutual trust and care and by just socio-economic and political-cultural relations" among the nations.[34] However grandiose this global perspective might have appeared, such a blanket rejection of nationalism and invocation of trust defied the canons of realism in international relations.

The 1987 Roundtable Conference returned to the "disastrous" concept of strategic defense. That subject had also arisen at an international anti-nuclear forum in Moscow the previous month, chaired by Metropolitan Yuvenaly of Krutitsky and Kolomna. At the Roundtable, 215 religious leaders from fifty-six countries heard the usual pro-Soviet speeches replete with attacks on the supposedly bellicose intentions of the United States. In his summary of the proceedings, Metropolitan Paulos Mar Gregorios, a bishop of the Syrian Orthodox Church in India (an Oriental Orthodox communion), reported that the assembled delegates insisted that "outer space and the high seas . . . be kept free from all weapons, including nuclear, laser, particle beam or other devices."[35]

While it was business as usual in the religious sector of the peace-and-disarmament campaign, genuine progress was occurring in the political realm. On December 7, 1987, President Ronald Reagan and Mikhail Gorbachev signed what has become known as the "INF [Intermediate-range Nuclear Forces] Treaty" — the first genuine mutual elimination, instead of mere numerical limitation, of an entire class of nuclear weapons. The treaty committed the signatories to eliminate all intermediate-range missiles (that is, those with a range of 300 to 3,000 miles), together with their launchers and support equipment. (The fissionable nuclear material in the warheads could be transferred to other warheads.) Another distinctive feature of this diplomatic breakthrough was the system of verification and on-site inspections to which both parties agreed.

Thus the Soviets promised to eliminate some 1,766 missiles including 405 SS-20s already deployed in European Russia and 249 scheduled for deployment. The Reagan administration pledged to remove from U.S. bases in Western Europe 120 Pershing II ballistic missiles (with a mere six-minute flight time from launch to detonation over Soviet targets) and 322 ground-launched "cruise" missiles (with a more "comfortable" twenty- to thirty-minute flight time). In addition, the Americans would forgo the deployment of an additional 114 Pershing II missiles and 121 cruise missiles.[36] Whether Mikhail Gorbachev or Ronald Reagan had earned the "bragging rights" for this extraordinary diplomatic achievement, the INF Treaty did eliminate far more Soviet than American nuclear-capable missiles from the European continent.

In the moral debate over intermediate-range nuclear forces, the Moscow Patriarchate had, as usual, played a partisan and morally dubious role. Even before NATO decided in December 1979 to deploy these missiles in Europe, the propaganda machinery within the Patriarchate was fully operational. In November 1979 at a public meeting in Moscow, Metropolitan Aleksii of Tallinn and Estonia— the future Patriarch Aleksii II—warned the gathering that

> a new death-carrying danger hangs over our continent: the United States nurtures plans to deploy medium-range missiles in a number of NATO countries, which will lead to the disruption of the balance of power on the continent, and will undermine the process of disarmament in Europe and start a new spiral in the arms race, fraught with many dangers.[37]

Aleksii neglected to mention the hundreds of already deployed Soviet "medium-range missiles," the SS-20s, to which the United States was merely responding.

This was a veritable clarion call to the Moscow Patriarchate and its allies in the peace-and-disarmament campaign. In June 1981, Patriarch Pimen tried to argue that the Soviet missiles in question were, in fact, "strategic," not intermediate-range—a pretense abandoned eventually by the Soviet political leaders themselves.[38] A CPC consultation in Budapest in May 1983 considered it "essential" that NATO postpone its anticipated deployment of intermediate-range missiles "to gain more time for negotiations on real steps toward disarmament."[39] A special anti-nuclear "World Assembly" in Moscow in June 1983 declared: "We say NO to Pershing 2 and Cruise Missiles on European soil. To break through the spiral of the arms race, unilateral first steps could lead to multilateral agreements."[40] The "unilateral" action was expected to come from the United States, of course, not from the Soviet Union.

Gradually the rhetoric became more shrill. In November 1983, the Orthodox Church in Czechoslovakia formally entered the fray when its primate, Metropolitan Dorotej of Prague, bewailed the "aggressive policy of the NATO countries" against the "peace-loving socialist countries." If NATO's new missiles were not deployed, Dorotej assured his clergy, "a catastrophe can be prevented."[41] By 1984 Patriarch Pimen was applying to the latest U.S./NATO policy such adjectives as "notorious," "unreasonable," "dangerous," and "reckless."[42] Similarly, Metropolitan Aleksii of Tallinn and Estonia told a January 1984 conference of the Soviet Peace Fund that "this irresponsible act" of the Reagan administration betrayed an intent "to tip the scales in the balance of power and attain military superiority over the Soviet Union and to bring to nought all the positive results of the policy of détente established with such difficulty over the last decades."[43]

All this one-sided rhetoric was swept away by one signature—that of Mikhail Gorbachev on the celebrated INF Treaty. The public moral witness of the leaders of the Moscow Patriarchate on issues of nuclear war has never been the same since that embarrassing disavowal by the state that they had served so faithfully.

The Romanian Orthodox Church

The Romanian Orthodox Church joined the anti-nuclear campaign rather late. In November 1981, the Democratic and Socialist Unity Front issued an "Appeal for Disarmament and Peace." This forum responded to Ceaușescu's call by bringing together the various popular organizations and all the recognized religious bodies in Romania to implement immediately "the urgent objectives of security, detente and international cooperation."[44]

The first "great Assembly" occurred in Bucharest with 235 delegates and 42 foreign guests in attendance. The delegates pledged themselves to urge all governments and the United Nations "to act unabatedly" against the arms race and for general disarmament, particularly nuclear disarmament; to reduce military expenditures; to halt the deployment of intermediate-range nuclear forces in Europe and to remove and destroy the existing (that is, Soviet) weapons; and to prohibit the production and use of the "neutron bomb." In his address to the delegates Patriarch Justin of Romania declared that gradual but total "disarmament . . . is the only radical solution to stop war and establish a lasting peace." The first step in this direction would entail the cessation of the nuclear-arms race.[45]

At the June 1982 meeting of the Holy Synod of Bishops, Bishop Roman Ialomiteanul, assistant to the patriarch, presented an appeal addressed to the United Nations General Assembly's second special session on disarmament. This appeal was subsequently signed by all the bishops and purportedly by some 18 million clergy and laity—an unlikely number in a total population of 23 million. The plank in this appeal pertaining to intermediate-range nuclear forces was far more balanced than the corresponding statements produced under Moscow's aegis:

> The same as the other European peoples, the Romanian people resolutely demands that the deployment and development of new medium-range nuclear missiles be cancelled, that the existing missiles be destroyed and nuclear armament be completely removed from the Continent.[46]

Fulfillment of this demand for a nuclear-free Europe would still have served the interests of the Warsaw Pact by forcing NATO to rely only on its vastly outnumbered conventional forces to deter a Soviet-led invasion of Western Europe.

Also at the 1982 conference, one working group dealt with the "catastrophic consequences" of the nuclear-arms race using the customary apocalyptic language, while another, on "new doctrines" of nuclear war, denounced the doctrine of limited nuclear war as irrational and irresponsible. During the deliberations of the latter,

Metropolitan Nestor of Oltenia declared the accumulation of nuclear weapons "a crime against mankind." He continued: "The utilization of these diabolical weapons is a heavy sin against God, man, against every creature, and the future generations."[47]

In his reflections on the deliberations at the April 1983 Christian World Conference on Life and Peace, held in Uppsala, Sweden, Metropolitan Nestor averred that all the religions agree that "nuclear war can never be justified, under any circumstance." The moral imperative for him was clear: "The religious workers in the world must firmly condemn as a moral evil the development, the production, the testing, the deployment, and the use of any nuclear weapon by anybody."[48] This was a definitive expression of what is known as "nuclear pacifism." To be sure, since Romania as a rather small nation did not have a nuclear arsenal, Nestor's plea was hardly magnanimous.

The Assembly of the Religions in Romania for Disarmament and Peace met in Bucharest in June 1984 at the initiative of the Orthodox Patriarchate. The delegates followed the lead of Moscow on several issues but with some deviation in keeping with Romania's position as a maverick member of the Warsaw Pact. The assembly insisted that nations "freeze and reduce the military expenses," thus implicitly subscribing to the so-called nuclear freeze. It lauded Ceauşescu for trying to stop both U.S. deployment of intermediate-range nuclear missiles in Western Europe and "the nuclear counter-measures announced by the Soviet Union."[49] The mere mention of Soviet missiles in a critical vein—albeit incorrectly in this context as "counter-measures"—represented an advance over the thoroughly one-sided pronouncements emanating from the peace events staged by the Moscow Patriarchate.

Another priority of the assembly was to persuade the superpowers to recognize the Balkans, together with North and Central Europe and certain other regions, as a nuclear-free zone. A more radical demand called for the elimination of "foreign military bases" in the Balkans—an obvious reference to the Soviets.[50]

Another mild challenge to the Warsaw Pact came in May 1985 from the National Council of the Socialist Democracy and Unity Front. The delegates called on the "socialist" governments to reduce "unilaterally their strengths by ten per cent." This military tithe to peace would not obviously affect the "necessary balance of forces." But it would, the delegates hoped, prove a powerful symbol of the "peace-loving" intentions of the peoples in Warsaw Pact countries.[51] Before the dramatic changes that swept through Eastern Europe in 1989, however, no Warsaw Pact government had picked up this gauntlet.

THE 1986 "MESSAGE"

The Roman Catholic bishops in the United States established a dramatic precedent in May 1983 with the final draft of a controversial "pastoral letter" on war and peace.[52] Addressed to their American Catholic flock and U.S. defense policymakers alike, this document quickly became the starting point of serious discussion of the moral dimensions of U.S. nuclear defense policy. The national Catholic bishops' conferences in West Germany and France soon followed suit, in part to counteract the perceived liberal trend among their colleagues in the United States.[53]

In the worldwide Orthodox community there is nothing comparable in breadth or depth to the American Catholic bishops' document. Occasional missives on peace bear the name of individual hierarchs of the Moscow Patriarchate. In July 1985, for example, Metropolitan Filaret of Kiev and Galich delivered a report to the sixth All-Christian Peace Assembly in Prague. This superficial "attempt at a theological assessment" of the global threats to peace propounded the familiar themes of nuclear apocalypticism, nuclear winter, the infeasibility of "limited" nuclear war, the evils of the U.S. policy of nuclear deterrence, the need for international "trust," and the nuclear freeze, plus a raft of specific proposals on such things as weapons in space and nuclear-free zones.[54]

An even more superficial booklet put out in 1987 by Metropolitan Filaret of Minsk, entitled *We Choose Life,* was significant mainly for the name of the publisher: Novosti Press Agency Publishing House in Moscow, the official government press.[55]

The only document remotely resembling the ambitious venture of the U.S. Catholic bishops was the "Message of the Holy Synod of the Russian Orthodox Church on War and Peace in a Nuclear Age." The text of this pastoral letter, dated February 7, 1986, occupied sixteen double-column pages in the *Journal of the Moscow Patriarchate.*[56] It is an uneven work, given to moments of brilliance mitigated by ideological boilerplate. However, as the only substantive product of *any* Orthodox Church on peace and security in the nuclear age, this "Message" warrants closer scrutiny.

Pointed political statements appear at the beginning and end of the document like brackets around the real content. An early section assigns blame for the international tension to "the policy pursued today by the US ruling circles." This "policy of confrontation" is grounded in the Americans' "search for military superiority," which has aggravated the arms race and "increased the danger of a nuclear war."[57] In contrast, socialist society "creates real conditions" for international cooperation in peace with justice. "The USSR has," the document asserts, "built its relations with all countries on the principle of mutual respect for international legal norms." In particular, the "peace policy of our Motherland" is "perfectly consistent with the Christian approach to the problem of war and peace in a nuclear age."[58]

Five Features

The real content of the "Message," within these political brackets, has several distinguishing features. First, it repeatedly sounds *an apocalyptic alarm.* At the outset, the bishops warn that in the nuclear age "the whole of creation runs the risk of being fully destroyed and the earth being turned into a lifeless desert."[59] They enumerate the disastrous physical and psychological consequences of a nuclear war, accepting uncritically the "latest estimates" of physicists concerning the "nuclear winter" effect of detonating a small number of nuclear weapons.[60] These prognoses lead the bishops to urge a wholesale rethinking of the relations among war, peace, and justice.

Second, the Message propounds *an uncompromising nuclear pacifism,* rejecting as inherently unjustified a nuclear exchange at any level. Although "war is evil," Christians, who have "had to face the vital need of fighting in wars," were not, until now, constrained to regard war as an "absolute" evil. Always recognizing "the right and the duty of the state to use force to remove evil from the life of society," the Church has "had a deep respect for the soldiers who protected the life and security of their neighbors at the price of their own lives." In

Russia, for example, the Church frequently bestowed her blessing on "warriors defending their Motherland from enemies."[61]

But neither the Western just-war tradition nor the Orthodox justifiable-war ethic envisioned war with a potential for total destruction. And so the bishops declare that the nuclear era has rendered obsolete and "senseless" the requirements of that ethic. To support this dramatic conclusion, the Message assembles a series of essentially prudential judgments. Like the American Catholic bishops, the Romanian Orthodox bishops slide back and forth between prudential and moral judgments without carefully distinguishing the two, and without acknowledging the possibility of error in facts or reasoning in the former. Nonetheless, the Russian bishops do offer some useful insights.

The just-war requirement that a nation pursue a right intent in its decision to resort to war cannot be fulfilled, the Message argues, by a retaliatory nuclear blow, much less a "first strike." (By "first strike" the bishops mean, presumably, a large-scale attack with strategic— that is, intercontinental—forces, since that is the conventional usage among deterrence theorists. Still, the bishops' lack of precision on this score may dilute their argument.) The late Paul Ramsey, a distinguished Protestant ethicist at Princeton University, argued forcefully in 1961 that a massive nuclear retaliation would be merely vengeful, politically and militarily pointless, and an immoral act of wanton destruction.[62] If the Russian bishops do indeed share this reasonable premise concerning massive nuclear attacks, their rejection of any and all anticipated uses of nuclear weapons still constitutes a quantum leap in logic: "Not to be the first to use nuclear weapons is the only morally justified position where such weapons exist."[63] "First use" *could* entail a limited launching of strategic, intermediate, or, as was most likely before 1991, tactical missiles or other nuclear-armed devices such as field artillery. But the Russian bishops arbitrarily ruled out such possible nuclear scenarios.

Nuclear war also obviates the classic Western just-war requirement of an official declaration of war. Here the bishops are on solid ground. For such a formal declaration would, in light of the speed of nuclear delivery vehicles, be "tantamount to suicide for the party which declares war." Further, nuclear war (again, presumably, on the strategic level) can neither safeguard noncombatant immunity nor promise an "equitable proportion of war damage to be done to the opposite party," especially if "all life on the planet is at risk."[64] This is a reasonable, even persuasive proposition at the strategic level, but not necessarily at the tactical level. Again, however, the bishops either fail to make these distinctions or simply presume that they have no relevance.

In view of the likely consequences, which the Russian bishops presume axiomatically, "the use of nuclear weapons in a war can only be regarded as a murder, a genocide of a terrifying dimension," "a crime against humanity," "a senseless fruit of sin, a terrible sin against God." More compelling, however, is another conclusion: "But to be ready to destroy entire humanity for one's own ideological presuppositions is criminal and inadmissible."[65]

What ultimately drives the bishops in this direction is their conviction — grounded in one side of a technical theoretical debate — that nuclear war can under no circumstances be "limited." They simply assert that most military experts believe a nuclear exchange at any level would inevitably escalate into a global catastrophe. Thus any notion of a limited nuclear war is, "according to scientific conclusions," merely "a delusion and a fiction."[66]

Third, the Russian Orthodox bishops, unlike their American Catholic counterparts, offer a categoric *rejection of nuclear deterrence as "basically evil."* They describe deterrence in an unusual way: a lack of confidence in one's opponent generates fear, which fosters "the desire to acquire military superiority," which, finally, leads to "reciprocal fear" and "reciprocal armament" in a spiraling arms race.

The bishops pronounce nuclear deterrence evil, because "it is built on the assumption that nuclear war is possible" and thus paves the way for annihilation of all life on earth. Further, the doctrine, as they misperceive it, "assumes that the destruction of God's creation is possible and admissible." Suspicions about a rival's willingness to initiate a nuclear war increase feelings of "alienation and distrust among nations." Deterrence policies also encourage the arms race, which squanders valuable natural, material, human, and intellectual resources. Finally, deterrence exploits the resources of developing countries, diverting them from using these resources to meet the social and economic needs of their people.

Ironically, the bishops propose an alternative that would, in any other political context, be called "deterrence." Deterrence, they aver, can be replaced as an international arms-control regime "only through parity, a balance of armaments that ensure equal security" among nations. But this balance may be justified only as a temporary measure "on the way to a lower level of parity and gradual disarmament, above all, nuclear disarmament." That way should begin with a freeze on the current nuclear arsenals.[67] Notwithstanding their use of the term "evil," the Russian bishops in effect echo the "strictly conditioned moral acceptance of nuclear deterrence" by the American Catholic bishops.[68]

A fourth aspect of the Russian bishops' Message is the *agenda of "urgent tasks"* that they set forth for implementing disarmament. Most of the tasks on this list have a familiar ring. They include the "prevention of the militarization of outer space" (that is, the Reagan administration's SDI program), a no-first-use pledge concerning nuclear weapons, creation of "nuclear free zones," and "establishment of effective international control over the nuclear power engineering for peace"—an ominous, albeit awkwardly phrased, prospect.[69] Once again, there is no attempt to distinguish these prudential policy preferences from moral obligations derived from the Orthodox religious perspective.

Finally, the Russian bishops present *a theology of peace,* but not till the third (and longest) section of the document—an unusual methodological decision, especially in light of the more logical sequence of topics in the American Catholic bishops' pastoral letter that preceded their Message (bishops would be expected to state their moral theology before applying it to specific cases). This section does offer, however, a solid explication of the meanings of peace in the Bible, particularly the linkage between peace and justice not only within the souls of individual persons but also among nations. Peacemaking, the bishops insist correctly, is not only an internal Church matter but "also a general Christian and ecumenical problem."[70] Moreover, the same principles that undergird Christian peacemaking are required for peaceful relations among nations. One statement in particular resonates well with the views of many advocates of freedom and reasonable policies of national security in the West:

This implies the right of peoples to self-determination, non-exploitation of poorer and weaker states by richer and stronger ones, recognition of political equality in relations between states, respect for territorial integrity and sovereignty of other states, non-aggression, and non-interference into the internal affairs of others.[71]

Conspicuously absent are the favorite biblical verses usually cited by the peace movements—Isaiah 2:4, Exodus 20:3, Deuteronomy 30:19, and Jeremiah 21:8.

TWO CASE STUDIES: ERW AND SDI

A closer look at two controversial developments in the nuclear-arms race may help to frame the public moral witness of the Russian and Romanian Orthodox Churches on issues of peace and security in the nuclear age. On the first, the "neutron bomb," these Churches, together with their governments and various European peace movements, greatly influenced the direction of the public debate and the ultimate disposition of the weapon system. On the other issue, the Strategic Defense Initiative, the forceful witness of the Patriarchates of Moscow and Romania may yet be overtaken by events.

The Neutron Bomb

The public debate over the so-called neutron bomb peaked on both sides of the Atlantic between 1977 and 1981, with harmonics continuing, at least in Moscow and Bucharest, through 1984.

The idea of an "enhanced radiation warhead" (ERW)—the proper name of the weapon—was hardly new on the nuclear scene.[72] Born in the early 1950s in connection with the Korean War, the ERW finally achieved headline status in 1977-78 when President Jimmy Carter publicly vacillated on the issue before finally authorizing production of the components of the bomb a year later. In August 1981, the Reagan administration announced that the ERW would be produced but would not be deployed in Europe without the consent of the European allies. In Europe massive protest marches greeted this decision, including demonstrations by some 300,000 anti-U.S. protesters in Bucharest.

By October 1983, however, the U.S. Congress had begun a retrenchment that stopped the production of ERW warheads, terminated some ERW-capable artillery shells, and dismantled all ERW warheads save those originally designated for the increasingly obsolescent Lance tactical missile. (If there are any of these warheads left in the U.S. arsenal, they are at the Pantex facility near Amarillo, Texas, awaiting disassembly in accordance with former President Bush's revised policy pertaining to tactical nuclear warheads.) The U.S. ERW project was essentially defunct long before the dissolution of the Warsaw Pact in 1990 and the virtual disappearance of the Soviet threat to Western Europe.

This embattled nuclear weapon had held promise of a genuine tactical and moral improvement in any nuclear war-fighting scenario. If detonated at an altitude of 3,000 to 5,000 feet, the ERW would theoretically release 80 per cent of its destructive energy as neutron-based radiation compared to the blast and heat that constitute 85 per cent of a fission nuclear warhead's destructive capability. The ERW presumably would function as a "death ray" that would incapacitate tank crews and other enemy military personnel without harming the civilian population beyond the immediate battlefield and the surounding countryside with its infrastructure. It would even preserve essentially intact the equipment and vehicles of the targeted military personnel.

To be sure, actual use of the ERW in combat might have lowered the nuclear "threshold" by blurring the distinction between nuclear and conventional warfare at the battlefield level. This might have increased the probability of escalation to higher levels of nuclear exchange at an even earlier stage of hostilities between the nuclear superpowers. And so a weapon designed to fulfill a military mission in accordance with the *continuity* school of nuclear deterrence might, ironically, have proved the merit of the *apocalyptic* argument.

But this reasonable line of rebuttal was not the one usually pursued by the leaders of the Orthodox Churches in Eastern Europe. From the outset of the international public moral debate over the "neutron bomb," they preferred hyperbole and bombast. For every reasonable statement like the "message" to the world's churches by the fifth All-Christian Peace Assembly in June 1978—the ERW "brings closer the threat of a new war by blurring the distinction between conventional and nuclear weapons"[73]—there were dozens like the following samples.

Patriarch Pimen kicked off the anti-ERW campaign of the Moscow Patriarchate in August 1977 by labeling the neutron bomb "the most terrible weapon of mass destruction of all that have ever been made previously for military use." He particularly railed against ERW advocates as "apologists of misanthropical wars, who find it possible to vindicate the making of a truly satanic weapon—the neutron bomb —and even call it 'clean.'"[74] (The last term had been used to distinguish the ERW's low blast and heat effects from those of so-called dirty nuclear-fission weapons.)

The following month, the Christian Peace Conference issued its first statement on the ERW, which Metropolitan Nikodim of Leningrad signed as CPC president. The CPC, together with the usual "peace forces," condemned the plan of the Carter administration to produce the ERW as a "perversion of reason." The "very possession" of what the CPC indicated had been "blasphemously called 'the doomsday weapon'" (the "blasphemers" were not identified) would signify "aggressive intentions of annihilating humanity and the whole of creation."[75]

The CPC was off and running on this issue. (The World Council of Churches was not far behind; it held an anti-ERW conference in Geneva in January 1978.) A resolution of the CPC working committee in November added to the previous CPC statement an objection that would prove to be a highly effective tool of propaganda. "The neutron bomb," the CPC averred, "contradicts all such endeavors for the 'humanization' of war. It is designed to destroy human lives with the greatest possible preservation of material values."[76] Ignoring the positive potential of the ERW for minimizing civilian casualties, this emotional appeal eventually metamorphosed into the full-fledged canard that the ERW destroys people while preserving property.

The Moscow Patriarchate showcased its anti-ERW outrage at a special inter-religious conference at Trinity–St. Sergius Monastery on December 14, 1977. In speech after speech, Patriarch Pimen and other religious leaders in the Soviet Union denounced the ERW as "a new weapon of mass destruction." The conference's "Appeal" to the religious leaders of the world warned that every human being's "right to live" would be jeopardized by deployment of "the neutron danger" on West European territory.[77]

In his keynote speech at this conference, Patriarch Pimen attempted to elucidate the technical features of the ERW. He reported that "a number of eminent specialists" regarded the weapon as strategic instead of tactical, because its "one and only purpose is to destroy enemy manpower, i.e., to kill people." His understanding of "strategic" here was obviously muddled. Pimen also emotionally denounced the proposed use of the weapon as a response to the "Soviet threat," calling it "a blasphemy against the memory" of the twenty million Soviet victims in the Second World War—a non-sequitur to which the bishops of the Patriarchate have resorted frequently in the absence of compelling counter-arguments. Pimen did, however, proffer one reasonable argument to the advocates of the ERW in the West. Introduction of the ERW to the European continent would, Pimen predicted, change the "balance of strategic equilibrium" there in favor of NATO. This would elicit a reaction from the Warsaw Pact countries. And, as "a new stage in the contest to build up and perfect weapons," the ERW would pose an "unsurmountable hindrance" to the process of halting the arms race and commencing disarmament.[78]

In his closing speech at this December 1977 conference, Pimen made opposition to this weapon mandatory for the Russian Orthodox faithful by declaring, "We are fulfilling our religious and patriotic duty in repudiating the neutron bomb."[79]

The leaders of the Romanian Orthodox Church also took an anti-ERW stand. The ambitious October 1981 "Appeal" of the religions in Romania—the first great statement on disarmament in that country—urged the world to work toward "the prohibition of production and use of the neutron bomb and of other weapons of mass killing."[80] During an extraordinary meeting of the Holy Synod in Bucharest, Bishop Vasile Tîrgovişteanul, assistant to Patriarch Justin, opined with rhetorical excess, "The new mass destruction weapons, medium range missiles and neutron bomb are seriously threatening the very existence of our whole planet."[81] The Assembly of the Religions in Romania for Disarmament and Peace, meeting in Bucharest in June 1984, expressed a desire that the superpowers "turn the atomic arsenals into granaries and the ballistic missiles into our daily bread, necessary to millions of starving people, and the neutron bomb into medicines."[82] Whatever merit this desire may have had as a reflection of the biblical ideal expressed, for example, in Isaiah 2:4 ("they shall beat their swords into plowshares, and their spears into pruning hooks"), it certainly could not be considered the basis for a realistic defense policy by either of the superpowers.

Strategic Defense

The second major policy debate that warrants closer scrutiny concerns the concept of strategic defense. The issue centers on President Reagan's Strategic Defense Initiative (SDI)—the nucleus of what we have called the *fortress* approach to nuclear deterrence. In February 1994, as he prepared to end his exile from Russia, Aleksandr Solzhenitsyn attributed the end of the Cold War to President Reagan and his SDI program, which finally convinced Mikhail Gorbachev that the Soviets could no longer sustain the high economic cost of the arms race with the United States.[83] But throughout the life of this particular nuclear debate, the public moral witness of the Russian and Romanian Orthodox Churches was, once again, directed at the United States alone, as if the Americans had a sinister purpose and the Soviet Union no strategic-defense research and development program of its own.

President Reagan's surprise announcement in March 1983 of a new defensive orientation in U.S. nuclear deterrence policy was intended to lead the country between the Scylla of the apocalyptic school and the Charybdis of the continuity school. That speech simply launched —in the vaguest, most nuanced language, to be sure—"a long term research and development program to begin to achieve our ultimate goal of eliminating the threat posed by strategic nuclear missiles." The specific task of pursuing "defensive technologies" would "give us the means of rendering these nuclear weapons impotent and obsolete."[84]

President Reagan's proposal met with a withering barrage of criticism from scientists, international security experts, and policymakers in both the Soviet Union and the United States. Opponents effectively painted a picture of SDI as "Star Wars"—a pseudo-scientific delusion and a waste of taxpayers' money. Consequently, the president's initial vision of "a space shield against ballistic missiles"[85] has undergone a metamorphosis. Even before the startling international developments in late 1989, the Bush administration downgraded the program, lowering its requests for funding to mere maintenance of the research and development phase alone. The U.S. Congress, especially the House of Representatives, has further eroded the appropriation for SDI. Moreover, the original intention, the defense of population centers, was eclipsed in the Bush administration by another one: enhancement of the nation's strategic counterforce capability—that is, the protection of military targets such as ballistic-missile silos and command centers.[86] After the success of the Patriot anti-missile missile in the Persian Gulf War, the U.S. Congress appeared to be moving toward a reduction of SDI to "ALPS," an Accidental Launch Protection System in case of a "mistake" by those who control the formerly Soviet arsenal or the launch of isolated strategic missiles from renegade nations such as Saddam Hussein's Iraq or Muammar Qaddafi's Libya. Either of these "limited" versions of strategic defense is little more than an adjunct to the continuity school of deterrence.

The scientific and technological pursuits of SDI have, however, remained fairly constant. The exotic high-tech devices under investigation include early-warning satellites, ground-based radars, airborne optical sensors using lasers, pop-up infrared sensors to be launched into space in crises, exoatmospheric homing interceptors, ultraviolet laser imaging on satellites, space-based mirrors for the relay and aiming of defensive weapons, ground-based battle-management computers, space-based battle-management systems, space-based chemical lasers, space-based particle beams, and nuclear-driven directed-energy weapons such as the X-ray laser. Among the non-nuclear kinetic-energy weapons envisioned by SDI officials are interceptor missiles and electromagnetic "gun" systems employing "smart rocks" or "brilliant pebbles"—precision-guided, high-velocity projectiles that disable enemy warheads and their vehicles by penetrating their complex mechanisms.[87]

"Complex" and "ambitious" aptly describe this grandiose vision, even within its more restricted parameters. And this list pertains only to the U.S. strategic-defense program. Whatever research the Soviets pursued and the Russians may still be pursuing is, of course, cloaked in secrecy. But the announcement in May 1990 by the Gorbachev regime that the Soviets planned to dismantle the controversial phased-array radar system in Krasnoyarsk, Siberia, was a tacit admission that the Soviet Union had indeed violated the provisions of the 1972 Strategic Arms Limitation Treaty concerning strategic defenses and had had a strategic-defense initiative of its own.

The 1984 Roundtable. The Russian and Romanian Orthodox Churches orchestrated an energetic public moral witness against the

American SDI program. The Moscow Patriarchate's campaign against the "militarization of outer space" by the United States was launched in April 1984, when the International Roundtable Conference in Moscow that year was entitled "Space Without Weapons." As usual at these events, Patriarch Pimen provided the keynote address. He suggested that the nations of the world conclude a treaty that would "put an insurmountable barrier to any use of outer space for non-peaceful purposes and give a new impetus to the scientific and practical exploration of outer space beneficial for all nations of the world."[88]

The final report of this 1984 conference was somewhat more balanced than its previous counterparts had been.[89] A space-based strategic defense represented for the assembled religious leaders "a sign of supreme human arrogance." If humanity had always looked to the heavens for life-giving sunlight and rain, the dawning of the SDI era would force humanity to "face the threat of space becoming the source of death and destruction." This would have been disingenuous had the report not contained an important qualification: "The militarization of space is not new." The delegates conceded the role played by space-based satellites in the current regimes of nuclear deterrence; they also spoke of the reliance of modern conventional forces on space-based objects for their command and control.

What the delegates did not acknowledge was that tens of thousands of ballistic missiles then in the arsenals of both superpowers had exoatmospheric trajectories; in theory at least, these nuclear warheads already represented a "militarization of outer space." And yet the delegates contended that "the new extension into space" of the U.S.-Soviet military confrontation "poses yet a new threat." They also declared that "security has taken on idolatrous proportions for some nations." Nor were they impressed by the claims of SDI advocates that potential space-based systems would be defensive. "Defence and offense are today inseparably interwoven," they said.

Conceding the feasibility of strategic defensive systems, the Roundtable delegates adduced three additional reasons for opposing deployment of such devices. First, "it is impossible to create an absolutely reliable system," so "all such attempts serve only to breed illusions about the possibility of victory in a nuclear war." Space-based weapons would "only intensify" the "dangerous trend" toward nuclear war-fighting strategies, which, of course, the apocalyptic school of nuclear deterrence rejects *a priori*.

Second, the delegates estimated that the costs of some space-based systems would exceed $500 billion—an "excessive expenditure" that "cannot be justified in the light of the enormous suffering and needs of people throughout the world today." Meanwhile, the "continuing militarization of space . . . would hamper the utilization of space for peaceful purposes." This would, in turn, "hurt the aspirations of all people, especially peoples of the Third World, to derive the benefits from space technology for their own accelerated development." The delegates did not explain how strategic defense and the "peaceful" use of space are disproportionately related; they did assume, however, that military expenditures could be transferred automatically to social welfare.

Third, the Roundtable—probably correctly—linked SDI "closely" to the current nuclear-arms race. As an innovation—if indeed the Soviet Union did not already have a similar program—the American SDI program would probably have triggered what the Roundtable delegates described as the "usual mechanism of the arms race: system, counter-system, counter-counter-system, etc., pushing towards redundancies in arms build-up." International security experts call this "escalation dominance."

Other Statements. Subsequent statements by assemblies and individuals in the Russian and Romanian Orthodox Churches have not really advanced the debate. A meeting of the Presidential Committee of the World Peace Council in Moscow in March 1985, for example, employed the usual language of the pro-Soviet peace movement: "No to 'star wars'! is the common call of all peace forces. Outer space must serve peace and progress!"[90] At the sixth All-Christian Peace Assembly in Moscow in June 1985, Patriarch Pimen described President Reagan's SDI program as "absolute insanity."[91] Two years later the representatives at a dialogue in Odessa between the Moscow Patriarchate and Pax Christi International urged, rather cryptically, that the "militarization of space and the 'stars wars' project should be opposed by the programme of 'star peace.'"[92] Metropolitan Nicolae of Banat in Romania denounced SDI at the 1987 Roundtable Conference in Moscow as "a threat to the life and progress of the human race" and "an obstacle to the desire of every nation to raise its living standards."[93]

The Russian and Romanian Orthodox Patriarchates were no doubt influential in the anti-SDI positions taken by the international ecumenical organizations. The 1987 meeting of the Central Committee of the World Council of Churches in Geneva in a statement on nuclear disarmament recommended "all necessary steps to prevent the development of space weapons." But the appeals to the two superpowers betrayed a bias: the Soviet Union was merely asked to resume its moratorium on nuclear testing, while the United States was urged to "respond positively" to Soviet initiatives on testing and to reconsider the decision to develop SDI.[94]

Not surprisingly, the pro-Soviet Christian Peace Conference was diligent in opposing SDI. The November 1985 communiqué of the CPC's International Secretariat Meeting at Piestany, Czechoslovakia, expressed a unanimous conviction in favor of "a decisive rejection and practical prevention of the SDI project of the US Government."[95] The next month at Budapest, the CPC Presidential Board, on which Metropolitan Filaret of Kiev was the most prominent Russian Orthodox representative, registered this objection: "SDI will only benefit those corporations which profit from the enormous expenditure of the military budget and will feed the military industrial complex for years to come."[96] The CPC's International Secretariat felt confident enough in September 1986 to declare that "*the* Christian position can only be an unequivocal . . . 'No' to the costly and dangerous SDI programme"[97](italics added). Finally, two months later, the Presidential Board expressed to Mikhail Gorbachev its opinion that "President Reagan's absurd adherence to SDI is, at present, the only big obstacle on the road to disarmament. Most of the American people do not share President Reagan's illusion regarding its effectiveness and usefulness." The CPC leaders were certain that they had divined the American president's real motives: "The true purpose of SDI is becoming ever more evident, namely: to secure an easy and guaranteed profit for some corporations and to slow down socialist development by exerting economic pressure upon socialist countries."[98]

There were some notable exceptions to this simplistic partisanship. The 1986 Message of the Holy Synod of the Moscow Patriarchate questioned the feasibility of an anti-missile defense system, noting that "many Soviet and other experts" have predicted that such a regime would be "70 to 95 per cent effective at the most." But the Russian bishops also registered an important caveat:

> It is generally known as well that every time a system becomes more complex technologically, the human factor in its control is reduced and accidents and errors in its operation become more significant. With reference to the so-called space defence system this means only a growing risk of creating a situation in which human beings with the best will in the world will not be able to prevent a nuclear disaster.[99]

The 1987 Roundtable Conference in Moscow raised another objection to SDI as the system seemed to be evolving. The delegates observed that in 1985 the United States had abandoned the original strategy of "star wars," which they took to mean "a sort of 'Maginot Line' in space," in favor of "star wars II"—a term lifted from a statement by former U.S. secretary of defense Robert S. McNamara.[100] The "new concept" emphasized "zonal" or "point shields" to protect the U.S. strategic nuclear arsenal and the command-and-control centers instead of the civilian population. The Soviet religious leaders attributed this supposed shift in policy to the sinister intentions they had perceived all along among U.S. defense policymakers: SDI was not a defensive shield but rather a cover for an aggressive, opportunistic strategy in which a U.S. "decapitating first strike" against the Soviets' nuclear arsenal could be followed by a successful parrying of what little retaliation the Soviets would be able to muster.[101]

This statement contained two factual errors. The shift in U.S. policy did not occur in 1985, if President Reagan's protestations to the contrary the following year have any credibility. Nor was the Maginot Line simile appropriate: President Reagan did not envision a perfect, impregnable wall of defensive systems in space but rather a shield of earth- and space-based devices sufficient to deter any strategic nuclear first strike by the Soviets. But the statement did underscore the chief moral problem entailed in any shift in the SDI program from population defense to "point defense" of military hardware. As noted earlier, such a shift did indeed begin in the Bush administration. Enhancing the U.S. strategic nuclear arsenal represents only a continuation of the *continuity* school of nuclear deterrence. No longer may advocates claim that SDI promises a new, more moral *fortress* approach based on pure anti-missile population defense. It matters not whether the intentions of the United States toward the nuclear successor states of the former Soviet Union are, in truth, honorable or aggressive. The Russians—and perhaps the Ukrainians, if they elect to retain control over the Soviet nuclear weapons on their territory—may reasonably presume the worst and prepare for it accordingly. For this insight, at least, the Moscow Patriarchate, deserves credit.

THE ORTHODOX IN AMERICA: A PIECEMEAL WITNESS

The Orthodox Churches in the United States were late in joining the nuclear debate. Prior to the massive strategic arms build-up during the first Reagan administration, and the revival of popular interest in nuclear issues, none of the jurisdictions had issued a single statement on nuclear defense.

Resolutions of the Churches

The first explicit discussion by a clergy-laity congress of the Greek Orthodox Archdiocese occurred in 1982. The following is from its statement on "Nuclear Disarmament Concerns:"

We believe that the peace of Christ makes nuclear war simply unthinkable. The current peace, Pax Americana and Pax Sovietica, is unacceptable because it is based on the principle of overkill and deterrents and not on positive human development. It is costly, dangerous and impossible to maintain in the long view. We agree that only through a mutual freeze and reversal of the arms race can we hope to arrive to that level of disarmament which signals the presence of the Kingdom of God. In this time of serious spiritual and political activity, as good stewards of God's creation, we should be employing the world's resources in social and economic development for humankind, instead of armaments.

While we do not condemn reasonable actions taken by governments to insure their sovereignty and territorial integrity from unlawful attack, . . . [t]he Church as peacemaker supports those policies which seek mutual arms reductions. . . . The Church as peacemaker must educate for peace and provide understanding and support of its members whose conscience condemns the sin of violence and war.[102]

This statement presumed as empirical fact several debatable hypotheses: (1) the apocalypticists' belief in the "unthinkable" nature of any nuclear war, with no possibility of a limited exchange of strategic or tactical nuclear weapons; (2) the virtual moral equivalence of the United States and the Soviet Union as world powers and enforcers of "pax" (peace), without distinguishing between the historical experiences of "peace" by peoples under the authority of the two governments; (3) the principle of "overkill," a hyperbolic slogan that oversimplifies the complexities of warfare, particularly the possibility of misfired or inaccurate weapons and confusion in command-and-control; (4) the value of a "mutual freeze" in the arms race, at a time when the Soviet Union enjoyed a distinct advantage in the number and magnitude of nuclear weapons; (5) the assertion that some particular "level of disarmament" would signify "the presence of the Kingdom of God"; and (6) a "zero-sum" relation between defense spending and domestic social spending by the federal government, which ignores the bureaucratic and institutional complexity of the U.S. federal budget. In addition, the statement included a blanket endorsement of arms-reduction policies in isolation from other relevant factors in the formation of a moral and prudent policy of national defense. Finally, the statement urged "understanding and support" for conscientious objectors, who were, as noted in chapter 5, the targets of *ad hominem* attacks at the 1966 and 1968 clergy-laity congresses.[103]

The resolution on nuclear defense by the 1983 clergy-laity assembly of the Greek Orthodox Diocese of Pittsburgh was more carefully nuanced. But it, too, reflected the political bias of its framers—in this case, conservative—more than they would probably care to admit.[104] This document identified "the right to self-defense from unjust aggression" as one of the "demands of the natural law." But is there yet a genuine consensus about natural law among the American public to which the Church may effectively appeal? The delegates expressed rather pointed criticism of "the present tendencies of the anti-nuclear peace movement in the U.S. and Western Europe, particularly the naïveté, simplistic moralism, and one-sided criticism of the U.S. and the NATO Alliance that characterize many official pronouncements by religious organizations and personal statements by religious leaders." Further, the resolution explicitly rejected the "nuclear freeze" proposition of "the so-called peace movement." Finally, the assembly encouraged the U.S. president "to achieve a more stable balance of power and a verifiable mutual reduction in strategic nuclear weapons as a meaningful contribution toward realistic peaceful relations between the NATO and Warsaw Pact governments." In the national debate over nuclear deterrence in 1983, "reduction" was the term of choice for the Reagan administration and its supporters, especially in opposition to "freeze," the term preferred by most activists in the peace movements.

The Orthodox Church in America commented on nuclear defense only once. The resolution on "Justice and Peace" at the 1983 All-American Council posited nuclear war as "unthinkable." The delegates exercised prudent self-restraint, however, by supporting "realistic efforts aimed at the total elimination of nuclear weapons" without elucidating such measures. The delegates also invoked the "butter-not-guns" shibboleth: they suggested that the "phenomenal" public expenditures on nuclear (and conventional) weapons, "while a majority of the world population suffers deprivation, poverty, and hunger," prove the "madness which dominates human society." The "major obstacle" to any real progress toward disarmament, the delegates declared, was "a mutual lack of confidence" between the two superpowers. But the delegates tempered this rather naïve premise by insisting on "on-site verification" of any reductions in the nuclear arsenals of the superpowers. Finally, the OCA council pointed to the deeper causes of the international mistrust that leads to war and violence, specifically the barriers that "artificially separate human beings from each other" and the "suppression of religious and intellectual freedom," especially by Communist dictatorships.[105]

A striking indication of Orthodox moral confusion on nuclear defense occurred in 1984, when official pronouncements from two Orthodox jurisdictions seemed to have been informed by the platforms of the opposing candidates in the presidential campaign.

First, the Greek Orthodox clergy-laity congress produced a statement that treated technical hypotheses as empirically verifiable fact and partisan political sentiment as Orthodox moral tradition. This is the statement, in full:

It's our conviction and intent that the entire human family of our planet earth cannot under any circumstances consider nuclear war to resolve conflicts between nations, or be subjected to any kind or level of nuclear war. Foremost in our thoughts is the survival of the human race. We must, therefore, begin now to boldly reestablish love, trust, and understanding among the superpower states.

Orthodox Christians have always viewed nuclear war as an evil, and sought its termination with prayer. Nuclear war would be an unprecedented evil in the history of the human race. It is unthinkable and its use is totally unacceptable. Nuclear war must never be permitted to begin. A nuclear conflagration would certainly cause the extinction of all creation.

The threat of total destruction by nuclear weapons and its cost in human lives, economic resources, culture and society, devastation of the environment, and its lingering and permanent residual impact on life of all kinds make nuclear war unacceptable. International tensions and the proliferation of nuclear weapons among all countries greatly increase the potential of total destruction.

Therefore, it is a moral and theological imperative that the superpowers of this earth immediately and sincerely embark upon meaningful and substantive negotiations to stop the increase of nuclear weaponry, to reduce nuclear arsenals, and to resume serious negotiations to eliminate their use. Moreover, it is the responsibility of the superpowers to prevent the proliferation of nuclear weapons by all nations.

Pending the complete prohibition and thorough destruction of nuclear weapons, all nuclear weapon states must, as a first step, unconditionally pledge not to use or threaten to use nuclear weapons against each other for any reason.

We have reached a level of nuclear armament beyond any morally defensible limits. We must stop this madness now. Therefore, we endorse, support, and encourage the following:

1. Verifiable limitations on nuclear arms.

2. The re-establishment of serious arms reduction negotiations between the superpowers.

3. Peaceful movements in the direction of de-escalation rather than proliferation.

4. The elimination of nuclear weaponry in space.[106]

The nuances of the 1982 Greek Orthodox document were swept away by this series of absolutist declarations: nuclear war of "any kind or level" is proscribed; "its use is totally unacceptable"; a nuclear conflagration "would certainly cause the extinction of all creation." These hypotheses proffered by the *apocalyptic* approach to nuclear deterrence apparently became for the Greek Orthodox Archdiocese articles of faith.

This document bore a marked resemblance to the 1984 National Democratic Party platform statement on "Arms Control and Disarmament."[107] Other features were a spiritually soothing but politically naïve summons to "love, trust, and understanding" between the international superpowers; a call for what amounts to a "no first use" pledge and, indeed, a pledge not to use nuclear weapons against an enemy state "for any reason"—a radical call, in effect, for nuclear pacifism; and the elimination of nuclear weapons in space. The last item may have represented a veiled rejection of President (and then candidate for reelection) Reagan's SDI, or it may have been intended as a call for the abandonment only of the space-based portion of the strategic-defense project. In either case, the use of the phrase thrust the Greek Archdiocese into the political debate concerning SDI in that election year, without sufficiently grounding its position in the Orthodox moral tradition. The simple assertion that "Orthodox Christians have always viewed nuclear war as evil" does not lead automatically to any moral position on "nuclear weaponry in space."

The second statement, a much briefer one, came out of the triennial *sabor* of the Serbian Orthodox Church in the U.S.A and Canada, in September 1984:

> On the global level, we are deeply disturbed by the moral problems of *nuclear proliferation,* particularly the nuclear arms race between the U.S. and the U.S.S.R., which threatens the life of everyone on this planet. But on the basis of the classic Orthodox *just war* tradition, this Sabor opposes any policies such as the "nuclear freeze" proposition that might jeopardize the reasonable self-defense of the Free World from unjust aggression, and hence endanger the lives and freedom of millions of people in the world.[108]

Like its Greek Orthodox counterpart, this statement expressed unease about the proliferation of nuclear weapons and the resultant threat to human life. But here these concerns were couched in more nuanced, less certain terms. The Serbian delegates counterbalanced the risk to human life posed by the nuclear-arms race to the danger to life and freedom that "unjust aggression" could cause. The explicit invocation of the "just war tradition"—equated here with "reasonable self-defense"—is rare in such documents. But it was cited here as the ground for rejecting the "nuclear freeze" proposition. Whether the freeze might or might not have jeopardized the Free World (an ideologically colored term certain to be absent from statements issued by the Moscow and Romanian Patriarchates), criticism of this defense policy betrayed the political provenance of the Serbs' moral thinking on this issue. If the Greek Orthodox delegates seem to have been heavily influenced by Democrat-endorsed policies, the Serbian Orthodox representatives appear to have imbibed the spirit of Republican thinking on defense issues.

The 1984 Serbian Orthodox paragraph is reminiscent of the hawkish, militaristic tone and orientation of the 1966 Greek Orthodox statement on the Vietnam War discussed in chapter 5. Had the Greek Orthodox deviated so far and so quickly from that original position, or were the Serbian Orthodox simply two decades behind the times?

The Greek Orthodox Archdiocese refined its position on nuclear weapons in space at the 1986 clergy-laity congress. The delegates resolved to "advise" the U.S. president "that the Strategic Defense Initiative, commonly known as 'Star Wars' be limited to a strategy of deterrence and defense of this country." This had been precisely the policy of the Reagan administration from the moment the president announced the program. However, the congress also resolved to advise the president "to condemn the use of nuclear weapons against non-nuclear countries and nuclear free zones."[109] Would such a self-imposed restraint preclude, for example, the use of tactical nuclear weapons against a North Korean invasion of South Korea? And would the United States be morally bound to oblige every nation, region, or city that declared itself, however arbitrarily or capriciously, a "nuclear free zone"?

The 1990 Greek Orthodox clergy-laity congress proposed a new metaphor. The "stockpiling of nuclear arsenals," it said, is "a form of 'substance abuse' for our planet, as morally wrong as the destruction of our human potential through drug abuse."[110]

Another unusual turn of phrase came out of the 1986 convention of the Ukrainian Orthodox League. After praying "for the end of the global nuclear arms race which is affecting our lives and this beautiful earth," the Ukrainians added that "we should not replace our love" for Christ "with the maniacal fear or love of the bomb."[111]

The National Council of Churches

The political partisanship and ideological leanings of the NCC have an older pedigree than those of the several Orthodox deliberative bodies. Generally the Orthodox delegates to the NCC's Governing Board (General Board since 1990) have gone with the anti-nuclear flow in this ecumenical organization.

Although several earlier resolutions had expressed reservations about U.S. nuclear-defense measures, not until a September 12, 1968, policy statement did the NCC call for a sea change in nuclear policy. Specific recommendations included a halt in the development of an anti-ballistic-missile system, the precursor of President Reagan's SDI.[112]

The NCC's anti-nuclear witness is firmly grounded in the *apocalyptic* school of nuclear deterrence. A resolution in May 1980, for example, observed that "it is becoming increasingly recognized that massive armaments buildup diverts resources away from human needs, does *not* provide national security, and endangers the survival of civlization."[113] Similarly, in March 1980, prominent NCC officials including Archpriest Vladimir Berzonsky of the OCA (who also signed the March 1979 "Choose Life" statement discussed above) sent a letter to Metropolitan Yuvenaly of Krutitsy and Kolomna lamenting the "increased militarism and greater danger" to humanity wrought by the development of "still more terrible weapons." That reasonable proposition, however, was mitigated by a questionable prudential judgment that the arms race has brought "fear, suspicion and an escalation of terror rather than the establishment of security."[114]

The NCC has pronounced on all manner of specific nuclear-policy issues. A resolution in May 1983 praised the Roman Catholic bishops in America, because in their pastoral letter they had assumed "the burden of risk in applying Christian principles" to the public debates concerning first use, counterpopulation warfare, first-strike weapons, nuclear war-fighting strategies, limited nuclear war, and the nuclear-freeze proposition.[115] On these and other technical dimensions of nuclear deterrence and nuclear defense, the NCC itself has weighed in mightily, usually in criticism of prevailing U.S. policy. The NCC was particularly vocal in its support of the freeze proposal and the Strategic Arms Limitation Treaty (SALT II) negotiated by President Carter but rejected by the U.S. Senate after the Soviet invasion of Afghanistan.[116]

Perhaps the most one-sided NCC statement on a nuclear issue was "A Message Concerning Arms Negotiations following the Reagan-Gorbachev Meeting at Reykjavik," adopted by the Governing Board on November 6, 1986. Three weeks earlier, the leaders of the two nuclear superpowers had held their surprising summit in Iceland. The NCC message closely reflected the testimony before the board on the previous day by Alan Geyer, a liberal United Methodist ethicist at Wesley Theological Seminary in Washington, D.C. Immediately striking is the willingness of the NCC to commit itself on technical empirical matters, such as the numerous ways that the Soviets could "thwart the intent of SDI."

The message attributed the failure to achieve an agreement at the summit solely to President Reagan's unwillingness to "give up his 'Star Wars'/SDI dream." The language was sharper than usual. The Governing Board said it was dismayed "by the President's intransigent trust in SDI," "deeply disturbed at the prospect of militarizing space, which is the inevitable result of proceeding with SDI," and "like-wise disturbed at President Reagan's failure to consider the cost of the major emphasis placed on this program." Woven among these personal attacks on the U.S. president were such ostensibly "reliable scientific estimates" as the projected cost of SDI—said to be at *least* one trillion dollars![117]

A more recent meeting of the NCC General Board demonstrated the NCC's inability to perceive a nuclear threat when it is real instead of imagined. A "Resolution on the Peace and Reunification of Korea" adopted on November 12, 1993, fretted about "talk of using military means to resolve a situation of apparent diplomatic impasse" and urged the Clinton administration to initiate "such confidence-building measures as the normalization of relations with the Democratic People's Republic of Korea (DPRK)" and "to take all appropriate measures to lessen the highly-charged atmosphere of confrontation with the DPRK." The problem with such irenic sentiments is the extreme naïveté they reveal in the face of the unrelenting militarism that makes the North Korea of Communist dictator Kim Il-sung (and son Kim Jong-il) one of the most dangerous, unstable states in the post–Cold War world. The NCC statement refers gingerly to "the DPRK's dispute with the International Atomic Energy Agency," as if the issue were merely forensic.[118] Conspicuously missing is any mention, much less prophetic moral judgment, of the North Koreans' nuclear program, their flaunting of international regimes against nuclear proliferation, and the enormous threat that nuclear weapons in the hands of the "DPRK" would pose to international peace.

Among the eight members of the "Reference Committee" that recommended adoption of this statement by the General Board in plenary session was Fr. Robert Stephanopoulos, dean of the Holy Trinity Cathedral of the Greek Orthodox Archdiocese in New York. By spring 1994, however, the Clinton administration, in which Fr. Robert's son George has a prominent advisory role, showed no signs of heeding the advice of the elder Stephanopoulos and his colleagues at the NCC. As the United States and the rest of the members of the United Nations—including, presumably, the People's Republic of China—continued to press the government in Pyongyang to allow international inspections of its nuclear facilities or to prepare for possible military action, the NCC once again seemed to have seriously misdiagnosed a crucial nuclear issue.

THE PRICE OF PROPHECY

If the record of the Greek Orthodox Archdiocese on the Vietnam War shows how one Orthodox jurisdiction can contradict its own public moral witness over time, the conflicting statements on the "nuclear freeze" proposition by the Greek (1982) and Serbian (1984) jurisdictions illustrate the risk of moral contradiction in different parts of the same Church. The temptation is ever present for religious leaders, both clergy and laity, to attempt to provide moral guidance for their churches and for the larger society on technical issues beyond their competence. Nowhere is this more evident than in the rarefied nuclear realm. Which was *the* Orthodox position on the "freeze," the Greek or the Serbian? The more important question is, Why should Orthodox Christians in America be forced to make such a choice?

A personal confession is necessary. I played a major role in shaping the 1984 Serbian Orthodox resolution that rejected the nuclear freeze proposal. Archpriest Milan Markovina of Milwaukee, the other principal drafter of the statement, vigorously opposed any reference to the nuclear freeze by name. I insisted that the plenary session of the *sabor* vote on the matter, and there was a nearly unanimous decision to include this reference. It is now painfully obvious to me that Fr. Milan's caution reflected a prudence that I, along with most of the other delegates, lacked.

However, by rejecting one particular policy, the Serbian Orthodox *sabor* did not commit itself to any alternative and so further erode its moral credibility. Moreover, the next *sabor,* in 1987, adopted a report by the Committee on Social and Moral Issues that eschewed such detailed statements on the vital issues of the day. The *sabor* displayed a newfound prudence by declaring that it "questions the effectiveness of the past practice of issuing resolutions that are soon forgotten." The delegates approved instead a permanent commission that would produce documents on moral issues with the direct guidance of the hierarchy.[119]

But the collective public moral witness on issues of nuclear-defense policy by the Orthodox Churches in the former Soviet Union, Romania, and the United States remains, on balance, tragically flawed. Hierarchs, priests, and laity alike have plunged fearlessly into the byzantine maze of nuclear deterrence. The result has been an abundance of resolutions, encyclicals, and other messages that, with rare exceptions, reflect an uncritical faith in the apocalyptic school, that claim to know more than their authors are capable of knowing, that tend to echo the clichés and slogans of the anti-nuclear "peace" movements instead of reflecting careful technical analysis, and that more often than not betray political pedigrees unbecoming to Orthodox Churches, which are supposedly above all that.

The slavish devotion of the Moscow Patriarchate to the vicissitudes of Soviet nuclear-defense policy was especially embarrassing, particularly when this crude propaganda took a more sinister turn by denouncing the United States in the person of its president. The Romanian Orthodox leadership, however, has not lagged far behind in its version of simplistic anti-nuclear moralism. In both of these cases, the Orthodox spokesmen frequently uttered extreme anti-nuclear rhetoric while conveniently either justifying the nuclear arsenal of the Soviet Union or advocating a "nuclear free zone" in the Balkans. Nor have the Orthodox performed with honor in the politically left-wing ecumenical forums of the WCC, NCC, and CPC. The 1986 "Message" of the Holy Synod of the Moscow Patriarchate is the best Orthodox commentary on nuclear matters, but it, too, as we saw above, is seriously flawed.

If the Orthodox Churches hope to make a meaningful contribution to the nuclear debate, they will first have to develop their own experts in this field to advise the bishops, and then exercise self-restraint so as to refrain from endorsing or rejecting specific weapons systems, theories of nuclear deterrence, or government policies. That does not leave much room to flex their moral muscle. But Orthodox leaders would then demonstrate by their caution that they are willing to pay the price of prophecy.

7

Conclusions: Dilemmas of the Orthodox Witness

The encyclicals, resolutions, and other proclamations on peace, freedom, and security issued by leaders of the Orthodox Churches in the former Soviet Union, Romania, and the United States have, on the whole, been woefully deficient as expressions of authentic Orthodox moral tradition.

These Orthodox hierarchs and national representative bodies, like their prolific Roman Catholic and Protestant counterparts, manifest a desire to engage the world and its problems. The Orthodox have contributed whatever moral and prudential solutions they could from the depths of their religious experience. However, the actual product has not, as we have seen in the preceding chapters, matched expectations. Instead of employing cogent moral reasoning based on unmistakable Orthodox virtues to reach morally sound conclusions, cautiously free at once from empirical error and from ideological contagion, these mostly brief, pungent statements have been marred by superficiality, acute historical conditioning and hence a lack of universal relevance, and distinct ideological bias. All too often they have expressed unfounded opinion based on presumed "facts."

St. Paul's epistles in the New Testament masterfully blend concrete, situational, contingent moral prescriptions with universal moral and spiritual insight, but the contemporary Orthodox missives to Churches and to governments mix the same ingredients far less successfully. Whereas the Apostle's inspired teachings and prescriptions do indeed reflect the "grace" and "peace" of God with which

321

he greets the readers of each of his epistles, the Orthodox documents on peace, freedom, and security seem, on the whole, uninspired, and destined to have little impact on either the present generation of political leaders or future leaders of the Church.

To be sure, the Orthodox do not suffer alone from this ineffectiveness. Critics have challenged the efficacy of the prevalent modes of public moral witness in the other American religious communities also. Michael Novak, for example, is one of many American Catholics who charged that the Roman Catholic bishops confused moral and prudential judgments in their celebrated 1983 pastoral letter on war and peace in the nuclear age, *The Challenge of Peace*. Moral judgments, when properly derived, are presumed universally binding, but prudential judgments, though they may conform to the virtue of prudence, are still subject to empirical error and faulty reasoning and hence do not carry the same moral weight for faithful Catholics.[1]

Among American Protestants, Paul Ramsey, in his seminal 1967 book *Who Speaks For the Church?*, questioned the modern tendency of denominational leaders to represent their personal moral views on all manner of complicated public-policy issues as the positions of their religious communities.[2] More recently, in a concise but potent commentary in *Christianity Today*, Mark R. Amstutz of Wheaton College outlined six reasons for minimizing the number and scope of church resolutions. Such resolutions, he said,

1. "are simplistic, offering categorical pronouncements on complex foreign-policy problems";

2. "are typically based on the political predilections of clergy and other church officials, rather than on careful moral analysis";

3. "seldom illuminate biblical perspectives on public-policy problems";

4. "tend to be moralistic—in part because public-policy making is regarded as a contest between justice and injustice, good and evil";

5. "seldom represent denominations' constituencies"; and

6. "are divisive." Amstutz contends that if churches wish to "offer redemptive leaven," instead of issuing simplistic pronouncements as if they were mere political lobbies, they ought to "cultivate moral analysis of issues."[3] Orthodox leaders could only benefit by heeding the advice of Novak, Ramsey, and Amstutz.

MORAL, POLITICAL, AND ECCLESIAL DILEMMAS

Approaching the collective Orthodox public moral witness on issues of peace, freedom, and security more systematically, we discover three dilemmas that must be resolved if that witness is to have any hope of credibility and utility. The dilemmas are moral, political, and ecclesial.

The Moral Dilemma

We may reasonably posit that moral pronouncements are a proper prophetic function of the Church. The dilemma that confronts any socially conscious hierarchy concerns not *whether* the Church ought to witness on behalf of its divinely revealed moral tradition, but rather *how* that witness ought to be communicated and on *which* issues the Church ought to focus its limited energies.

The Church cannot expect to speak with equal force, conviction, and effectiveness on every pressing social or moral problem. To avoid a futile dissipation of energy, critical choices must be made. Further, mere affirmations or denunciations, however confidently expressed, are seldom persuasive without compelling moral argument and tend to erode further the credibility of those who utter them.

A precarious balance obtains between saying too much and saying too little in the presentation of moral positions. In an attempt to be comprehensive, a statement may smother the point with extraneous details or lapse into stilted, jargon-filled academic language. An excessively long, over-amplified moral pronouncement risks being widely ignored by its intended audience of policymakers and other citizens. Extreme conciseness also has its risks. If the case for a particular moral position is too brief and underdeveloped, or consists merely of scriptural or patristic "proof texts" for an otherwise arbitrary conclusion, that position may be discounted or dismissed as unsubstantiated. The vast majority of the Orthodox moral pronouncements discussed in the previous chapters clearly tend toward the latter extreme. Bullet-like opinions, rather than comprehensive reflection papers such as the "Message" on war and peace in the nuclear age issued by the Holy Synod of Bishops of the Moscow Patriarchate, have been the order of the day.

Balance is also needed in the Church's assessment of which moral and social issues warrant serious comment. Should the Church confine its attention to broad, general questions or get involved in specific policy disputes? Contemporary Roman Catholic moral theology distinguishes formal from material norms. The "formal" category denotes moral virtues that Christians—indeed, all human beings—ought to embody in their lives. These are presumably universal qualities of human *being* such as generosity, patience, unselfishness, and forgiveness. "Material" norms, however, refer to how persons ought to act—what they ought to *do*—in concrete situations. They may lack the universal moral force of formal norms but attempt to shape moral living in specific, realistic contexts. The Orthodox Churches may profit from this useful distinction as they attempt to witness morally to their governments and societies.

By appealing to *formal* norms governing issues of peace, freedom, and security, the Church may play it safe. Who would object on principle, for example, to a fervent plea for humility, love, and forgiveness in international relations, or to a categorical denunciation of violence as ungodly and anti-human? The 1975 OCA resolution on violence comes readily to mind. But such highly generalized resolutions prove virtually meaningless to public policymakers and other citizens, whose moral decision-making is invariably constrained by practical considerations in concrete, real-world situations. The danger entailed in these general moral pronouncements is the further marginalization of the role of the Church in society, resulting from an increasingly widespread perception of the Church as a purveyor of empty, ineffectual platitudes.

By proclaiming certain *material* norms as the authentic voice of Orthodox Christianity, the Church may succeed in sharply focusing its moral scope and addressing the existential decisions that public policymakers and other citizens must confront in their daily political lives. But the trade-off here is equally grave. The Church runs the risk of ethical micro-management—of plunging headfirst into the minutiae of public policymaking, or attempting in vain to make the tough policy decisions *for* rather than *with* the policymakers and citizenry. Further, it does not take long in such cases for Church leaders to exceed their competence in defense policy or political theory. The net result is usually devastating for the Church, which is widely perceived as a bunch of rank amateurs intruding in technical, professional matters beyond their ken. Under this rubric one may include, for example, the numerous pronouncements of the Moscow Patriarchate on specific nuclear weapons systems such as the neutron bomb or on specific concepts of nuclear deterrence such as President Reagan's Strategic Defense Initiative. Alternatively, by blessing or cursing specific weapons systems, defense strategies, forms of political governance, theories of human rights, and the like that are similarly in favor or disfavor with the government, the Church risks being dismissed as a tool of the state—a voice of propaganda rather than prophecy.

In either case, the more specific the issue or the more concrete the situation addressed, the greater the risk of moral or empirical error: the Church may become guilty quite simply of teaching falsely! This peculiar danger will be assessed below. Suffice it to say here that the cardinal virtue of prudence dictates that the Church effect a balance between the "general" and the "specific" in selecting issues for critical comment, and between proper "amplification" and practical "conciseness" in elucidating its moral positions. Instead of squandering their moral capital on all manner of particular moral and social issues, Orthodox hierarchies would be well advised to confront only the most pressing challenges to the well-being of the faithful by (1) conducting careful, painstakingly documented studies, (2) deliberating in synod with complete candor and freedom of opinion in exhaustive debates, and (3) issuing two-part formal pronouncements that include a detailed study document accompanied by a carefully crafted précis. The formal—if not necessarily material—model for this procedure is the pair of "pastoral letters" issued by the National Conference of Catholic Bishops on war and peace (1983) and economic justice (1986).

The Political Dilemma

The political dilemma is both more obvious and somewhat easier to resolve.

Whatever the particular moral methodology the Orthodox Churches use, whether they seek to maximize certain virtues, the proportionality of proper means to good ends, universally binding principles, or desirable consequences, Orthodox Tradition must be the primary source of their inspiration and moral reasoning. Concerning peace, freedom, and security issues in particular, a firm, explicit grounding in the rich Orthodox heritage of teachings such as those summarized in chapter 1 is a *sine qua non* for an authentic public moral witness. Despite their currency among the several Orthodox hierarchies considered in this book, Marxist-Leninist theories of imperialism, modern varieties of nationalism and militarism, and bald ethnic prejudice do not qualify as appropriate sources of Orthodox moral pronouncements.

The problem in all this is how to avoid the taint of ideology or tribalism without witnessing to some mythical "humanity" devoid of particular histories and cultures. In a sense, this dilemma is a variation of the "general" vs. "specific" dichotomy.

Remaining faithful to its fundamental mission of mediating salvation to all of humanity irrespective of contingent circumstances, the Orthodox Church in every nation must transcend parochial interests, political ideologies, and social prejudices. That may be easier said than done. But with some diligence the more flagrant violations can be avoided. The Communist-inspired rhetoric of Metropolitan Nikodim of Leningrad and Patriarch Justinian of Romania, the entire Romanian Orthodox "social apostolate" with its unique blend of socialism and Orthodoxy, the preoccupation of most Orthodox jurisdictions in the United States with human rights in their own ethnic or national homelands often to the exclusion of appropriate concern for other nations: these are only a few of the most blatant abuses of the universal appeal of the Gospel of Jesus Christ. Neither should the Greek Orthodox Archdiocese squander its moral capital in a semantic battle over the name of the new Republic of Macedonia based in Skopje, nor the Serbian Orthodox Church in the former Yugoslavia and the United States risk identifying too closely with Serbian nationalist aspirations in Croatia and Bosnia-Hercegovina, nor the Antiochian Archdiocese—and its parent Patriarchate based in Damascus—stake its moral credibility on the political fortunes of the PLO in the Israeli-occupied territories. Orthodox hierarchies can at least comb their prospective moral statements for such obvious partisanship and eliminate any language that might be perceived as needlessly political, parochial, or ideological.

Conversely, too wide a focus on humanity "in general" might lead to a disembodied moral outlook. One may fall prey to a kind of "I love humanity; it's people I can't stand" fallacy. National Orthodox Churches such as those in the Russia, Ukraine, Romania, and Serbia, or even the fragmented Orthodox jurisdictions in the United States, can hardly ignore their own geographic circumstances and cultural histories. But a properly circumscribed national or ethnic pride need not entail national or ethnic self-glorification or, worse, phyletism or ethnoracism. The manifest hatred of some leaders of the Ukrainian Orthodox Church of the U.S.A. for all things Russian clearly exceeds this limit. So does the anti-Zionist (and sometimes explicitly anti-Jewish) rhetoric of both the Antiochian Orthodox Archdiocese and the "Red-Brown" faction in the Moscow Patriarchate led by Metropolitan Ioann of St. Petersburg and Ladoga. Particular Churches might sidestep this moral pitfall by balancing the number and scope of their public moral statements between local and universal concerns.

Speaking positively, we may insist, for example, that a national Orthodox Church ground its support of any international military action by its government squarely and minimally in the Orthodox justifiable-war ethic (the disavowal of the latter by the Holy Synod of the OCA notwithstanding). The specific requirement of a "proper spiritual ethos" — the unique Orthodox version of "legitimate authority" in the Western just-war tradition — would seem to exclude *a priori* any support, much less jingoistic championing, by an Orthodox Church for military action by a totalitarian, anti-Christian regime such as the brutal Communist governments of the Soviet Union and Romania. Similarly, advocacy of religious freedom and human rights commensurate with Orthodox Tradition does not allow the Churches to make self-serving exceptions to the principle, such as the Greek Catholic ("Uniate") communities in Ukraine and Romania. Indeed, the rationalizations proffered by leaders of the Orthodox Patriarchates in those countries for the systematic liquidation of the Greek Catholic communities by the Communists remain acutely odious, especially now that the Soviet regime has collapsed and the current Romanian government has reversed the oppressive policies of its predecessor. Serious Orthodox pronouncements on religious freedom and human rights must be rooted instead in the traditional Orthodox virtue of "tolerance," which the Church Fathers derived from their anthropological doctrine of free will. Given the rich moral heritage of Orthodoxy, there is simply no need to import any of the foreign doctrines or worldviews that prevail in the modern world.

The Ecclesial Dilemma

Perhaps the most serious question for the Orthodox Churches concerns their very identity as the Church: what has been the effect on their ecclesial claims of the dubious public moral witnessing that we have been examining?

The problem of proper authority arises whenever a public statement is issued. With synods of bishops, individual bishops, and clergy-laity assemblies all vying for attention as spokesmen for Orthodoxy, who—to echo Paul Ramsey's question—speaks for the Orthodox Churches? Fr. Stanley Harakas has already conceded, for example, that the biennial clergy-laity congress of the Greek Orthodox Archdiocese has no authority to pronounce on doctrinal matters. Doctrine is the proper purview only of an Ecumenical Council of all the Orthodox bishops throughout the world. The last undisputed council of this sort met in A.D. 787, and the last Orthodox councils that defined theological doctrine occurred in the fourteenth century. Orthodoxy is not described as conservative for nothing.

The only matters, therefore, on which the various clergy-laity congresses (and their counterparts in the other jurisdictions in the United States, the ancient Patriarchates, and the national Orthodox Churches in Eastern Europe) may profitably deliberate involve the financial and organizational life of the parishes. It was under the latter rubric that the biennial congresses of the Greek Archdiocese began in 1954 to introduce statements and resolutions on social and moral issues, culminating in the formal establishment in 1966 of a Social and Moral Issues Committee. The expressed purpose of that committee is to propose a coherent document to the plenary session of each congress. Each committee report, Fr. Harakas insists, "reflects the concrete concerns and views of those who prepare it." Consequently, "it is possible to discern differing emphases, terminology, approaches and, in some issues, even varying ethical stances." Fr. Harakas contends that these committee documents nonetheless "form a coherent body of teaching and moral pronouncement" (a dubious proposition in light of the glaring contradictions we have noted above). The ultimate decisions of each congress on contemporary moral and social issues, he says, are designed to express "the mind of the Church in this place," to influence the society in which the Church is situated, and to afford the membership of the Church "an exercise in spiritual nurture."[4]

With all due respect to this valiant attempt to justify a dangerous practice, I must take exeption to such language. It is not the "mind of the Church in this place" that ought to matter, but rather the mind of Christ as interpreted preeminently by the Church Fathers. Influencing society is too modest a goal for a Church that deems itself the sole source of salvation from sin, death, and Satan: this Church has far more to offer its social environments than merely another "input" into society's ethical matrix. Similarly, the members of any Orthodox Church have no business engaging in self-indulgent intellectual "exercises" when the product is flabby at best or even threatening to the Church's spiritual health.

The dilemma, though shared by other religious bodies, is particularly acute for the Orthodox, owing to the risk of proclaiming an admixture of truth and error. The twin dangers of incorporating incorrect empirical data or faulty logic and moral reasoning, on the one hand, or of confusing prudential judgments (in which error is possible) with moral judgments (supposedly normative) await any clergy-laity assembly that feels so moved to "exercise" its freedom of expression. Whatever minimal gains or influence might be expected from such a process would seem to be outweighed by the possibly irreversible damage of a soiled public moral witness.

For Protestant communions, by contrast, the risks to their credibility are minimal and the potential gains significant. Unlike the Orthodox Churches, these "denominations" do not claim to be the one, undivided, continuing Church of Christ, spiritually guided and indwelled by the Holy Spirit and hence not subject to doctrinal or moral error in its collective witness. As churches "reformed and ever reforming," to cite the Calvinist self-understanding, the Protestant denominations may issue official pronouncements through their representative bodies that are in no way deemed infallible or even universally applicable. If these pronouncements happen to change radically in style and substance from era to era, or even from year to year, there is usually no adverse effect on the identity, authority, or sense of purpose of the Protestant churches.

For the Orthodox Churches, shifting positions on contemporary moral and social issues and, worse, clearly discernible moral error are theoretically impossible. Otherwise the Church would lapse into the heresy of what Vladimir Lossky termed a "Nestorian ecclesiology." This fifth-century distortion of the Church's identity, named after an errant archbishop of Constantinople, would divide the Church into two "beings," as it were: a heavenly, invisible, absolutely true Church, and an earthly, imperfect, relative, shadowy human Church, or, more properly, "churches."[5] Any risk of creating this ecclesial heresy, or even the appearance of it, must be avoided, even if it means circumscribing official involvement of the Orthodox Churches in particular issues of moral and social concern.

The now classic negative examples must be, first, the contradictory positions of the Greek Orthodox Archdiocese clergy-laity congresses pertaining to the U.S. involvement in the Vietnam War, and, second, the contradictory resolutions on the "nuclear freeze" proposition produced by the Greek Orthodox congress and the Serbian Orthodox *sabor* in 1984. Other qualms may arise concerning the peculiarly pro-Soviet and anti-American coloration of the numerous "peace assemblies" organized by the Moscow Patriarchate during the Communist era, and the battle for the soil and soul of the new Republic of Moldova still being waged by the Russian and Romanian Orthodox Churches.

This perilous process of formulating a public moral witness by plebiscite may have reached its *reductio ad absurdam* at the 1989 All-American Council of the OCA. The approximately 750 delegates had to vote twice on a resolution committing the OCA to a moral rejection of capital punishment—the first vote was deemed by the chairman "too close to call"![6] Thus on so grave a moral issue, the OCA, by the narrowest of democratic margins, now feels confident that it is proclaiming moral truth. This incident epitomizes the folly of such resolutions. Any Orthodox clergy-laity assembly would better serve the Church by refraining from the attempt to address complex moral and social problems through so-called moral resolutions or statements. These concerns are the proper domain of the hierarchs, who alone, as archpastors and apostolic teachers, ought to initiate the "official" public moral witness of the Orthodox Church.

Happily, the 1992 OCA council may prove a watershed in this jurisdiction's public moral witness. Eschewing the usual mode of moral proclamation by plebiscite, the Holy Synod of Bishops, as we noted in chapter 4, issued a coherent and truly prophetic statement of "affirmations" on marriage, family, sexuality, and the sanctity of life. Rather than submitting this statement to the assembled clergy and lay delegates for a vote, Metropolitan Theodosius simply announced the decision of the Holy Synod to issue this moral edict and moved to the next item on the agenda. The Holy Synod's May 1993 statement on the civil war in the former Yugoslavia—an exemplary, moderate, even-handed moral pronouncement on an excruciatingly complex moral issue—also betokens a positive trend in the OCA.

To be sure, the bishops themselves are not immune from the twin dangers of error and confusion mentioned above. The disavowal of the justifiable-war ethic by the same OCA bishops in March 1992 comes immediately to mind. While imploring the guidance of the Holy Spirit, the bishops might also welcome the views of their flock on various issues—expressed privately, individually, and unofficially. The calculus of the "moral dilemma" applies perforce here as well: the more specific the particular moral or social issue and the more concrete their moral position, the greater the danger that Orthodox bishops may incorporate empirical error, subjective opinion, and moral misjudgment instead of presenting solely the objective moral truth of Christ and His Church applied to existential problems judiciously, cautiously, and without fear of contradiction.

THE PRICE OF PROPHECY

As the benighted Orthodox Patriarchates in Russia, Ukraine, and Romania emerge ever so gingerly from decades of collaboration with their erstwhile Communist persecutors, we may expect more prophecy and less propaganda in their public moral pronouncements. Signs of such a shift are evident: in the collective statements of these hierarchies since 1990; in the actions of individual bishops such as Metropolitan Daniel of Moldova and Bukovina, Archbishop Khrizostom of Vilnius and Lithuania, Metropolitan Nicolae of Timişoara and the Banat, Metropolitan Kirill of Smolensk and Kaliningrad, and, lately, Patriarch Aleksii II himself; in the election of former dissident priest Vasyl Romaniuk as Patriarch Volodymyr of Kyyiv and All-

Ukraine (at least according to one of the rival Ukrainian Orthodox factions); and in significant publications such as the *Journal of the Moscow Patriarchate* and *Romanian Orthodox Church News*. Now that the price of prophecy is no longer so high in their native lands, more and more Russian, Ukrainian, and Romanian Church leaders appear willing to pay it.

But while a profound revision of the usual modes of public moral witnessing is, at last, under way, it still lags behind the remarkable social and political changes. Distinguished American observers have begun to notice the historic social significance and promising propects of Orthodoxy in Russia and the rest of Eastern Europe. For example, in what may prove to be a seminal essay in the summer 1993 issue of *Foreign Affairs* entitled "The Clash of Civilizations," Harvard political scientist Samuel P. Huntington suggested that a "Slavic Orthodox" civilization occupies a significant middle ground between the Western European and Islamic civilizations.[7] In a February 1994 issue of the *Wall Street Journal,* Jewish social commentator Irving Kristol pronounced "the re-emergence" of the Russian Orthodox Church "probably the most important single fact about post-Gorbachev Russia."[8] And in a May 1994 issue of *The New Republic,* Librarian of Congress James H. Billington—a long-time friend of the Russian Orthodox Church—waxed hopeful about its potential to fill the political and moral void left by Soviet Communism.[9] The question that must occupy us, however, is this: Will the Orthodox Churches rise to the occasion?

More specifically, having revived the truly representative *sobor* for the election of Patriarch Aleksii II in June 1990, will the Moscow Patriarchate find itself tempted, like its sister Orthodox jurisdictions in the United States, to achieve moral consensus by plebiscite? Will the ancient Orthodox Churches of Russia, Ukraine, and Romania, flexing their new democratic muscles, also seek unwisely to scatter their moral wisdom shotgun-like over a wide array of social issues, most of which are beyond their competence or proper moral purview? Will they swing from one extreme to another: from debilitating propaganda to pseudo-prophecy? We can only hope that restraint, selectivity, and prudence will be the watchwords in their new prophetic endeavors. Surely their recent history affords them a wealth of experiences of what to avoid at all costs in the new era.

The Orthodox jurisdictions in the United States have yet to demonstrate moral maturity. The remarkable solidarity and force of argument they demonstrated concerning the civil war in the former Yugoslavia may yet constitute for them a moral rite of passage. But scandalously divided and at odds with one another over petty concerns, these Churches usually find it easier to mimic their Protestant and Catholic counterparts than to achieve administrative unity through genuine humility and hard work. Only this kind of unity, it seems, would enable them to develop the institutional confidence based on strength of numbers to witness forcefully, prophetically, and consistently to the wider society. An American Orthodox Church with a membership in excess of four million would dwarf most Protestant denominations. It would no longer need the cobwebbed halls of the National Council of Churches to establish its "mainline" credentials. It would not feel a compulsive need to prove its "relevance" or its Americanism by trying to "influence" American society tangentially through numerous misbegotten "moral resolutions."

Until such administrative unity is achieved by the Orthodox jurisdictions in the United States, the temptation of a "Nestorian ecclesiology" will probably continue to prove irresistible. It would be profoundly ironic, indeed, if the morally reborn Orthodox Patriarchates in Russia, Ukraine, and Romania were to surpass the Orthodox in America as genuinely prophetic voices of Orthodox moral tradition.

Key to Notes

Notes

INTRODUCTION

1. Serge Schmemann, "Pre-1917 Ghosts Haunt a Bolshevik Holiday," *New York Times,* November 7, 1991, p. A1.

2. The undisputed autocephalous Churches include the ancient Patriarchates of Constantinople, Alexandria, Antioch, and Jerusalem, and the national Churches of Russia, Georgia, Serbia, Romania, Bulgaria, Cyprus, Greece, Albania, Poland, and the Czech Republic and Republic of Slovakia. Still lacking universal recognition are the Orthodox Church in America — to which Moscow granted independence in 1970 — and the Ukrainian Autocephalous Orthodox Church based in Kyyiv, which proclaimed its own independence, declared its primate a patriarch in 1990, and split into two competing factions, each with its own "patriarch of Kyyiv," in the autumn of 1993.

3. Bishop Nifon currently heads the diocese of Buzau. Before this assignment he was known as Nifon Ploieşteanul. Suffragan (or assistant) bishops in Romania are commonly identified by their titular see — in this case the city of Ploieşti.

4. Alexander F. C. Webster, "Orthodox Church Is Rent Over Dukakis," *Wall Street Journal,* October 13, 1988, p. A22.

5. See, for example, Alexander F. C. Webster, "Orthodox Battle of the Patriarchs," *Washington Times,* July 2, 1990, p. D3.

6. National Conference of Catholic Bishops, *The Challenge of Peace: God's Promise and Our Response (A Pastoral Letter on War and Peace)* (Washington, D.C.: United States Catholic Conference, 1983).

7. United Methodist Council of Bishops, *In Defense of Creation: The Nuclear Crisis and a Just Peace* (Nashville: Graded Press, 1986).

8. National Association of Evangelicals, *Guidelines: Peace, Freedom and Security Studies* (Wheaton, Ill.: National Association of Evangelicals, 1987), p. 3.

9. Stanley S. Harakas, *Toward Transfigured Life: The Theoria of Eastern Orthodox Ethics* (Minneapolis: Light and Life Publishing Co., 1983), p. 136.

10. See, for example, Alexander F. C. Webster, "More Than a Whisper," *National Catholic Register,* LXVII, no. 39 (September 29, 1991), 5.

11. For insights on the debate currently raging among Protestants and Roman Catholics over how to deal now with the collaboration of their churches with the East German secret police, the "Stasi," see Richard E. Koenig, "The Churches and the Stasi," *The Christian Century,* CIX, no. 13 (April 15, 1992), 396-99.

12. Allegation of Fr. Gleb Yakunin at a March 20, 1992, press conference in

Washington, D.C., co-sponsored by the Ethics and Public Policy Center and the Jamestown Foundation. This event is discussed in chapter 2. To be sure, in April 1992 the All-Russian Council of Bishops appointed a special commission chaired by 35-year-old Bishop Aleksandr of Kostroma to investigate the alleged KGB connections of Orthodox clergy. By November 1993, however, only one person, the scholarly monk-priest Damaskin Orlovsky, was actually delving into the KGB archives in pursuit of evidence. So reports Dimitry V. Pospielovsky, "The Russian Orthodox Church in the Post-Communist CIS" (paper presented at the Conference on Religion and Politics of the Russian Littoral Project, University of Maryland at College Park, November 10, 1993), p. 32.

CHAPTER 1

1. John Meyendorff, *Living Tradition: Orthodox Witness in the Contemporary World* (Crestwood, N.Y.: St. Vladimir's Seminary Press, 1978), pp. 7f.

2. Christos Yannaras, *The Freedom of Morality,* trans. Elizabeth Briere (Crestwood, N.Y.: St. Vladimir's Seminary Press, 1984), pp. 215, 216, 217f.

3. George W. Peters, *A Biblical Theology of Missions* (Chicago: Moody Press, 1972), pp. 21-31.

4. Sergius Bulgakov, *The Orthodox Church,* trans. Elizabeth S. Cram (New York: Morehouse Publishing Co. [1935]), p. 179.

5. Dumitru Staniloae, "Witness Through 'Holiness' of Life," in Ion Bria, ed., *Martyria/Mission: The Witness of the Orthodox Churches* (Geneva: World Council of Churches, 1980), pp. 47, 49.

6. Ion Bria, "The Church's Role in Evangelism: Icon or Platform?" *International Review of Mission,* LXIV (1975), 243-50.

7. Favorable assessments of the WCC by "insiders" include Philip Potter, *What in the World Is the World Council of Churches?* (Geneva: World Council of Churches, 1978), and Marlin VanElderen, *Introducing the World Council of Churches* (Geneva: World Council of Churches, 1990). Sharply critical views may be found in J. A. Emerson Vermaat, *The World Council of Churches and Politics* (New York: Freedom House, 1989), and Ernest W. Lefever's two-part critique, *Amsterdam to Nairobi: The World Council of Churches and the Third World* and *Nairobi to Vancouver: The World Council of Churches and the World, 1975-87* (Washington, D.C.: Ethics and Public Policy Center, 1979 and 1987).

8. I myself can attest, however, to the occasional value of WCC "consultations," having participated in one on the island of Rhodes, Greece, in October 1991 on the theme "Justice, Peace and the Integrity of Creation"—provided, that is, the Orthodox witness is firm, resolute, and authentic.

9. Detlef Urban, "A Crisis from the Beginning: Reflections on the 25th Anniversary of the Christian Peace Conference," *Occasional Papers on Religion in Eastern Europe,* V, no. 3 (May 1985), 19.

10. P. I. David, "The Christian Ecumenical Organizations in the Active Front for Defending Life and Peace," *Romanian Orthodox Church News,* XIII, no. 4 (October-December 1983), 73.

11. Quoted in Laslo .Revesz, *The Christian Peace Conference: Human Rights and*

Religion in the USSR, Conflict Studies no. 91 (London: Institute for the Study of Conflict, 1978), p. 4.

12. For a positive assessment of the CPC, see Ingo Roer, *Christian Peace Conference: A Place of Ecumenical Peace Work* (Prague: Information Department, Christian Peace Conference, 1974). A stinging denunciation is provided in Revesz, *The Christian Peace Conference.* For reluctant but firm criticisms from two American Protestants who are generally sympathetic to the aims of the CPC, see Wayne H. Cowan, "In Prague, Too Many One-Way Streets," *Christianity and Crisis,* XLV, no. 16 (October 16, 1985), 398-400, and Paul Mojzes, "Editorial," *Occasional Papers on Religion in Eastern Europe,* V, no. 3 (May 1985), i-iv.

13. Vitaly Borovoi, "The Problem of Co-Existence, as a 'Covenant of Life and Peace,'" *Christian Peace Conference,* nos. 11-12 (September 1964), p. 279.

14. William Yoder, "The Christian Peace Conference Is Facing Hard Times," *Occasional Papers on Religion in Eastern Europe,* XII, no. 3 (June 1992), 43f.

15. Sarah Vilankulu, ed., *Toward a Community of Communions: Triennial Report 1985-1987* (New York: Office of Information, National Council of Churches of Christ in the U.S.A., n.d.), inside front cover.

16. For one unrelentingly critical assessment, see Lloyd Billingsley, *From Mainline to Sideline: The Social Witness of the National Council of Churches* (Washington, D.C.: Ethics and Public Policy Center, 1990).

17. For an earlier, more hopeful assessment of this bold move, see my article, "Greek Orthodox Give Notice," *National Catholic Register,* LXVII, no. 32 (August 11, 1991), 5.

18. Larry Witham, "Church Councils Ask Carter's Help—and Reagan's, Too," *Washington Times,* June 26, 1993, p. A4.

19. Quoted in Larry Witham, "A State of Grace at NCC: Church Group Has Clinton's Attention," *Washington Times,* October 25, 1993, p. A1.

20. Quoted *ibid.,* pp. A1, A14.

21. Alexander Schmemann, *Church, World, Mission* (Crestwood, N.Y.: St. Vladimir's Seminary Press, 1979), pp. 193-208.

22. A strong case in favor of Orthodox ecumenism may be found in Gregory Wingenbach, *Broken, Yet Never Sundered* (Brookline, Mass.: Holy Cross Orthodox Press, 1978). For a corresponding argument against ecumenism, see George P. Macris, *The Orthodox Church and the Ecumenical Movement During the Period 1920-1969* (Seattle: St. Nectarios Press, 1986).

23. Text in Constantin G. Patelos, ed., *The Orthodox Church in the Ecumenical Movement: Documents and Statements 1902-1975* (Geneva: World Council of Churches, 1978), p. 89.

24. Synod of Bishops, Orthodox Church in America, *Christian Unity and Ecumenism* (New York: 1973), p. 9.

25. For more detailed explanations of these themes, see Alexander F. C. Webster, "The Pacifist Option: An Eastern Orthodox Moral Perspective on War in the Nuclear Age" (Ph.D. diss., University of Pittsburgh, 1988), pp. 198-218, and *idem,* "'Non-Revisionist' Orthodox Reflections on Justice, Peace, and the Integrity of Creation," *Greek Orthodox Theological Review,* XXXVII, nos. 3-4 (1992), 259-73.

26. Stanley S. Harakas, "The Morality of War," in Joseph J. Allen, ed., *Orthodox Synthesis: The Unity of Theological Thought* (Crestwood, N.Y.: St. Vladimir's Seminary Press, 1981), p. 87.

27. For a strong Orthodox affirmation of this position, see Stanley S. Harakas, "The N.C.C.B. Pastoral Letter, *The Challenge of Peace:* An Eastern Orthodox Response," in Charles J. Reid, Jr., *Peace in a Nuclear Age: The Bishops' Pastoral Letter in Perspective* (Washington, D.C.: Catholic University of America Press, 1986), p. 259. The original proponent of the term "justified war" in lieu of the more familiar "just war" was the Princeton University theologian Paul Ramsey. See, for example, his seminal work, *War and the Christian Conscience: How Shall Modern War Be Conducted Justly?* (Durham, N.C.: Duke University Press, 1961), p. 15.

28. Alexander F. C. Webster, "Just War and Holy War: Two Case Studies in Comparative Christian Ethics," *Christian Scholar's Review,* XV, no. 4 (1986), 358-61.

29. Other *jus ad bellum* conditions include a just cause, right intent, last resort, formal declaration of war, proportionality of violent means to desired ends, and a reasonable chance of success.

30. Stanley S. Harakas, *Contemporary Moral Issues Facing the Orthodox Christian,* 2d rev. ed. (Minneapolis: Light and Life Publishing Co., 1982), p. 130.

31. Stanley S. Harakas, "Human Rights: An Eastern Orthodox Perspective," *Journal of Ecumenical Studies,* XIX, no. 3 (Summer 1982), 14-16.

32. J. Roland Pennock, "Rights, Natural Rights, and Human Rights—A General View," in Pennock and John W. Chapman, eds., *Human Rights (NOMOS XXIII)* (New York: New York University Press, 1981), p. 7.

33. Harakas, "Human Rights," pp. 18, 19.

34. John W. Chapman, "Natural Rights and Justice in Liberalism," in D. D. Raphael, ed., *Political Theory and the Rights of Man* (Bloomington: Indiana University Press, 1967), p. 42.

35. Harakas, "Human Rights," p. 18.

36. *Ep.* 262 in Saint Basil, *The Letters,* IV, trans. Roy J. Deferrari (Cambridge: Harvard University Press, 1970), 85.

37. Harakas, *Contemporary Moral Issues,* p. 134.

38. *Ep. ad Diog.,* 7.4. English translation: Cyril C. Richardson, trans. and ed., *Early Christian Fathers* (New York: Macmillan Co., 1970), p. 219.

39. Lactantius, *Divinae Institutiones,* V.19. English translation: Lactantius, *The Divine Institutes,* trans. Sr. Mary Francis McDonald, O.P., The Fathers of the Church, vol. 49 (Washington, D.C.: Catholic University of America Press, 1964), p. 378.

40. Quoted in Jerome I. Cotsonis, "Freedom and Coercion in the Propagation of the Faith," *Greek Orthodox Theological Review,* IX, no. 1 (Summer 1963), 98.

41. *Ibid.*

42. St. Gregory of Nyssa, *De Opificio Hominis,* XVII.11. English translation: Gregory of Nyssa, "On the Making of Man," in Philip Schaff and Henry Wace, eds., *A Select Library of Nicene and Post-Nicene Fathers of the Christian Church,* V, 2d ser. (Grand Rapids: Eerdmans Publishing Co., 1975), p. 405.

43. Quoted in Archimandrite Vasileios, *Hymn of Entry: Liturgy and Life in the Orthodox Church* (Crestwood, N.Y.: St. Vladimir's Seminary Press, 1984), pp. 48-49.

44. *Ibid.,* p. 49.

45. Demetrios J. Constantelos, "Religious Minorities and the State in Sixth Century Byzantium," *St. Vladimir's Seminary Quarterly,* VII, no. 4 (1963), 198; Cotsonis, "Freedom and Coercion," p. 110; John S. Romanides, "The Orthodox

Churches on Church-State Relations and Religious Liberty," *Journal of Church and State,* VI (1964), 178-79.

46. Vasileios, *Hymn of Entry,* p. 49.

47. St. Athenagoras of Athens, *Presbeia peri Christianōn,* 2. English translation: Athenagoras, "A Plea for the Christians," in Alexander Roberts and James Donaldson, eds., *The Ante-Nicene Fathers,* II, American Reprint of the Edinburgh Edition (Grand Rapids: Eerdmans Publishing Co., 1956), 130.

48. Amos A. Jordan and William J. Taylor, Jr., *American National Security: Policy and Process* (Baltimore: Johns Hopkins University Press, 1981), p. 3.

49. *Ibid.,* p. 14.

50. Stanley S. Harakas, "Orthodox Church-State Theory and American Democracy," *Greek Orthodox Theological Review,* XXI, no. 4 (Winter 1976), 399.

51. *Epanagogē,* Titulus II and III. English translation in Ernest Barker, *Social and Political Thought in Byzantium: From Justinian I to the Last Palaeologus* (Oxford: Clarendon Press, 1957), pp. 89-93.

52. Steven Runciman, *The Byzantine Theocracy* (Cambridge: Cambridge University Press, 1977), p. 95.

53. Michael Azkoul, *Sacred Monarchy and the Modern Secular State* (Montreal: Monastery Press, 1984), pp. 13-14; Bulgakov, *The Orthodox Church,* pp. 185-86; Stanley S. Harakas, "The Orthodox Approach to Modern Trends," *St. Vladimir's Theological Quarterly,* XIII, no. 4 (1969), 7-8. I explored the propects of revived Orthodox monarchies in Bulgaria, Romania, and Serbia in a panel presentation at the January 1993 meeting of the Society of Christian Ethics. See the published text of my readers in "Kingdoms of God in the Balkans?" *East European Quarterly,* XXVII, no. 4 (Winter 1993), pp. 437-51.

54. John Meyendorff, *Byzantine Theology* (New York: Fordham University Press, 1974), p. 193.

55. Runciman, *The Byzantine Theocracy,* pp. 5-25. Cf. Alexander F. C. Webster, "Varieties of Christian Military Saints: From Martyrs Under Caesar to Warrior Princes," *St. Vladimir's Theological Quarterly,* XXIV, no. 1 (1980), 15-17.

56. This term was laid to rest in Deno Geanakoplos, "Church and State in the Byzantine Empire: A Reconsideration of the Problem of Caesaropapism," *Byzantine East and Latin West* (New York: Harper Torchbooks, 1966), pp. 57-83.

CHAPTER 2

1. See, for example, George Huntston Williams and Alexander F. C. Webster, "The Revolutionary Plight of Russian Orthodoxy," *The Unitarian Universalist Christian,* XXXI, nos. 3-4 (Autumn/Winter 1976), 71-109; Eugene B. Shirley, Jr., and Michael Rowe, eds., *Candle in the Wind: Religion in the Soviet Union* (Washington, D.C.: Ethics and Public Policy Center, 1989); and Kent Hill, *The Soviet Union on the Brink: An Inside Look at Christianity and Glasnost,* 2d rev. ed. (Portland, Ore.: Multnomah Press, 1991).

2. *JMP,* 1988, no. 7, p. 2.

3. *Ibid.,* p. 5.

4. Quoted in David Remnick, "Lenin's Birthday Less than Happy," *Washington Post,* April 22, 1991, p. A14.

5. Bill Keller, "Cult of the Last Czar Takes Root in Russia," *New York Times,* November 21, 1990, p. A1.

6. Serge Schmemann, "Pre-1917 Ghosts Haunt a Bolshevik Holiday," *New York Times,* November 7, 1991, p. A18.

7. Communiqué from the Permanent Mission of the U.S.S.R. at the United Nations to Angelo Vidal d'Almeida Ribeiro, Special Rapporteur to the Commission on Human Rights, cited in Third Annual Report, December 30, 1988, p. 45; Serge Schmemann, "A Moment of Rapture as a Saint Is Marched Home," *New York Times,* February 8, 1991, p. A4.

8. Pedro Ramet, "Gorbachev's Reforms and Religion," in Shirley and Rowe, *Candle in the Wind,* pp. 282-87; "Soviet Religious Growth Continues," *National Catholic Register,* LXVI, no. 44 (November 4, 1990), 9; Eugenia Ordynsky, "The Persecution of the Russian Orthodox Church and the Rise of 'Russian Nationalism,' " *Russian-American Review* (quarterly publication of the Congress of Russian Americans, Washington, D.C.), Fall 1990, pp. 1f; Serge Schmemann, "One Weight Rolls Away, and Russia Rejoices," *New York Times,* April 8, 1991, p. A5.

9. *Time,* April 10, 1989, p. 55; "Priests Elected for First Time to Parliament," *Report on the USSR* (Radio Liberty), I, no. 13 (March 31, 1989), 33; KNS no. 369 (February 21, 1991), p. 14.

10. "Church Council Meets," *TOC,* XXIV, no. 8 (August 1988), 4; Helen Bell and Jane Ellis, "The Millennium Celebrations of 1988 in the USSR," *RCL,* XVI, no. 4 (Winter 1988), 308-11.

11. Communiqué from the Permanent Representative of the Soviet Union at the United Nations to Angelo Vidal d'Almeida Ribeiro, Special Rapporteur to the Commission on Human Rights, quoted in Second Annual Report, January 6, 1988, p. 14. For the text of the 1929 Law, see "Religion in the USSR: Law, Policy, and Propaganda" (Appendix I), *The Orthodox Monitor* (Washington, D.C.), no. 15 (January-July 1983), 74-84.

12. See, for example, the early analyses in KNS no. 359 (September 27, 1990), pp. 15f., and KNS no. 365 (December 20, 1990), pp. 17-20.

13. "Agreement Between the Church and the State," *JMP,* 1993, no. 2, p. 9.

14. Coelestin Patock, O.S.A., "The Bishops of the Moscow Patriarchate Today," *RCL,* XV, no. 3 (Winter 1987), 279f; *Pravoslavni Tserkovni Kalendar 1992* (Moskva: Moskovskoï Patriarkhii, 1991), insert; updated figure in May 1994 by John B. Dunlop of the Hoover Institution.

15. Victor Orlov, "Putting the KGB in a Cassock: Why Moscow Is Infiltrating the Soviet Orthodox Church," *Washington Post,* July 17, 1988, p. C5.

16. Zoya Krakhmalnikova identified Patriarch Aleksii II as KGB agent "Drozdov" in *Novoe Russkoe Slovo,* March 3, 1992, p. 5 See also Michael Dobbs, "Business as Usual for Ex-KGB Agents," *Washington Post,* February 11, 1992, p. A11, and Fen Montaigne, "Orthodox Patriarch Said to be KGB Agent," *Philadelphia Inquirer,* May 3, 1992, p. A1. The first public interview with Fr. Gleb while the investigation was still in progress appeared in the January 1992 issue of the Russian monthly *Argumenti i Fakti.* For an English translation, see "Father Yakunin Says 20 Percent of USSR Clergy Worked for KGB," FBIS-USR-92-024 (March 5, 1992), p. 122. The March 20 press conference in Washington was reported the same day by Carl Rochelle of Cable News Network and John Roberts of Voice of America. Other stories were

filed within a week by Bill Bole of Religious News Service, Marcia Kunstel of Cox Newspapers, and Ted Okada of News Network International.

17. Quoted in Fr. Victor S. Potapov, "The Religious Revival in the USSR on the Eve of the Millennium," *RCDA*, XXVI, no. 2 (Spring 1987), 38. Archbishop John was scheduled to be canonized in July 1994 by the Russian Orthodox Church Outside Russia and known henceforth as St. John of Shanghai (China).

18. The portion of the Furov Report relevant to this chapter appeared as V. Furov, "Cadres of the Church and Legal Measures to Curtail Their Activities: A Report by the Council on Religious Affairs," *RCDA*, XIX, nos. 10-12 (1980), 149-61.

19. "Record of a Conversation with Synod Member Archbishop Alexis (Held at the Council on February 20, 1967)," *Glasnost Information Bulletin*, nos. 13-15 (October 1988), p. 5.

20. A. S. Plekhanov, "Report on Pimen, Metropolitan of Leningrad and Ladoga," *Glasnost Information Bulletin*, nos. 13-15 (October 1988), pp. 3f.

21. "Record of a Conversation with Synod Member Archbishop Alexis," p. 5.

22. Dmitry Pospielovsky, *The Russian Church Under the Soviet Regime 1917-1982*, II (Crestwood, N.Y.: St. Vladimir's Seminary Press, 1984), p. 392.

23. Williams and Webster, "The Revolutionary Plight of Russian Orthodoxy," pp. 77-79.

24. See his official biography in *JMP*, 1990, no. 9, pp. 40-43.

25. See his official biography in *JMP*, 1979, no. 4, pp. 25-31.

26. "Orthodox Metropolitan a Catholic Bishop?" KNS no. 291 (January 7, 1988), p. 4.

27. Cited in Michael Bourdeaux, *Patriarchs and Prophets: Persecution of the Russian Orthodox Church* (London: Mowbray and Co., 1970), pp. 153f., 172f., 284, 331f.

28. "Metropolitan Nikodim Remembered," *RCL*, VI, no. 4 (1978), 229f.

29. John B. Dunlop, "KGB Subversion of Russian Orthodox Church," *RFE/RL Research Report*, I, no. 12 (March 20, 1992), 52; Anthony Ugolnik, "The Orthodox Church and Contemporary Politics in the USSR: A Special Report to the National Council of Soviet and East European Research" (unpublished report, November 1991), p. 43.

30. Quoted in *Time*, June 18, 1990, p. 71.

31. Fax from Moscow of Russian text: "Opredelenie Arkhiereïskogo Sobora Russkoï Pravoslavnoï Tserkvi" (April 2, 1992). The crucial language is "blagoslovil nesti episkopskoe sluzhenie na drugoï kafedre Ukrainskoï Pravoslavnoï Tserkvi." An incorrect report overstating the severity of the *sobor*'s action apparently was furnished by Professor Dimitry Pospielovsky to Larry Witham, "Russian Church Leader 'Retired' for Bad Behavior," *Washington Times*, April 11, 1992, p. D4.

32. Telegram from Patriarch Aleksii II to Metropolitan Theodosius in New York printed in *Orthodox Church in America (OCA) News* (Syosset, N.Y.), July 17, 1992, p. 2. Though previously silent about Filaret's immoral lifestyle, Dmitry V. Pospielovsky, a Canadian member of the Orthodox Church in America who fervently supports the Moscow Patriarchate, cited it publicly in "The Russian Orthodox Church in the Post-Communist CIS" (unpublished paper presented at the Conference on Religion and Politics of the Russian Littoral Project, University of Maryland at College Park, November 10, 1993), pp. 16f.

33. Jim Forest, "Bishop Blasts Russian Orthodox Mediocrity," *National Catholic Reporter*, XXVI, no. 30 (May 18, 1990), 11f.

34. English translation of text in Matthew Spinka, *The Church in Soviet Russia* (New York: Oxford University Press, 1956), pp. 161-65.

35. Alexander F. C. Webster, "Concerning Christians in the Soviet Military: Several Russian Orthodox Views," *Diakonia*, XIII, no. 2 (1978), 148.

36. Quoted in Stanley Evans, *The Churches in the U.S.S.R.* (London: Cobbett Publishing Co., 1943), p. 122.

37. Quoted in William C. Fletcher, *A Study in Survival: The Church in Russia 1927-1943* (New York: Macmillan Co., 1965), pp. 109f. Italics added.

38. *JMP*, 1984, no. 1, p. 4.

39. *JMP*, 1984, no. 3, p. 3.

40. *JMP*, 1988, no. 7, pp. 4f.

41. *JMP*, 1985, no. 8, p. 17.

42. Alexander F. C. Webster, "The Canonical Validity of Military Service by Orthodox Christians," *Greek Orthodox Theological Review*, XXIII, nos. 3-4 (Fall/Winter 1978), 257-81.

43. William Van Den Bercken, "Holy Russia and the Soviet Fatherland," *RCL*, XV, no. 3 (Winter 1987), 270-73.

44. Text in Pospielovsky, *The Russian Church*, p. 492 (Appendix 5).

45. *JMP*, 1977, no. 12, p. 4.

46. *JMP*, 1987, no. 11, p. 2.

47. *Ibid.*, p. 6.

48. Archbishop Nikodim, "Peace and Freedom," *Christian Peace Conference*, no. 4 (May 1963), pp. 98-100.

49. Aleksii Osipov, "Theological Aspects of Human Rights," *JMP*, 1984, no. 5, pp. 51-56.

50. Valery Lobachev and Vladimir Pravotorov, *A Millennium of Russian Orthodoxy* (Moscow: Novosti Press Agency Publishing House, 1988), p. 107.

51. Quoted in Fletcher, *A Study in Survival*, p. 49.

52. Quoted in "Russian Hierarchs Deny Religious Persecution," *TOC*, XVI, no. 5 (May 1980), 2.

53. Patriarch Pimen, *The Baptism of Rus 1000 Years Ago Determined, to a Large Extent, the Development of the Peoples of Our Country,* Expert Opinion series (Moscow: Novosti Press Agency Publishing House, n.d.), p. 9.

54. "Statement by Metropolitan Yuvenaly," *RCL*, III, nos. 1-3 (January-June 1975), 24.

55. See, for example, Ernest W. Lefever, *Nairobi to Vancouver: The World Council of Churches and the World, 1975-87* (Washington, D.C.: Ethics and Public Policy Center, 1987), pp. 63-70, and J. A. Emerson Vermaat, *The World Council of Churches and Politics* (New York: Freedom House, 1989), pp. 9-25.

56. Quoted in Pospielovsky, *The Russian Church*, p. 446.

57. Quoted in Pospielovsky, "Metropolitan Nikodim Remembered," p. 230.

58. FBIS-SOV-90-235 (December 6, 1990), p. 49.

59. Joint Publications Research Service, Soviet Union Political Affairs (JPRS-UPA), 91-042 (October 7, 1991), p. 69.

60. Fax of "provisional" English translation of text from Moscow Patriarchate to Chancery of Orthodox Church in America, Syosset, N.Y., September 13, 1991, p. 3.

61. Untitled text furnished by Georgetown University in special press packet.

62. *Information Bulletin* (Department of External Relations, Moscow Patriarchate), no. 5 (March 15, 1993).

63. News items in *Path*, XXVI, no. 2 (February 1991), 10, and *TOC*, XXVII, no. 1 (January 1991), 10.

64. The patriarch's refusal to repent eventually led to a schism within the Bulgarian Holy Synod. The pro-Maksim faction on July 22, 1992, even excommunicated Fr. Khristofor — now Bishop Khristofor of Makaripol and an elected member of parliament. The anti-Maksim faction, led by Metropolitan Pimen of Novrokop is — as of June 1994 — clearly on the defensive, as the primates of several autocephalous Orthodox Churches including Patriarch Aleksii II of Moscow have closed ranks behind the embattled Maksim. Reports questioning Khristofor's mental stability have also surfaced among unimpeachable observers of the Bulgarian scene. See, for example, Spas Raikin, "Schism in the Bulgarian Orthodox Church," *Religion in Eastern Europe* (formerly *Occasional Papers on Religion in Eastern Europe*), XIII, no. 1 (February 1993), 19-25.

65. For documentation on this case, see Bourdeaux, *Patriarchs and Prophets*, pp. 221-23, 239-41, 247-54.

66. *JMP*, 1975, no. 5, p. 4.

67. Pospielovsky, *The Russian Church*, p. 448.

68. V. Furov, "Cadres of the Church and Legal Measures to Curtail Their Activities," *RCDA*, XX, nos. 1-3 (1981), 11.

69. "Moscow Patriarchate Against Solzhenitsyn," *RCDA*, XIII, nos. 3-4 (March-April 1974), 39f.

70. "Two Responses of Moscow Patriarchate Defend Solzhenitsyn," *RCDA*, XIII, nos. 3-4 (March-April 1974), 41.

71. Personal interview in College Park, Maryland, November 11, 1993. Cf. the contrasting coverage in Kim A. Lawton, "Russian Orthodox Church Defrocks Fr. Gleb Yakunin," *News Network International*, November 14, 1993, p. 6f., and "Dissident Russian Priest Deposed," *OCA News*, November 1993, p. 3. Fr. Gleb issued a press release on November 5, 1993, that also cites a decision of the All-Russian Orthodox *Sobor* on August 15, 1918, permitting a priest to engage in political activities as a civic duty on his own behalf but not in the name of the Church. But that *sobor* met under extreme duress, with the Bolsheviks about to crush the Church. In the current precarious — but not dire — political climate of Russia, the Holy Synod has seized the higher moral ground by endeavoring to keep active priests out of political office, where their spiritual and moral leadership would invariably be compromised. For an analysis of the Church canons on this issue, see my essay cited in n. 42 above.

72. Figures provided by Metropolitan Nikodim of Lvov and Ternopol in *JMP*, 1986, no. 8, p. 15.

73. "Statement on Religious Freedom in Eastern Europe and the Soviet Union," *Origins: NC Documentary Service*, XVIII, no. 26 (December 8, 1988), 420. For a more detailed history of recent events by a Ukrainian Catholic scholar, see Bohdan R. Bociurkiw, "The Ukrainian Catholic Church in the USSR Under Gorbachev," *Problems of Communism*, XXXIX, no. 6 (November-December 1990), 1-19, and *idem*, "Politics and Religion in Ukraine: The Orthodox and the Greek Catholics" (unpublished paper presented at the Conference on Religion and Politics of the Russian Littoral Project, University of Maryland at College Park, November 11, 1993).

74. Quoted in "Statement on Religious Freedom in Eastern Europe and the Soviet Union," p. 420.

75. *JMP*, 1986, no. 7, p. 5.

76. *JMP*, 1986, no. 8, p. 5.

77. *Ibid.*, p. 6.

78. *JMP*, 1986, no. 7, p. 3.

79. *Ibid.*, p. 6.

80. Myroslaw Tataryn, "Russian Orthodox Attitudes Towards the Ukrainian Catholic Church," *RCL*, XVII, no. 4 (Winter 1989), 323.

81. Quoted in Patricia Lefevre, "Ecumenical Movement Best Place for Orthodox/Uniate Talks," *Occasional Papers on Religion in Eastern Europe,* IX, no. 6 (November 1989), 35.

82. "Statement of the Hierarchy of the Ukrainian Greek Catholic Church in Ukraine," *ABN Correspondence* (Bulletin of the Anti-Bolshevik Bloc of Nations), XLI, no. 3 (May-June 1990), 25-28.

83. "Dialogues," *National Catholic Reporter,* LXVI, no. 21 (May 27, 1990), 9.

84. Ugolnik, "The Orthodox Church and Contemporary Politics," pp. 56-57.

85. Reported in Moscow by TASS in English, December 27, 1989. Text reprinted in FBIS-SOV-90-003, (January 4, 1990), pp. 95f. This charge was renewed by the Patriarchate in an April 11, 1990, statement by the Department of External Church Relations. Fax printed in *OCA News* (Syosset, N.Y.), May 5, 1990, p. 2. More details of the violence were reported by Patriarch Aleksii himself on August 29, 1990, in another fax to Metropolitan Theodosius of the Orthodox Church in America. Text in *OCA News,* September 7, 1990, p. 1. Ugolnik, "The Orthodox Church and Contemporary Politics," pp. 4, 47f., reports that he "saw firsthand" several battles in Ukraine — particularly in Druhabych — over church property.

86. At a conference in Washington, D.C., sponsored by the United States Institute of Peace as recently as June 1990, Jane Ellis still insisted that "no specific case of actual violence has emerged." See the report and analysis of this event (at which I offered a critical response) in David Little, *Ukraine: The Legacy of Intolerance* (Washington, D.C.: U.S. Institute of Peace, 1991), pp. 43f.

87. Quoted in Patricia Lefevre, "Vatican Ecumenist Says Catholics to Play Second Fiddle in Ukraine," *National Catholic Reporter,* XXVIII, no. 18 (March 6, 1992), 2. Metropolitan Spyridon Papagheorghiou of Venice, who did attend on behalf of the Ecumenical Patriarchate, read a stinging rebuke of Catholic proselytism, which surprised the assembled bishops. For the text of this speech, see "Orthodox Metropolitan Reports on Orthodox-Catholic Conflict," *Origins: CNS Documentary Service,* XXL, no. 29 (December 26, 1991), 466f.

88. Final text in English furnished by Fr. Miltiades Efthimiou of the Greek Orthodox Archdiocese in New York.

89. "Thousands Greet Ukrainian Orthodox Patriarch," *The Ukrainian Review,* XXXVIII, no. 4 (Winter 1990), 72f.; KNS no. 363 (November 22, 1990), pp. 15-17; KNS no. 365 (December 20, 1990), pp. 7f.; JPRS-UPA-91-005 (January 29, 1991), pp. 73-77.

90. English translation of text provided by Fr. Serge Kelleher of Keston College, Oxford, England. The Ukrainian original of these controversial remarks reads as follows: "Vy zberehly tserkovne sokrovyshche, jake nalezhyt' do vsikh nas. Vash synod

je spadkojemtsem Kyivs'kykh Mytropolytiv." See also Leila Preloc, "Ukrainian Church Seeks Bridge-Building Role," *National Catholic Register,* LXVIII, no. 26 (July 5, 1992), 1.

91. Peter Hebblethwaite, "Ukrainians Bickering Toward Ecumenism," *National Catholic Register,* XXXVIII, no. 37 (August 28, 1992), 12.

92. Among the attendees at the funeral rites for Mstyslav on June 21-23 at the headquarters of the Ukrainian Orthodox Church of the U.S.A. in South Bound Brook, New Jersey, were Bishop Vsevolod Majdanski of the Ukrainian Orthodox Church of America (Ecumenical Patriarchate), Bishop Nicholas Smisko of the American Carpatho-Russian Orthodox Diocese (Ecumenical Patriarchate), and four Ukrainian Catholic bishops based in the United States, who represented Cardinal Myroslav Lyubachevskij of Lviv. *UOW,* XXVI, no. 5 (July-August 1993), 1.

93. For these somewhat conflicting numerical claims, see "Metropolitan Volodymyr on Interdenominational Conflicts," FBIS-USR-94-013 (February 14, 1994), p. 52; Marta Kolomayets, "UOC Enthrones Patriarch Volodymyr," *The Ukrainian Weekly* (Jersey City, N.J.), LXI, no. 44 (October 31, 1993), 1; Bociurkiw, "Politics and Religion in Ukraine," p. 25.

94. Quoted in Hebblethwaite, "Ukrainians Bickering Toward Ecumenism," p. 12.

95. "The Grace of a New Beginning" (Papal Address to the Ukrainian Bishops), *Catholic International,* I, no. 2 (October 16-31, 1990), 68.

96. Quoted in KNS no. 366 (January 10, 1991), p. 11. To be sure, Keston College reported subsequently that a source in the Moscow Patriarchate contends that Patriarch Aleksii did not sign the letter in its final form. But there has been no official disavowal of the signature. KNS no. 369 (February 21, 1991), p. 5.

97. *JMP,* 1989, no. 9, p. 6.

98. *JMP,* 1990, no. 9, p. 26.

99. FBIS-SOV-90-125 (June 28, 1990), p. 101.

100. *JMP,* 1990, no. 9, pp. 9-11.

101. FBIS-SOV-91-161 (August 10, 1991), pp. 57f.

102. Fax of "Statement" from Moscow Patriarchate to Chancery of Orthodox Church in America, Syosset, N.Y., September 13, 1991.

103. Fax of Patriarch Aleksii's "Appeal" from Moscow Patriarchate to Chancery of Orthodox Church in America, Syosset, N.Y., September 13, 1991. Cf. David Remnick, "Russians Wondering: 'Who Are We Now?'" *Washington Post,* December 30, 1991, p. A10.

104. *JMP,* 1993, no. 3, p. 8.

105. The principal source for this quote and the chronology of events is *OCA News,* October 10, 1993, pp. 3f.

106. An earlier version of portions of this section appeared in Williams and Webster, "The Revolutionary Plight of Russian Orthodoxy," pp. 85-89.

107. Aleksandr Solzhenitsyn, *A Lenten Letter to Patriarch Pimen of All Russia* (Minneapolis: Burgess Publishing Co., 1972).

108. David Remnick, "KGB Plot to Assassinate Solzhenitsyn Reported," *Washington Post,* April 21, 1992, p. D1.

109. See, for example, Valery Chalidze, "Solzhenitsyn's Authoritarian Russian Nationalism," *Russia,* 1981, no. 3, pp. 13-24, and Mihajlo Mihajlov, "The Return of

the Grand Inquisitor: A Critique of Solzhenitsyn," *Journal of Interdisciplinary Studies,* I, no. 1-2 (1989), 85-100.

110. For excerpts of this text in translation, see *New York Times,* September 19, 1990, p. A8.

111. English translation of text in *The Orthodox Monitor* (Washington, D.C.), no. 16 (August 1984), pp. 64-67.

112. *Ibid.,* p. 67.

113. Quoted in "Senator Robert Kasten on the Krakhmalnikova Case," *The Orthodox Monitor,* no. 15 (January-July 1983), p. 29.

114. Felix Svetov, "Appeal to Primates of All Orthodox Churches," *The Orthodox Monitor,* no. 15 (1983), p. 20.

115. Dimitry Pospielovsky, "Russian Nationalism and the Orthodox Revival," *RCL,* XV, no. 3 (Winter 1987), 300f.

116. Zoya Krakhmalnikova, "Orthodox Christians Must Still Carry a Soviet Cross," *Glasnost,* II, no. 5 (January-March 1990), 24-28.

117. English translation of Russian original (in *Ogonyek,* nos. 18-19 [1992]) in John B. Dunlop, "The Russian Orthodox Church as an 'Empire-Saving' Institution" (paper presented at the Conference on Religion and Politics of the Russian Littoral Project, University of Maryland at College Park, November 10, 1993), p. 24.

118. For a more detailed account of the witness of the dissidents, see the magisterial work by Jane Ellis, *The Russian Orthodox Church: A Contemporary History* (Bloomington: Indiana University Press, 1986), pp. 287-454.

119. For the text of this extraordinary appeal, see *RCDA,* XIV, nos. 10-12 (1975), 161-66.

120. Ellis, *The Russian Orthodox Church,* p. 379.

121. KNS no. 349 (May 3, 1990), p. 4.

122. Text in Bourdeaux, *Patriarchs and Prophets,* pp. 209, 210f.

123. Text in "Documents" section, *RCL,* VI, no. 1 (Spring 1978), 33f.

124. "Letter to Mikhail Gorbachev by Russian Orthodox Clergymen and Laymen," *RCDA,* XXVI, no. 3 (Summer 1987), 76.

125. Text in *TOC,* XXV, nos. 3-4 (March-April 1989), 10.

126. "Interview with Father Gleb Yakunin," *Uncaptive Minds,* V, no. 2 (Summer 1992), 35.

127. Quoted in "Russian Orthodox Legislator Urges U.S. Support for Yeltsin," *National Catholic Reporter,* XXIX, no. 43 (October 8, 1993), 6.

128. *JMP,* 1993, no. 2, p. 12. To be sure, the Patriarchate's anxieties about foreign missionaries are not without some foundation in fact. Cf., for example, the scurrilous disinformation contained in a "Russia Field Report" circulated in autumn 1993 by Mike Evans Ministries, a fundamentalist Protestant missionary group based in Texas:

> What you were not able to see in the news is that the Russian Orthodox Church is at the very center of the conflict in Russia. One of the greatest battles in history is being fought with the Russian Orthodox Church to take over the nation of Russia. They would be more than delighted to kill tens of millions of Bible-believing Christians in Russia. As shocking as it may sound, the majority of Russian Orthodox priests in leadership are also Communists. As you can see from the following paragraph from the Archbishop of the Russian Orthodox Church, it was his mobilization of 60 million Russian Orthodox that

convinced Parliament to unanimously pass a resolution to throw out all evangelicals in the nation.

In the controversy over the proposed legislation, the methods—not the motives—of the Patriarchate were questionable.

129. Quoted in "Russian Parliament Clamps Down on Foreign Missionaries," *TOC*, XXIX, nos. 7-8 (July/August 1993), 8.

130. Trevor Beeson, *Discretion and Valour: Religious Conditions in Russia and Eastern Europe*, 2d rev. ed. (Philadelphia: Fortress Press, 1982), p. 21.

131. Quoted in *Washington Post*, January 17, 1991, p. A18.

132. Quoted in "Arkhiepiskop Khrizostom: KGB Platil Komplimentami," *Rossiskaya Gazeta*, March 4, 1992, p. 7.

133. English translation in Mikhail Pozdnyayev, " 'I Cooperated With the KGB . . . But I Was Not an Informer': An Interview With Archbishop Khrizostom of Vilnius and Lithuania," *Religion, State and Society*, XXI, nos. 3-4 (1993), 347.

134. Archbishop Kirill of Smolensk and Vyazma, "Renewal of Humanity, Unity of the Church and the New Thinking," *Ecumenical Review*, XL, no. 2 (April 1988), 261.

135. *Ibid.*, p. 266.

136. JPRS-UPA-91-001-L (January 14, 1991), p. 33.

137. *JMP*, 1990, no. 6, p. 17.

138. This alleged incident was first reported in Lawrence Uzzell, "Patriarch Aleksii: The Last Soviet Man," *Wall Street Journal Europe*, January 7, 1992, p. 10. I have also obtained copies of the internal memoranda between the State Department and the U.S. Information Agency. These documents leave no doubt as to the accuracy of Uzzell's charge and the journalistic balance of Fr. Victor's broadcasts.

139. For a subsequent reaffirmation of this decision, see "Epistle of the Council of Bishops of the Russian Orthodox Church Outside Russia" (October 1991), *Orthodox Life*, XL, no. 6 (November-December 1991), 11. For a hard-hitting critique of the "schism" and "false teachings" that undergird what he deems the Russian Orthodox Church Outside Russia's untimely opportunism in Russia, see Fr. Robert Kondratick, "Why Deepen the Schism?" *TOC*, XXVI, no. 9-10 (September-October 1990), 3. Ironically, Fr. Victor Potapov also has criticized his own hierarchy for its "uncanonical" and "scandalous" role in establishing a rival jurisdiction in Russia that clearly implies that the Moscow Patriarchate is not a real Church instead of merely a "sick" Church. See the interview of him by Yulia Goryacheva, "Protiv ili Vmeste," *Nezavisimaya Gazeta*, January 27, 1994, p. 5.

140. "Epistle to the Children of the Free Russian Orthodox Church, Beloved in the Lord," in *Orthodox Life*, XL, no. 6 (November-December 1991), 27.

141. Pospielovsky, "The Russian Orthodox Church in the Post-Communist CIS," pp. 43, 50, 56.

142. Dunlop, "The Russian Orthodox Church as an 'Empire-Saving' Institution," p. 27. Nor is the Russian Orthodox Church Outside Russia immune from this political contagion. In his interview, "Protiv ili Vmeste," Fr. Victor Potapov also denounced the "flirtation with Pamjat" (an anti-Semitic neo-fascist organization) by some of his own bishops, which has "scandalized" many in that Church and elsewhere. According to Pospielovsky, "The Russian Orthodox Church in the Post-Com-

munist CIS," p. 40, Metropolitan Vitaly, primate of the Russian Orthodox Church Outside Russia, has subscribed in print to the notion of an international Zionist-Masonic conspiracy to destroy Russia and its Orthodox Church. To complicate matters further, Fr. Victor Potapov reported in a conversation with me on February 21, 1994, that in the autumn of 1993 Dmitry Vassiliev, head of Pamyat, joined the Moscow Patriarchate and even received holy communion from Patriarch Aleksii himself. Church life in Russia and Ukraine often defies rational explanation.

143. Furov, "Cadres of the Church," p. 150.

144. Text of interview in "Aleksiï II," *Moscow News,* no. 16 (April 17-24, 1994), p. II A.

CHAPTER 3

1. Keith Hitchins, "The Sacred Cult of Nationality: Rumanian Intellectuals and the Church in Transylvania, 1834-1869," in Stanley B. Winters and Joseph Held, eds., *Intellectual and Social Developments in the Habsburg Monarchy to World War I* (Boulder, Colo.: East European Quarterly, 1975), p. 148.

2. Alexander F. C. Webster, *The Romanian Legionary Movement: An Orthodox Christian Assessment of Anti-Semitism,* Carl Beck Papers, no. 502 (Pittsburgh: Center for Russian and East European Studies, University of Pittsburgh, 1986), pp. 38-42.

3. Walter M. Bacon, Jr., "Romania: Neo-Stalinism in Search of Legitimacy," *Current History,* LXXX, no. 465 (April 1981), 171; Vladimir Tismaneanu, "Byzantine Rites, Stalinist Follies: The Twilight of Dynastic Socialism in Romania," *Orbis,* XXX, no. 1 (Spring 1986), 83; Michael Shafir, "The Men of the Archangel Revisited: Anti-Semitic Formations Among Communist Romania's Intellectuals," *Studies in Comparative Communism,* XVI, no. 3 (Autumn 1983), 227, 237n.68; Eugen Weber, "Romania," in Weber and H. Rogger, eds., *The European Right* (Berkeley: University of California Press, 1966), p. 567.

4. Ion Mihai Pacepa, *Red Horizons: Chronicles of a Communist Spy Chief* (Washington, D.C.: Regnery Gateway, 1987), pp. 50, 181.

5. Mark Almond, *Decline Without Fall: Romania Under Ceauşescu,* European Security Studies, no. 6 (London: Institute for European Defence and Strategic Studies, 1988), p. 20.

6. Alexander F. C. Webster, "New Reign of Terror on the Danube," *The Wanderer,* CXXIII, no. 2 (January 11, 1990), 4+.

7. Almond, *Decline Without Fall,* p. 9.

8. Quoted *ibid.,* p. 13.

9. Dinu Giurescu, *The Razing of Romania's Past* (Washington, D.C.: U.S. Committee, International Council on Monuments and Sites, 1989), p. 67.

10. Srdjan Trifkovic, "Romanians Seek Sanctuary in Yugoslavia, Hungary," *Washington Times,* April 17, 1989, p. A7.

11. Jonas Bernstein, "Ceauşescu Remains Unrepentant," *Insight (On the News),* V, no. 29 (July 29, 1989), 26.

12. Bacon, "Romania: Neo-Stalinism," p. 169.

13. See, for example, Christine Bohlen, "Fight Against AIDS Lags in Romania," *New York Times,* May 9, 1990, p. A10, and Mary Battiata, "A Ceauşescu Legacy: Warehouses for Children," *Washington Post,* June 7, 1990, p. A1.

14. Tismaneanu, "Byzantine Rites," p. 74.

15. *Amnesty International Report 1988* (London: Amnesty International Publications, 1988), p. 210.

16. Bernstein, "Ceauşescu Remains Unrepentant," p. 28.

17. FBIS-EEU-90-247 (December 24, 1990), p. 43.

18. See, for example, her open letter to the FSN government published on June 2, 1990, in *România Liberă.* English translation in *Uncaptive Minds,* III, no. 3 (May-July 1990), 10.

19. Press conference at National Forum Foundation in Washington, D.C., April 11, 1991. For the initial "Declaration of the Civic Alliance," see *Uncaptive Minds,* IV, no. 1 (Spring 1991), 48-50.

20. David Binder, "U.S. Offers Measure of Approval to Romania," *New York Times,* April 1, 1992, p. A11. Cf. the more anxious views of William McPherson, "On Democracy's Edge," *Washington Post* (Outlook Section), March 22, 1992, p. C1+.

21. FBIS-EEU-94-021 (February 1, 1994), p. 27

22. FBIS-EEU-94-034 (February 18, 1994), p. 26.

23. "News in Brief: Romania," *RCL,* V, no. 2 (Summer 1977), 122.

24. Robert Tobias, *Communist-Christian Encounter in East Europe* (Indianapolis: School of Religion Press, 1956), p. 322.

25. Quoted *ibid.,* p. 324.

26. English translation of text *ibid.,* p. 342.

27. English translation of text *ibid.,* p. 339.

28. To be sure, in 1864 Prince Alexander Cuza of the newly united Romanian principalities announced that henceforth bishops would be nominated by the ministry of cults. Whatever machinations this political interference entailed, however, were nothing compared to the clearly enunciated aim of the Communist regime to extirpate religion in Romania. See Alf Johansen, "The Relations of the Rumanian Orthodox Church with Other Churches," *Occasional Papers on Religion in Eastern Europe,* V, no. 4 (August 1985), 4f.

29. English translation of text in Tobias, *Communist-Christian Encounter,* pp. 340-47.

30. English translation of text *ibid.,* pp. 349f.

31. Roman Braga and Gheorghe Calciu-Dumitreasa, "The Church in Romania Under Communist Rule," *Solia,* LI, no. 2 (February 1986), 7-9.

32. Trevor Beeson, *Discretion and Valour: Religious Conditions in Russia and Eastern Europe,* 2d rev. ed. (Philadelphia: Fortress Press, 1982), p. 368; Dionisie Ghermani, "The Orthodox Church in Romania," *RCDA,* XXVII, no. 1 (Winter 1988), 24.

33. Beeson, *Discretion and Valour,* p. 371; Ghermani, "The Orthodox Church in Romania," pp. 24f.

34. Earl A. Pope, "The Contemporary Religious Situation in Romania," in Dennis J. Dunn, ed., *Religion and Communist Society* (Berkeley: Berkeley Slavic Specialties, 1983), pp. 122, 148.

35. Ghermani, "The Orthodox Church in Romania," p. 25; Janice A. Broun, "Rumania's Churches Behind the Facade of Liberalism," *America,* CL, no. 9 (March 10, 1984), 167f.

36. Janice Broun, *Conscience and Captivity: Religion in Eastern Europe* (Washington, D.C.: Ethics and Public Policy Center, 1988), p. 219.

37. FBIS-EEU-90-223 (November 19, 1990), p. 64.

38. *ROCN,* XXI, no. 1 (January-February, 1991), 4.

39. Keith Hutchins, "The Romanian Orthodox Church and the State," in Bohdan R. Bociurkiw and John W. Strong, eds., *Religion and Atheism in the USSR and Eastern Europe* (London: Macmillan Press, 1975), p. 320.

40. Alan Scarfe, "Patriarch Justinian of Romania: His Early Social Thought," *RCL,* V, no. 3 (Autumn 1977), p. 169 no. 26.

41. *ROCN,* VII, no. 1 (January-March 1977), 6.

42. Ghermani, "The Orthodox Church in Romania," p. 25.

43. *JMP,* 1986, no. 11, p. 49.

44. According to Fr. Gheorghe Calciu in a personal interview in Washington, D.C., January 22, 1990. Officials of the Patriarchate denied this contention during my visit to Romania in September 1990.

45. Quoted in April 8 issue of *România Liberă.* FBIS-EEU-90-072 (April 13, 1990), p. 50.

46. *JMP,* 1987, no. 4, p. 39.

47. *ROCN,* XVI, no. 4 (October-December 1986), p. 62.

48. Earlier versions of this section appeared in Alexander F. C. Webster, "Romanian Church Seeks to Cleanse Itself," *The Christian Century,* CVIII, no. 11 (April 3, 1991), 358, and in *idem,* "Prophecy and Propaganda in the Romanian Orthodox Patriarchate," *East European Quarterly,* XXV, no. 4 (January 1992), 523f.

49. See, for example, Daniel Ciobotea, "The Problem of a Vital and Coherent Theology in the WCC," *ROCN,* XVIII, no. 2 (March-April 1989), 37-43, and *idem,* "The Task of Orthodox Theology Today," *St. Vladimir's Theological Quarterly,* XXXIII, no. 2 (1989), 117-26.

50. FBIS-EEU-90-124 (June 27, 1990), p. 71.

51. Dionisie Ghermani, "The Orthodox Church Press Under Balkan Communism," *RCDA,* XXIII, nos. 10-12 (1984), 156.

52. *ROCN,* IV, no. 3 (July-September 1974), 4.

53. *ROCN,* XIII, no. 1 (January-March 1983), 7.

54. *ROCN,* XV, no. 1 (January-March 1985), 5.

55. *ROCN,* VIII, no. 1 (January-March 1978), 9.

56. Quoted in Hutchins, "The Romanian Orthodox Church," p. 321.

57. Quoted in Tobias, *Communist-Christian Encounter,* p. 326.

58. Ghermani, "The Orthodox Church in Romania," p. 23.

59. *ROCN,* XVIII, no. 1 (January-February 1988), 4-6.

60. Quoted in Associated Press wire story in *Washington Times,* December 25, 1989, p. A10.

61. Quoted *ibid.,* p. A1.

62. Quoted in Andrew Borowiec, "Romanian Church Blesses Revolution," *Washington Times,* January 3, 1990, p. A7.

63. Vasile Tîrgovişteanul, "The Romanian Orthodox Church Today," in James E. Will, ed., *Must Walls Divide?* (New York: Friendship Press, 1981), p. 80. Bishop Vasile's surname is Costin. See Introduction, n. 3.

64. (Metropolitan) Antonie of Transylvania, "Ecuview: The Church in Romania," *Ecumenical Press Service* 86.03.41.

65. *ROCN,* IV, no. 3 (July-September 1974), 4.

66. *ROCN,* VIII, no. 1 (January-March 1978), 8. This language is repeated verbatim in *ROCN,* XIII, no. 1 (January-March 1983), 7.

67. *ROCN,* XVIII, no. 1 (January-March 1988), 6.

68. Antonie, "Ecuview."

69. Peter Keresztes, "The Bible as Romanian Toilet Paper," *Wall Street Journal,* June 14, 1985, p. 24.

70. Antonie, "Ecuview."

71. Patriarch Justinian of Romania, "Evangelical Humanism and Christian Responsibility," *The Ecumenical Review,* XIX, no. 2 (April 1967), 157-60.

72. *ROCN,* XII, no. 4 (October-December 1982), 4.

73. Quoted in Tobias, *Communist-Christian Encounter,* p. 351.

74. Bishop Antonie, "Church and State in Romania," *Church and State: Opening a New Ecumenical Discussion,* Faith and Order Paper, no. 85 (Geneva: World Council of Churches, 1978), pp. 95f.

75. Quoted in Tobias, *Communist-Christian Encounter,* p. 326.

76. Quoted in Ghermani, "The Orthodox Church in Romania," p. 23.

77. Bishop Antonie, "Church and State," p. 92

78. Quoted in Tobias, *Communist-Christian Encounter,* p. 326.

79. *ROCN,* XIV, no. 3 (July-September 1984), 12.

80. Quoted in Scarfe, "Patriarch Justinian," p. 166.

81. *ROCN,* XIV, no. 3 (July-September 1984), 3.

82. *ROCN,* XVIII, no. 4 (July-August 1988), 3-4.

83. *ROCN,* IV, nos. 1-2 (January-June 1974), 6-8.

84. Quoted in Scarfe, "Patriarch Justinian," p. 167.

85. Sr. Eileen Mary, S.L.G., "Orthodox Monasticism in Romania Today," *RCL,* VIII, no. 1 (Spring 1980), 25.

86. Quoted in translation in Gerald J. Bobango, *The Romanian Orthodox Episcopate of America: The First Half Century, 1929-1979* (Jackson, Mich.: Romanian-American Heritage Center, 1979), p. 187.

87. Quoted in *ROCN,* XV, no. 1 (January-March 1985), 14.

88. Constantin Galeriu, "The Romanian Patriarchate," in Ion Bria, ed., *Martyria/Mission: The Witness of the Orthodox Churches Today* (Geneva: World Council of Churches, 1980), p. 98.

89. Quoted in Bishop Antonie, "Church and State," p. 104.

90. Bishop Antonie, "Church and State," pp. 94-97, 101, 103; Bishop Antonie Ploieşteanul, "Interview (with BBC-London)," *ROCN,* VIII, no. 3 (July-September 1978), 116-17.

91. I have omitted discussion of the burgeoning dispute between evangelical Protestants and the Patriarchate in the post-Communist era. Charges by the former that the latter are in collusion with the DFSN's attempt to "suppress" the Protestant minority are exaggerated. To be sure, the Patriarchate does seem zealous to assert its historic identity as the Church of the vast majority of Romanians, currently some 85 per cent of the total population. But such a majoritarian approach to church-state relations, an approach that seems strange to most Americans with their considerably more varied religious landscape, need not necessarily translate into violations of "minority rights." Conversely, some evangelicals have raised the ire of the Orthodox by attempting—often aggressively and sometimes through the propagation of distor-

tions and falsehoods—to convert them to the Protestant gospel. For an ongoing debate on these issues between Kent Hill, former president of the Institute on Religion and Democracy, and myself, see my essay, "Evangelicals vs. Orthodox in Romania," *The Christian Century,* CVII, no. 18 (May 30–June 6, 1990), 560f., and the exchange in *The Christian Century,* CVII, no. 23 (August 8-15, 1990), 745-49. Ecumenical cooperation will not, in any event, be advanced by the public comments of Evangelical Alliance president Paul Negruţ, who has compared the Orthodox to Pharisees who lack "substance" and "a transformed life in Christ" (Interview with Ted Okada, *News Network International,* February 12, 1991, p. 32), or the remark by evangelist Josif Ţon that the *only* faith that can build a civil society in Romania is evangelical Protestantism (KNS no. 371, March 21, 1991, p. 17).

92. "Documents: Cardinal Laszlo Paskai," *RCL,* XVI, no. 4 (Winter 1988), 361f.

93. John V. Eibner, "Refugees from Romania in Hungary," *RCL,* XVI, no. 3 (Autumn 1988), pp. 254-56.

94. English translation in *ROCN,* XVII, no. 2 (April-June 1987), 81-83.

95. *Ibid.,* p. 82.

96. "WCC Committee Speaks on Romania" (Excerpt), *RCDA,* XXVII, no. 3 (Summer 1988), 93.

97. Associated Press wire service story in *New York Times,* February 25, 1992, p. A10.

98. See, for example, an interview with Salagean in the January 19, 1994, issue of *România Liberă* translated and reprinted in FBIS-EEU-94-016 (January 25, 1994), pp. 32-34.

99. Quoted in KNS no. 363 (November 22, 1990), pp. 4f.

100. Mircea Păcurariu, "Truths Unrevealed," *ROCN,* XX, no. 2 (March-April 1990), 7-9, and *idem, Pages From the History of the Romanian Church (The Uniatism in Transylvania)* (Bucharest: Romanian Orthodox Church Bible and Mission Institute Publishing House, 1991), esp. pp. 47-49. See also the more dispassionate analysis in Nicholas K. Apostola, "The Reemergence of the Greek-Catholic Church in Romania Following the December 1989 Revolution," *Greek Orthodox Theological Review,* XXXV, no. 4 (1990), 299-316, and the even-handed account in Ronald G. Roberson, CSP, "The Revolution of 1989 and the Catholic-Orthodox Dialogue," *Christian Orient,* XIII, no. 4 (December 1992), 195-211.

101. Quoted in Tobias, *Communist-Christian Encounter,* p. 330.

102. Text *ibid.,* p. 347.

103. Broun, *Conscience and Captivity,* p. 206.

104. Quoted in Pope, "The Contemporary Religious Situation," p. 126.

105. Kurt Hutten, *Iron Curtain Christians: The Church in Communist Countries Today,* trans. Walter G. Tillmans (Minneapolis: Augsburg Publishing House, 1967), p. 392.

106. Alexander Raţiu and William Virtue, *Stolen Church: Martyrdom in Communist Romania* (Huntington, Ind.: Our Sunday Visitor, 1979), pp. 77, 173.

107. *Ibid.,* p. 137.

108. Ghermani, "The Orthodox Church in Romania," p. 23.

109. Reuters News Agency story in *Washington Times,* January 9, 1990, p. A9.

110. This is the latest published figure according to Ronald G. Roberson, C.S.P., *The Eastern Christian Churches: A Brief Survey (1993 Edition)* (Rome: Edizioni "Orientalia Christiana," 1993), p. 119. There were no known additions by June 1994,

according to Fr. Roberson and Msgr. John M. Botean, Apostolic Administrator of the Romanian Catholic Diocese based in Canton, Ohio.

111. *ROCN,* XXI, no. 1 (January-February 1991), 5.

112. *ROCN,* XX, no. 1 (January-February 1990), 26.

113. Quoted in *Orthodox Observer,* LXI, no. 1060 (September 1991), 25. As recently as July 8, 1993, in a fervent *apologia pro vita sua* on behalf of his Church to Pope John Paul II, Bishop Guţiu repeated this strange Bulgarian thesis, which appears to retain quite a grip on the Uniate imagination. I wish to thank Fr. Ronald G. Roberson, C.S.P., for sharing his English translation of this "Letter to His Holiness Pope John Paul II," originally published in *Viaţa Creştina* in October 1993.

114. See also "Romanian Catholics May Go to Court," *National Catholic Register,* LXVI, no. 52 (December 30, 1990), 9.

115. See n. 113 above ("Letter to His Holiness Pope John Paul II").

116. Romanian Committee of Christian Solidarity International, "Truths Which Cannot Be Hidden," *RCL,* X, no. 2 (Summer 1982), 224.

117. Broun, *Conscience and Captivity,* p. 220.

118. Quoted in KNS no. 303 (June 23, 1988), p. 3. The names of other Orthodox priests persecuted merely for practicing their faith have been publicized by various champions in the West. Fr. Ştefan Gavrila and Fr. Costica Maftei are noteworthy in this respect. Another priest, Fr. Vasile Vasilachi, emigrated to the United States and serves, ironically, as a priest in the jurisdiction headed by the Patriarchate's exarch, Archbishop Victorin. For Vasilachi's candid, self-published recollections of prison life, see Fr. Dr. Vasile Vasilachi, *Another World: Memories from Communist Prisons* (New York: n.p., 1987).

119. The information in this section has been culled from Alan Scarfe, "Dismantling a Human Rights Movement: A Romanian Solution," *RCL,* VII, no. 3 (Autumn 1979), 168f.; Eugene Ionescu, "Outcry of a Rumanian Priest," *The Orthodox Monitor,* nos. 11-12 (January-June 1981), pp. 42f.; Doru Aurel Gheorghe Gaga, "Appeal to International Public Opinion from Rumanian Priest," *The Orthodox Monitor,* nos. 11-12 (January-June 1981), pp. 97-100; Paul Booth, "Father Calciu's First Year of 'Freedom,'" *RCL,* XIII, no. 3 (Winter 1985), 330f.; Vladimir Socor, "La repression religieuse en Roumanie," *Service Orthodoxe de Presse,* no. 102 (November 1985), 17-20; Ghermani, "The Orthodox Church in Romania," p. 26; Broun, *Conscience and Captivity,* pp. 212f., 235f.; and Gheorghe Calciu, "The Persecuted, the Persecutors, and the Church" (unpublished memoirs, hereafter cited as Calciu, "Memoirs").

120. Calciu, "Memoirs," p. 6.

121. *Ibid.,* p. 26.

122. Letter from Fr. Gheorghe Calciu-Dumitreasa to His Sanctity John-Paul II. Bucharest: October 17, 1978. (Typescript of English translation of Romanian original by Fr. Gheorghe, available from Keston College.)

123. Letter from Fr. Gheorghe Calciu-Dumitreasa to C.I.E.L. Bucharest: October 17, 1978. (Typescript of English translation of Romanian original by Fr. Gheorghe, available from Keston College.)

124. Dumitru Popescu *et al.,* "Letter from Romanian Orthodox Priests," *RCL,* VII, no. 3 (Autumn 1979), 176.

125. *ROCN,* XV, no. 2 (April-June, 1983), 46.

126. Calciu, "Memoirs," p. 52.

127. *Ibid.,* p. 53.

128. Randy Tift, "Orthodox Church Given Preferential Status in Proposed Religion Law," *News Network International,* November 24, 1993, pp. 12f. The current rift may undermine the ecumenical progress between Orthodox and Baptists in Romania that reached a high-water mark in May 1993, when the rectors of the Orthodox and Baptist theological faculties at the University of Bucharest lectured each other's students on the prospects of a common evangelistic witness in Romania. Ecumenical Press Service story in *Orthodox Observer,* LVIII, no. 1082 (August 1993), 20.

129. Church news item in *National Catholic Reporter,* XXX, no. 13 (January 28, 1994), 4. To be sure, Teoctist also issued a public appeal in September 1990 on behalf of the children of Romania, including the sick, the handicapped, the orphaned, and "those whose lives were stilled before they even saw the light of day." For the original Romanian text, see "Apelul," *Vestitorul,* II, nos. 17-18 (September 1990), 1. But such oblique references to abortion have now been surpassed by the clear condemnation in the most recent public appeal.

CHAPTER 4

1. Richard John Neuhaus, *The Naked Public Square: Religion and Democracy in America* (Grand Rapids: Eerdmans Publishing Co., 1984), p. 263.

2. "Amicus Curiae Brief of the Holy Orthodox Church in the Supreme Court of the United States, October Term, 1988: William L. Webster, State of Missouri, v. Reproductive Health Services, et al." (February 21, 1989). See also my reflections on this brief — in which I, too, was privileged to be asked to endorse — in "Orthodox Church Enters Public Debate Over Abortion," *The Greek Star* (Chicago), August 17, 1989, p. 3+.

3. For the historical development of Orthodoxy in America, see Constance J. Tarasar, ed., *Orthodox America 1794-1976: Development of the Orthodox Church in America* (Syosset, N.Y.: Orthodox Church in America, Department of History and Archives (1975); Archimandrite Serafim [Surrency], *The Quest for Orthodox Church Unity in America: A History of the Orthodox Church in North America in the Twentieth Century* (New York: Saints Boris and Gleb Press, 1973); and George Papaioannou, *From Mars Hill to Manhattan: The Greek Orthodox in America Under Patriarch Athenagoras I* (Minneapolis: Light and Life Publishing Co., 1976).

4. Paul Schneirla, "Report of Department of Inter-Orthodox and Inter-Faith Relations," *Word,* XXIX, no. 9 (November 1985), 8.

5. Kenneth Bedell, ed., *Yearbook of American and Canadian Churches 1994* (Nashville: Abingdon Press, 1994).

6. Statistics concerning the financial contributions and delegations from the respective Orthodox member jurisdictions were provided by Metropolitan Christopher Kovacevich (SOC) and Frs. Miltiades Efthimiou (Greek Archdiocese), Rodion Kondratick (OCA), Paul Schneirla (AOCA), and Rastko Trbuhovich (SOC). The figures are the most current that these spokesmen have disclosed to me.

7. As late as May 1962, SCOBA was willing to accept the UOC into its ranks provided that the latter's hierarchs and other clergy applied to the Ecumenical Patriarchate for "regularization" and received anew the holy mysteries (the preferred

Orthodox term for "sacraments") of chrismation and holy orders. For this SCOBA resolution, see Serafim [Surrency], *The Quest for Orthodox Church Unity*, pp. A148f.

8. The selection also reflects which jurisdictions responded to requests for documentary materials. The American Carpatho-Russian Orthodox Greek Catholic Diocese, the Ukrainian Orthodox Church of America, and the Romanian Orthodox Missionary Archdiocese failed to provide any assistance. Bishop Hilarion Kapral of the Russian Orthodox Church Outside Russia indicated that his jurisdiction has not produced ad hoc resolutions on issues of peace, freedom, and security.

9. These documents in Greek and/or English may be found in *EAD*, pp. 95f, 666-68, 703.

10. Quoted in *LMA*, p. 46

11. Quoted in Stanley S. Harakas, "Human Rights: An Eastern Orthodox Perspective," *Journal of Ecumenical Studies*, XIX, no. 3 (Summer 1982), 21.

12. *LMA*, p. 116.

13. *Ibid.*, p. 123.

14. *Ibid.*, p. 154.

15. *Ibid.*, pp. 155f.

16. Resolution on "Political and Racial Justice in the World," report of Resolutions Committee, 30th Biennial Clergy-Laity Congress (Washington, D.C., 1990), p. R-7.

17. *EAD*, p. 1248.

18. Quoted in *LMA*, p. 41.

19. *EAD*, p. 1252.

20. *Ibid.*, p. 1159.

21. *Ibid.*, p. 1202.

22. *Ibid.*, pp. 1180, 1182.

23. *Ibid.*, p. 1242.

24. *Ibid.*, pp. 1222-24.

25. *LMA*, p. 160.

26. Cited *ibid.*, p. 114.

27. *EAD*, pp. 1169f.

28. Quoted in *LMA*, p. 40.

29. *Ibid.*, p. 39.

30. Typescript in Hellenic College/Holy Cross Library, Brookline, Mass.

31. "Church's Positions on Current Issues," *Orthodox Observer*, LII, no. 975 (September 24, 1986), 1.

32. *Ibid.*

33. *Ibid.*, p. 4.

34. *EAD*, p. 1174.

35. *Ibid.*, p. 1195.

36. Quoted in *LMA*, p. 47.

37. Text in *Orthodox Observer*, LVII, no. 1066 (March 1992), 3.

38. The texts of the resolutions of the NCC's Governing Board (since late 1990 called the General Board) are not published in readily available volumes. A collection is maintained at the Ethics and Public Policy Center in Washington, D.C.

39. *LMA*, p. 104.

40. George Stephanopoulos, for example, has earned a special place in President

Bill Clinton's inner circle of advisors, and Fr. Robert Stephanopoulos — George's father and dean of the Archdiocese's cathedral in Manhattan — served as one of several honorary New York state chairmen of Clinton's campaign for the Democratic presidential nomination. When Archbishop Iakovos met with Clinton at the White House on March 25, 1993, for the annual presidential proclamation of "Greek Independence Day," the president mentioned the names of the six Greek Orthodox members of his staff. "Iakovos Visits President Clinton in Washington," *Orthodox Observer,* LVIII, no. 1078 (April 1993), 4.

41. *Ibid.,* p. 162.

42. *Ibid.,* p. 158.

43. *Ibid.,* p. 157.

44. "Church's Positions on Current Issues," p. 1

45. *Ibid.,* pp. 1, 4.

46. *Ibid.,* p. 4.

47. *Ibid.*

48. Typescript in Hellenic College/Holy Cross Library, Brookline, Mass.

49. *RCDA,* XIV, nos. 4-6 (1975), 87.

50. Quoted *LMA,* p. 40.

51. Quoted *ibid.,* p. 43.

52. Quoted in "Christian Leaders Protest Settlers," *TOC,* XXVI, nos. 7-8 (July-August 1990), 1, 3.

53. Text in *Orthodox Observer,* LVII, no. 1066 (March 1992), 1f.

54. "Thousands Insist: 'Macedonia Is Greek!!!'," *Orthodox Observer,* LVII, no. 1069 (June 1992), 1.

55. "Thousands Rally in NYC for Macedonia," *Orthodox Observer,* LVIII, no. 1076 (February 1993), 1f.

56. Texts in "Recognition of Skopje Outrages His Eminence," *Orthodox Observer,* LVIII, no. 1089 (March 1994), 3, 23.

57. *News From Greece* (Newsletter of the Embassy of Greece, Washington, D.C.), March 9, 1994, pp. 3f.

58. *RCDA,* XIV, nos. 4-6 (1975), 87.

59. *RCDA,* X, nos. 1-2 (January 1971), 7.

60. "OCA Primate Appeals on Behalf of Fr. D. Dudko," *The Orthodox Monitor,* nos. 7-8 (January-June 1980), p. 26.

61. Quoted in "Serbian Orthodox Church Holds Triennial Clergy-Laity Assembly in Libertyville," *TOC,* XX, no. 12 (December 1984), 2.

62. "Statement on the 50th Anniversary of the Famine of 1932-33 in the USSR," *RCDA,* XXII, nos. 10-12 (1983), 190.

63. "Bishops Designate October for Prayer for Persecuted," *TOC,* XXI, no. 12 (December 1985), 3.

64. Quoted in "Metropolitan Voices Problems of Church on American Scene," *TOC,* XXIII, no. 4 (April 1987), 1.

65. Metropolitan Theodosius, "The Millennium: A Challenge and an Opportunity," *RCDA,* XXVI, no. 2 (Spring 1987), 35.

66. "Message of Metropolitan Theodosius to the NCC," *TOC,* XXIV, no. 1 (January 1988), 3. Italics in original.

67. Official Minutes of the Eighth All-American Council of the Orthodox

Church in America in Washington, D.C., August 1986 (OCA Chancery, Syosset, N.Y.), p. 31. Hereafter the official minutes of councils will be cited as OCA-M with the year and page number.

68. OCA-M 1975, Attachment I, p. 2.

69. "On the Death Penalty," *TOC,* XXV, nos. 9-10 (September-October 1989), 11.

70. OCA-M 1986, p. 34.

71. *Ibid.,* pp. 35, 36.

72. *Ibid.,* pp. 23f, 39f.

73. OCA-M 1975, Attachment VI.

74. OCA-M 1983, p. 13.

75. *Ibid.,* pp. 14f.

76. *Ibid.,* p. 21.

77. OCA-M 1980, p. 18.

78. OCA-M 1986, pp. 41f.

79. *Ibid.,* p. 42.

80. OCA-M 1973, p. 3.

81. OCA-M 1975, p. 1.

82. OCA-M 1977, p. 6.

83. OCA-M 1980, p. 17.

84. OCA-M 1986, pp. 25-29.

85. K. L. Billingsley, *From Mainline to Sideline: The Social Witness of the National Council of Churches* (Washington, D.C.: Ethics and Public Policy Center, 1990); Ernest W. Lefever, *Amsterdam to Nairobi: The World Council of Churches and the Third World* and *Nairobi to Vancouver: The World Council of Churches and the World, 1975-1987* (Washington, D.C.: Ethics and Public Policy Center, 1979 and 1987).

86. Text in *RCDA,* XXII, nos. 7-9 (1983), 109.

87. John Meyendorff, "The WCC in Vancouver: A Preliminary Evaluation," *RCDA,* XXII, nos. 10-12 (1983), 154.

88. "Primate of Ukraine Guest of Metropolitan Theodosius," *TOC,* XXX, no. 2 (February 1994), 1.

89. "Metropolitan at White House Dialogue," *TOC,* XXIX, nos. 4-5 (April-May 1993), 1f.

90. Text in *TOC,* XXVIII, nos. 8-9 (August-September 1992), 13. A personal note: as a priest-delegate to this council, I declined for reasons of conscience to vote in favor of this resolution, which passed on a voice vote without audible dissent.

91. For a detailed history of this rivalry, see Gerald J. Bobango, *The Romanian Orthodox Episcopate: The First Half Century, 1929-1979* (Jackson, Mich.: Romanian-American Heritage Center, 1979), pp. 168-229.

92. Text in *Solia,* LVIII, no. 8 (August 1993), 7.

93. *RCDA,* IX, nos. 21-22 (November 1970), 181.

94. Ion Mihai Pacepa, *Red Horizons: Chronicles of a Communist Spy Chief* (Washington, D.C.: Regnery Gateway, 1987), pp. 286-90. For another view of Rabbi Rosen's controversial collaboration with the Ceauşescu regime, see the syndicated column of Jack Anderson and Dale Van Atta, "Ransom for Romania's Jews," *Washington Post,* October 20, 1991, p. C7.

95. Gerald P. Bobango, *Religion and Politics: Bishop Valerian Trifa and His Times* (Boulder, Colo.: East European Monographs, 1981), esp. pp. 173-78.

96. *Solia,* LIV, no. 7 (July 1989), 10.

97. "Resolution Concerning Destruction of Villages and Churches in Romania," *TOC,* XXIV, no. 10 (October 1988), 4.

98. Text still unpublished as of spring 1994. I was one of the dissenters—an unenviable role for a priest who is otherwise committed to enhancing the dignity of the Romanian people.

99. Text of letter to Patriarch Aleksii in *Solia,* LIX, no. 1 (January 1994), 4; response of Archpriest Victor Peliuchenko on behalf of Aleksii in *Solia,* LIX, no. 6 (June 1994), 6.

100. *The Word,* XXV, no. 9 (November 1981), 11f. The minutes of each convention appear in the November (or, in early years, October) issue of this organ. Hereafter resolutions, reports, or episcopal messages will be cited as *Word* with year and page number.

101. Quoted in *Word* 1977, p. 19.

102. *Word* 1972, p. 20.

103. *Word* 1989, p. 39.

104. *Word* 1979, p. 34.

105. *Word* 1974, p. 46.

106. *Word* 1978, p. 39.

107. *Word* 1983, p. 33.

108. *Word* 1979, p. 34.

109. *Word* 1985, p. 29.

110. *Word* 1987, p. 31.

111. *Word* 1978, p. 39.

112. *Word* 1985, pp. 29, 32.

113. *Word* 1972, p. 33.

114. "Religious Leaders on Lebanon," *Solia,* LIV, no. 5 (May 1989), 11.

115. *Word* 1978, p. 22.

116. *Word* 1967, p. 20.

117. *Word* 1993, p. 50.

118. *Word* 1981, p. 25.

119. *Word* 1979, p. 18.

120. *Word* 1981, p. 26.

121. *Word* 1985, p. 31.

122. *Word* 1978, p. 39.

123. *Word* 1985, pp. 30f.

124. *Word* 1991, p. 40.

125. *Word* 1993, p. 52.

126. *Ibid.*

127. *Word* 1967, p. 18.

128. *Word* 1970, p. 23.

129. *Word* 1974, p. 47.

130. *Ibid.*

131. Neil C. Livingstone and David Halevy, *Inside the PLO* (New York: William Morrow and Co., 1990), p. 200. And now documents in the recently opened archives of the Communist Party of the Soviet Union apparently reveal that the KGB provided funds and arms to Habesh and the PFLP. "Russia to Reveal KGB Secrets," *Parade Magazine,* July 19, 1992, p.14.

132. *Word* 1975, p. 44.
133. *Word* 1979, p. 35.
134. *Word* 1981, p. 25.
135. *Word* 1987, p. 32.
136. *Word* 1989, p. 38.
137. *Ibid.*
138. "Peace Proposal Concerning Lebanon," *Solia*, LIV, no. 10 (October 1989), 11.
139. Text of remarks in "PLO-Israeli Accord Signed," *Origins: CNS Documentary Service*, XXIII, no. 15 (September 23, 1993), 251.
140. *Word* 1983, p. 7.
141. *Word* 1978, p. 9.
142. *Word* 1976, p. 12.
143. *Word* 1981, p. 6.
144. *Path*, XIII, no. 11 (November 1980), 1.
145. *Ibid.*
146. *Ibid.*, p. 9.
147. *Path*, XX, nos. 10-11 (October-November 1984), 10.
148. *Path*, XIX, no. 1 (January 1983), 8.
149. Minutes of Church National Assembly, Chicago, 1970 (CNA-16), in Archives of the Diocese of Eastern America, Serbian Orthodox Church in the U.S.A. and Canada, Edgeworth, Pennsylvania.
150. *Path*, XIII, no. 11 (November 1980), 1.
151. *Path*, XX, no. 12 (December 1984), 7.
152. *Ibid.*, p. 8.
153. For the other side of this religio-ethnic conflict, see the letter of Joseph J. DioGuardi, former U.S. congressman and current president of the Albanian American Civic League, "Rights and Wrongs in Balkan Upheaval," *Washington Times*, February 2, 1990, p. F2. For a more even-handed approach to human-rights violations in this region, see *Yugoslavia: Crisis in Kosovo* (n.p.: Helsinki Watch and the International Helsinki Federation for Human Rights, March 1990).
154. *Path*, XX, no. 12 (December 1984), p. 7.
155. *Path*, XIX, no. 1 (January 1983), 3.
156. *Ibid.*
157. *Ibid.*
158. Quoted in "State Dept. Responds to Resolution," *Path*, XIX, no. 3 (March 1983), 1.
159. *Path*, XXVII, no. 1 (January 1992), 3+.
160. Texts of both letters in *Path*, XXVIII, nos. 10-11 (October-November 1993), 15f.
161. *Path*, XXVIII, nos. 10-11 (October-November 1993), 3.
162. *Path*, XXIV, no. 12 (December 1988), 3.
163. *Path*, XV, no. 2 (February 1982), 1.
164. *Path*, XX, no. 2 (February 1984), 1, 8.
165. Text in *Path*, XXIV, no. 12 (December 1988), 3.
166. Text *ibid.*, p. 8.
167. Text *ibid.*

168. Personal letter from Milan Visnick, treasurer of Serb Net, Inc., McLean, Va., September 28, 1992.

169. "Serb Hierarchs Endorse Serb Net In Its Serbian National Umbrella Effort," *American Srbobran* (Pittsburgh, Pa.), September 16, 1992, p. 3.

170. *UOW,* XIV, no. 1 (January 1980), 15. Hereafter this publication, the first volume of which appeared in 1967, will be cited as UOW with month and year and page number.

171. *UOW,* September 1986, p. 21.

172. *UOW,* July 1987, p. 10.

173. *UOW,* January 1968, p. 6.

174. *UOW,* March 1968, p. 16.

175. "Ukrainian Orthodox Synod Appoints Bishop to Head UAOC," *ABN Correspondence* (Bulletin of the Anti-Bolshevik Bloc of Nations), XL, no. 6 (November-December 1989), 30.

176. The late Patriarch Dimitrios of Constantinople also pledged his full support to Patriarch Aleksii II of Moscow in the latter's struggles against the Ukrainian Catholics, denouncing the "anti-Christian activity of the Uniates" including "their seizure of holy churches, vandalism, sacrilege and so forth." Quoted in KNS no. 368 (February 7, 1991), p. 17.

177. See, for example, Anthony Ugolnik, "Unraveling Ukraine," *American Orthodoxy,* no. 3 (Spring 1993), 7-9, and *idem,* "Living at the Borders: Eastern Orthodoxy and World Disorder," *First Things,* no. 34 (June-July 1993), 18. Bishop Nathaniel, who edits *Calendarul Solia,* the official directory of parishes and clergy of the ROEA, pointedly included the hierarchy and seminary of the UOC in the 1994 edition's section on the Orthodox jurisdictions in North America.

178. *UOW,* April 1988, p. 3.

179. *UOW,* June 1968, pp. 1, 3.

180. *UOW,* January 1978, p. 5.

181. *UOW,* June 1985, p. 7.

182. *UOW,* January 1989, p. 3.

183. *UOW,* April 1978, p. 8.

184. *UOW,* November 1982, p. 3.

185. *UOW,* July 1988, p. 12.

186. *UOW,* January 1983, p. 3.

187. *UOW,* September 1993, p. 13

188. *UOW,* January 1994, p. 13.

189. *UOW,* July 1974, p. 9; September 1974, p. 13.

190. *UOW,* December 1974, p. 13.

191. *UOW,* February 1976, pp. 4f.

192. *UOW* January 1976, p. 19.

193. *UOW,* May 1986, p. 18.

194. *UOW,* July 1986, p. 16.

195. *UOW,* December 1986, p. 15.

196. *UOW,* May 1987, p. 9.

197. *UOW,* October-November 1992, p. 15.

198. *UOW,* January 1989, pp. 4, 7.

199. *UOW,* November-December 1990, p. 11.

200. *UOW,* July-August 1993, p. 4.

201. *UOW,* January 1989, p. 7.

202. *Ibid.,* p. 8.

203. *UOW,* May,1986, pp. 8f.

204. *UOW,* December 1988, p. 12.

205. William E. Schmidt, "Chicago Groups Aiding East European Homelands," *New York Times,* February 19, 1990, p. A9; telephone interview with Fr. Steven Zenchuch in Chicago, March 8, 1990.

206. *UOW,* July-August 1993, p. 10.

207. See my op-ed article, "What the Media Have Missed in Eastern Europe," *Washington Post,* July 31, 1990, p. A25.

208. (Bishop Kallistos) Timothy Ware, *The Orthodox Church* (Baltimore: Penguin Books, 1964), p. 86.

209. Ioannes N. Karmiris, "Nationalism in the Orthodox Church," *Greek Orthodox Theological Review,* XXVI, no. 3 (Fall 1981), 172f.

CHAPTER 5

1. Walter Laqueur, "From Russia With Hate," *The New Republic,* February 5, 1990, pp. 21-25. See my letter of protest in *The New Republic,* March 12, 1990, pp. 4+. The editors of this periodical demonstrated their insensitivity to Orthodox Christians yet again on the cover of the May 30, 1994, issue. To illustrate a generally positive article on Russian Orthodoxy by Librarian of Congress James H. Billington, the cover depicts the erstwhile Soviet hammer and sickle with a distinctive Orthodox triple-bar cross in place of the hammer.

2. Alexander F. C. Webster, "New Reign of Terror on the Danube," *The Wanderer,* CXXIII, no. 2 (January 11, 1990), 4+.

3. John Meyendorff, *Byzantine Theology* (New York: Fordham University Press, 1974), pp. 199f.; and Alexander Schmemann, *Historical Road of Eastern Orthodoxy* (Crestwood, N.Y.: St. Vladimir's Seminary Press, 1977), pp. 289-91.

4. Alfred Vagts, *A History of Militarism: Civilian and Military,* rev. ed. (New York: The Free Press, 1959), pp. 13, 14.

5. *Peace and Disarmament: Documents of the World Council of Churches and Roman Catholic Church* (Geneva: World Council of Churches, 1982), p. 92.

6. *JMP,* 1990, no. 9, p. 3.

7. English translation of text furnished by Eugenia Ordynsky, former Washington, D.C., director of the Congress of Russian Americans.

8. Quoted in George Lemopoulos, "The Prophetic Mission of Orthodoxy: A Witness to Love in Service," *The Ecumenical Review,* XL, no. 2 (April 1988), 176f.

9. Quoted in Alan Cowel, "World Religious Leaders Meet on Ethnic Strife," *New York Times,* February 10, 1994, p. A15.

10. Quoted in William C. Fletcher, *Nikolai: Portrait of a Dilemma* (New York: Macmillan Co., 1968), p. 102.

11. "Conference of the Soviet Peace Foundation," *RCDA,* VIII, nos. 17-18 (September 1969), 167.

12. Quoted in *JMP,* 1988, no. 10, p. 51.

13. *JMP*, 1983, no. 1, p. 52.

14. *JMP*, 1984, no. 8, p. 50.

15. *JMP*, 1979, no. 5, p. 54.

16. *JMP*, 1987, no. 2, p. 46.

17. *JMP*, 1987, no. 11, p. 43.

18. *JMP*, 1984, no. 8, pp. 50f.

19. *The "Vita" of St. Sergii of Radonezh,* trans. Michael Klimenko (Houston: Nordland Publishing International, 1980), p. 168.

20. *JMP*, 1981, no. 9, p. 49.

21. *JMP*, 1980, no. 12, p. 46.

22. *JMP*, 1980, no. 9, p. 5.

23. *JMP*, 1993, no. 2, p. 27.

24. Clyde Haberman, "Bulgaria Worried by Rising Hostility to Minority Turks," *New York Times,* January 8, 1990, p. 1.

25. *JMP*, 1978, no. 11, p. 57. By early 1992, however, the Bulgarians had worked through those problems satisfactorily. See, for example, the editorial, "Eastern Europe's Surprise," *Washington Post,* March 9, 1992, p. A16.

26. *JMP*, 1986, no. 6, p. 50.

27. *JMP*, 1978, no. 2, pp. 44, 50, 53.

28. *Ibid.,* p. 54.

29. *Ibid.,* pp. 57f.

30. *JMP*, 1977, no. 12, p. 47.

31. *JMP*, 1978, nos. 4-5, p. 68.

31. See my article, "The Canonical Validity of Military Service by Orthodox Christians," *Greek Orthodox Theological Review,* XXIII, nos. 3-4 (Fall-Winter 1978), 257-81.

32. *JMP*, 1985, no. 5, p. 4.

33. Quoted in *JMP*, 1983, no. 2, p. 67.

35. Quoted in *JMP*, 1986, no. 6, p. 46.

36. Quoted in *JMP*, 1985, no. 5, p. 37.

37. Boris Talantov, "Sergianism, the Leaven of Herod," *The Orthodox Word,* VII, no. 6 (1971), 278.

38. *JMP*, 1985, no. 6, p. 37.

39. Quoted in *JMP*, 1985, no. 3, p. 51.

40. *JMP*, 1987, no. 4, pp. 34, 35

41. Quoted in Stanley Evans, *The Churches in the U.S.S.R.* (London: Corbett Publishing Co., 1943), p. 122.

42. Quoted in *JMP*, 1980, no. 5, p. 38.

43. *JMP*, 1975, no. 7, p. 4.

44. *JMP*, 1980, no. 6, p. 40.

45. Quoted in *JMP*, 1984, no. 12, p. 51.

46. *JMP*, 1985, no. 5, p. 38.

47. *Ibid.,* p. 37.

48. *JMP*, 1975, no. 5, p. 5.

49. Quoted in *JMP*, 1980, no. 5, p. 38.

50. Quoted in *JMP*, 1984, no. 12, p. 51.

51. *JMP*, 1975, no. 8, p. 13.

52. See, for example, canon 5 of St. Gregory of Nyssa in Agapius and Nicodemus, *The Rudder,* trans. D. Cummings (Chicago: Orthodox Christian Educational Society, 1957), p. 876.

53. *JMP,* 1985, no. 5, pp. 46f.

54. *JMP,* 1985, no. 3, p. 49.

55. *JMP,* 1985, no. 8, p. 52.

56. Quoted in *JMP,* 1985, no. 6, p. 52.

57. *JMP,* 1975, no. 7, p. 8.

58. *Ibid.,* pp. 6f.

59. Quoted in *JMP,* 1983, no. 7, p. 32.

60. See, for example, William C. Fletcher, *Religion and Soviet Foreign Policy* (London: Oxford University Press, 1973), and John B. Dunlop, *The Recent Activities of the Moscow Patriarchate Abroad and in the U.S.S.R.* (Seattle: St. Nectarios Orthodox Press, 1974).

61. *JMP,* 1977, no. 8, p. 31.

62. *Ibid.,* pp. 20, 23.

63. Metropolitan David, *To Deliver the Oppressed from Their Bonds* (Moscow: Novosti Press Agency Publishing House, 1988), p. 39.

64. *JMP,* 1985, no. 1, p. 44.

65. *JMP,* 1977, no. 9, p. 42.

66. *RCDA,* XV, nos. 4-6 (1976), 82.

67. *JMP,* 1981, no. 6, p. 51.

68. *JMP,* 1978, no. 9, pp. 54, 55.

69. *RCDA,* XXII, nos. 1-3 (1983), 44.

70. *JMP,* 1983, no. 3, p. 42.

71. *JMP,* 1987, no. 1, p. 46.

72. *JMP,* 1980, no. 6, p. 50.

73. David Gill, ed., *Gathered for Life: Official Report, VI Assembly, World Council of Churches* (Geneva: WCC, 1983), pp. 157, 159.

74. *JMP,* 1987, no. 6, p. 55.

75. *RCDA,* IV, no. 10 (May 31, 1965), 79.

76. *RCDA,* V, no. 4 (February 28, 1966), 29, 30.

77. *RCDA,* VIII, nos. 19-20 (October 1969), 174.

78. *RCDA,* X, nos. 11-14 (June-July 1971), 100.

79. *JMP,* 1979, no. 3, p. 3.

80. *JMP,* 1979, no. 5, p. 60.

81. *RCDA,* VI, nos. 17-18 (September 15/30, 1967), 147.

82. *RCDA,* V, no. 5 (March 15, 1966), 38.

83. *JMP,* 1977, no. 6, p. 28.

84. *JMP,* 1979, no. 4, p. 59.

85. *JMP,* 1980, no. 6, p. 48

86. *New York Times,* December 28, 1989, p. A3.

87. *JMP,* 1980, no. 5, p. 5.

88. *JMP,* 1980, no. 8, p. 37.

89. *JMP,* 1980, no. 3, pp. 33f.

90. *RCDA,* XXII, nos. 1-3 (1983), 45.

91. Ernest W. Lefever, *Nairobi to Vancouver: The World Council of Churches and the*

World, 1975-87 (Washington, D.C.: Ethics and Public Policy Center, 1987), pp. 27-32, and J. A. Emerson Vermaat, *The World Council of Churches and Politics 1975-1986* (New York: Freedom House, 1989), pp. 39-50.

92. Vermaat, *The World Council,* pp. 40f.

93. Text in Gill, *Gathered for Life,* pp. 161f.

94. Quoted in Vermaat, *The World Council,* p. 48.

95. Quoted in Emil Varadi, "Russia's Patriarch Apologizes to Hungary for 1956," Reuter's wire story, March 4, 1994.

96. *ROCN,* XI, no. 4 (October-December 1984), 4.

97. *Ibid.,* p. 24.

98. *Ibid.,* pp. 24, 28.

99. *ROCN,* XV, no. 2 (April-June 1984), 16, 17.

100. *ROCN,* XV, no. 1 (January-March 1985), 19.

101. *ROCN,* XIV, no. 2 (April-June 1984), 23.

102. *ROCN,* XIV, no. 3 (July-September 1984), 47.

103. KNS no. 370 (March 7, 1991), p. 7.

104. *ROCN,* XIII, no. 4 (October-December 1983), 4.

105. *Ibid.,* p. 8.

106. *ROCN,* XVI, no. 4 (October-December 1986), 56.

107. *ROCN,* XIII, no. 4 (October-December 1983), 8.

108. *Ibid.,* p. 45.

109. *ROCN,* XIV, no. 2 (April-June 1984), 14.

110. *Ibid.,* p. 30.

111. "A Letter to Ceauşescu," *RCL,* XVII, no. 4 (Winter 1989), 365.

112. Quoted in *Official Documents Concerning the Legal Status of the Romanian Orthodox Episcopate of America and Its Relations with the Patriarchate of Romania* ([Jackson, Mich.:] Public Relations Office, Romanian Orthodox Episcopate of America, 1955), p. 22.

113. Quoted *ibid.,* p. 24.

114. Quoted *ibid.,* p. 25.

115. *RCDA,* VI, nos. 17-18 (September 15/30, 1967), 150.

116. *RCDA,* VIII, nos. 1-2 (January 15/31, 1969), 15.

117. "Letter to Dr. J. Hromadka, President of the Christian Peace Conference," *RCDA,* VIII, nos. 3-4 (February 1969), 28.

118. Quoted in Robert Tobias, *Communist-Christian Encounter in East Europe* (Indianapolis: School of Religion Press, 1956), p. 335.

119. Patriarch Justinian of Romania, "Evangelical Humanism and Christian Responsibility," in Constantin G. Patelos, ed., *The Orthodox Church in the Ecumenical Movement: Documents and Statements 1902-1975* (Geneva: World Council of Churches, 1978), p. 250.

120. Original Romanian text furnished by Fr. Ron Roberson, C.S.P.

121. *JMP,* 1993, no. 2, p. 5.

122. *Nezavisimaya Gazeta,* December 25, 1992, p. 1; *România Liberă,* December 30, 1992, p. 8.

123. "Church's Position on Current Issues," *Orthodox Observer,* LII, no. 975 (September 1986), 4.

124. *UOW,* December 1988, p. 27.

125. *Word,* 1975, p. 44.

126. OCA-M 1975, Attachment I, no. 7.

127. *Path,* XXV, no. 4 (April 1989), 7. Italics in original.

128. *UOW,* December 1986, p. 2.

129. *UOW,* January 1968, p. 6.

130. *EAD,* p. 1156.

131. *Ibid.,* pp. 1254f.

132. *Ibid.,* p. 1223.

133. *Ibid.,* p. 1242.

134. *Path,* XX, no. 12 (December 1984), 7.

135. *Path,* XXVI, no. 2 (February 1990), 8.

136. *UOW,* June, 1985, p. 8.

137. *LMA,* pp. 156f.

138. OCA-M 1983, pp. 18f.

139. K. L. Billingsley, *From Mainline to Sideline: The Social Witness of the National Council of Churches* (Washington, D.C.: Ethics and Public Policy Center, 1990), pp. 49-63, 79-131.

140. Quoted *ibid.,* p. 122.

141. *EAD,* p. 1182.

142. *Ibid.,* p. 1205.

143. *UOW,* January 1968, p. 6.

144. *Word* 1970, p. 25.

145. *LMA,* pp. 116f.

146. *Ibid.,* pp. 124f.

147. *Ibid.,* pp. 123f.

148. *Ibid.,* p. 129.

149. *Ibid.,* p. 140.

150. Dissenting opinions expressed privately, however, cannot be quoted here without violating confidences. In the former Soviet Union, Fr. Gleb Yakunin is one Russian Orthodox priest who refused to go along with the anti-military tide in his own Patriarchate. KNS no. 366 (January 10, 1991), p. 12.

151. Text in *Solia,* LVI, no. 1 (January 1991), 7+.

152. *Word* 1990, pp. 3f.

153. Dispatch from OCA Office of Public Information and Public Relations, Syosset, N.Y., January 17, 1991.

154. Text in *TOC,* XXVII, nos. 5-6 (May-June 1991), 4.

155. Quoted in *National Catholic Register,* LXX, no. 10 (March 6, 1994), 7.

156. "Message of Church Leaders on the Situation in the Former Yugoslavia," *Religion in Eastern Europe* [formerly *Occasional Papers on Religion in Eastern Europe*], XII, no. 3 (June 1993), 39, 40. None of the usual Eastern Orthodox signatories appeared on this rather moderate document, because it did call for a greater U.S. involvement in the conflict.

157. Text in *Path,* XXIX, nos. 2-3 (February-March 1994), 1.

158. *JMP,* 1993, no. 4, pp. 2f.

159. "Patriarch Denies 'Orthodox Axis' Linking Belgrade and Moscow," Ecumenical Press Service wire story, May 4, 1994.

160. English translation of text in FBIS-EEU-92-113 (June 11, 1992), pp. 54-57.

161. The SOC bishops issued their statement on August 6, 1992, and persuaded

Senator Mitch McConnell (R.-Ky.) to enter it into the record (*Congressional Record– Senate,* August 10, 1992, p. S12046).

162. Text in *Path,* XXVIII, no. 12 (December 1993), 1+.

163. Ibid.

164. See note 161.

165. Text in *Path,* XXVIII, nos. 10-11 (October-November 1993), 3.

166. Text in *Path,* XXIX, no. 5 (May 1994), 10.

167. Quoted in *Solia,* LVIII, no. 12 (December 1993), 13.

168. Quoted in *Orthodox Observer,* LVIII, no. 1080 (June 1993), 1+.

169. Texts provided by Fr. Miltiades Efthimiou, ecumenical officer of the Greek Orthodox Archdiocese and secretary of SCOBA.

170. Text in *TOC,* XXIX, no. 6 (June 1993), 1+. For the Appeal of Conscience event, see "Religious Leaders of Serbia, Bosnia and Croatia Issue Appeal for Peace," *Orthodox Observer,* LVIII, no. 1075 (January 1993), 3+.

171. "International Orthodox Christian Charities Expands Humanitarian Aid to Eastern Europe," *TOC,* XXIX, nos. 4-5 (April-May 1993), 8; "IOCC Continues Effort in Ex-Yugoslavia," *Orthodox Observer,* LVIII, no. 1081 (July 1993), 14; "Father Efthimiou Visit Solidifies IOCC/Serbian Church Relationship," *International Orthodox Christian Charities Newsletter* (Baltimore, Maryland), II, no. 1 (March 1994), 1.

172. Quoted in "Orthodox Bishops Counter Pittsburgh Appeal on B-H," *Path.* XXVIII, no. 4 (April 1994), 1+.

173. Text *ibid.*

CHAPTER 6

1. Text in *Washington Post,* September 27, 1991, p. A23.

2. Fred Hiatt, "Gorbachev Pledges Wide-Ranging Nuclear Cuts," *Washington Post,* October 6, 1991, p. A1+.

3. Steven Erlanger, "U.S. Agrees to Postpone Russia Games," *Washington Post,* June 1, 1994, p. A6.

4. James Sherr, "Russia's New Threat to Neighbors," *Wall Street Journal,* December 17, 1993, p. A14.

5. R. Jeffrey Smith, "Freeh Warns of a New Russian Threat," *Washington Post,* May 26, 1994, p. A1.

6. Robert J. Art, "To What Ends Military Power?" *International Security,* IV, no. 4 (Spring 1980), 6.

7. Michael E. Howard, "On Fighting a Nuclear War," *International Security,* V, no. 4 (Spring 1981), 16.

8. Michael E. Howard, "Reassurance and Deterrence: Western Defense in the 1980s," *Foreign Affairs,* LXI, no. 2 (Winter 1982-83), 317.

9. Bernard Brodie, ed., *The Absolute Weapon: Atomic Power and World Order* (New York: Harcourt, Brace and Co., 1946), p. 76.

10. William Borden, *There Will Be No Time: The Revolution in Strategy* (New York: Macmillan, 1946), pp. 72f.

11. Charles-Philippe David, *Debating Counterforce: A Conventional Approach in a Nuclear Age* (Boulder, Colo.: Westview Press, 1987), p. 18.

12. *JMP*, 1982, no. 9, p. 44.

13. *JMP*, 1982, no. 12, p. 53.

14. *JMP*, 1978, no. 8, pp. 66f.

15. *JMP*, 1979, no. 6, pp. 35-37.

16. *JMP*, 1978, no. 9, pp. 48-50.

17. *JMP*, 1981, no. 6, p. 45.

18. *JMP*, 1983, no. 3, p. 38.

19. *JMP*, 1985, no. 9, p. 61.

20. *JMP*, 1986, no. 4, p. 58.

21. Quoted in J. A. Vermaat, *The World Council of Churches and Politics 1975-1986* (New York: Freedom House, 1989), p. 90.

22. *Ibid.*

23. *JMP*, 1985, no. 3, p. 45.

24. *JMP*, 1982, no. 6, p. 15.

25. *Ibid.*, p. 16.

26. *RCDA*, nos. 1-3 (1983), pp. 24f.

27. *JMP*, 1983, no. 6, p. 55.

28. *JMP*, 1983, no. 8, pp. 47, 49.

29. *JMP*, 1982, no. 6, p. 20.

30. *JMP*, 1983, no. 10, p. 26.

31. *JMP*, 1983, no. 5, pp. 45f.

32. Metropolitan Filaret of Minsk and Byelorussia, *We Choose Life!* (Moscow: Novosti Press Agency Publishing House, 1987), p. 29.

33. The "nuclear winter" hypothesis has been effectively debunked by the M.I.T. scientist George Rathgens and the nuclear strategist Albert Wohlstetter. See Albert Wohlstetter, "Between an Unfree World and None: Increasing Our Choices," *Foreign Affairs*, LXIII, no. 5 (Summer 1985), 962-94, and Russell Seitz, "In From the Cold: 'Nuclear Winter' Melts Down," *The National Interest*, no. 5 (Fall 1986), 3-17.

34. *JMP*, 1986, no. 9, p. 49.

35. *JMP*, 1987, no. 5, p. 52.

36. For a surprisingly useful summary of the treaty's provisions, see *The First Anniversary of the INF Treaty* (Moscow: Novosti Press Agency Publishing House, 1989), esp. pp. 13f.

37. *JMP*, 1980, no. 2, p. 46.

38. *JMP*, 1981, no. 8, p. 62.

39. *JMP*, 1983, no. 10, p. 29.

40. *JMP*, 1983, no. 9, p. 29.

41. *JMP*, 1984, no. 3, pp. 37, 38.

42. *JMP*, 1984, no. 5, p. 37; *JMP*, 1984, no. 10, p. 31.

43. *JMP*, 1984, no. 5, p. 48.

44. *ROCN*, XI, no. 4 (October-December 1981), 4.

45. *Ibid.*, p. 27.

46. *ROCN*, XII, no. 2 (April-June 1982), 3.

47. *Ibid.*, p. 15.

48. *ROCN*, XIV, no. 3 (July-September 1984), 46, 47.

49. *ROCN*, XIV, no. 2 (April-June 1984), 6, 7.

50. *Ibid.*, p. 25.

51. *ROCN,* XV, no. 2 (April-June 1985), 7.

52. National Conference of Catholic Bishops, *The Challenge of Peace: God's Promise and Our Response (A Pastoral Letter on War and Peace)* (Washington, D.C.: United States Catholic Conference, 1983).

53. James V. Schall, S.J., ed., *Out of Justice, Peace/Winning the Peace* (San Francisco: Ignatius Press, 1984).

54. *JMP,* 1985, no. 10, pp. 29-34.

55. Filaret, *We Choose Life!,* p. 29.

56. *JMP,* 1986, no. 6, pp. 2-18.

57. *Ibid.,* p. 2.

58. *Ibid.,* p. 17.

59. *Ibid.,* p. 2.

60. *Ibid.,* p. 6.

61. *Ibid.,* pp. 3-5.

62. Paul Ramsey, *War and the Christian Conscience* (Durham, N.C.: Duke University Press, 1961), pp. 169f.

63. *JMP,* 1986, no. 6, p. 6.

64. *Ibid.*

65. *Ibid.,* p. 7.

66. *Ibid.*

67. *Ibid.,* pp. 7-8.

68. National Conference of Catholic Bishops, *The Challenge of Peace,* p. 59.

69. *JMP,* 1986, no. 6, p. 10.

70. *Ibid.,* p. 14.

71. *Ibid.,* p. 15.

72. For more details about the weapon and the international debate about it, see Alexander F. C. Webster, "Evaluating the Neutron Bomb," *Global Affairs,* IV, no. 2 (Spring 1989), 19-35.

73. *JMP,* 1978, no. 9, p. 45.

74. *JMP,* 1977, no. 10, p. 35.

75. *JMP,* 1977, no. 11, p. 45.

76. *JMP,* 1978, no. 3, p. 33.

77. *JMP,* 1978, no. 2, p. 36.

78. *Ibid.,* pp. 38, 39.

79. *Ibid.,* p. 43.

80. *ROCN,* XI, no. 4 (October-December 1981), 5.

81. *Ibid.,* p. 13.

82. *ROCN,* XIV, no. 2 (April-June 1984), 7.

83. John McCaslin, "'Star Wars' Victory," *Washington Times,* February 10, 1994, p. A6.

84. "President's Speech on Military Spending and a New Defense," *New York Times,* March 24, 1983, p. 8.

85. "Text of Reagan's Address to Nation," *Washington Post,* December 11, 1987, pp. A34f.

86. This was precisely the paradigm shift advocated during the Reagan years in Robert S. McNamara, "Reducing the Risk of Nuclear War: Is Star Wars the Answer?" in Craig Snyder, ed., *The Strategic Defense Debate: Can "Star Wars" Make Us Safe?*

(Philadelphia: University of Pennsylvania Press, 1986), p. 124, and Zbigniew Brzezinski, "Mutual Strategic Security and Strategic Defense," in Brzezinski *et al.*, eds., *Promise or Peril: The Strategic Defense Initiative* (Washington, D.C.: Ethics and Public Policy Center, 1986), pp. 61, 63, 65.

87. See, for example, Office of Technology Assessment, "Ballistic Missile Defense Technologies," in *Strategic Defenses (Two Reports by the Office of Technology Assessment)* (Princeton: Princeton University Press, 1986), pp. 197-210, and Craig Snyder, "Star Wars and Nuclear Ideologies," in Snyder, *The Strategic Defense Debate,* pp. 15-20.

88. *JMP,* 1984, no. 6, p. 48.

89. *Ibid.,* pp. 43-46.

90. *JMP,* 1985, no. 8, p. 44.

91. *JMP,* 1985, no. 9, p. 51.

92. *JMP,* 1986, no. 3, p. 40.

93. As summarized in *JMP,* 1987, no. 6, p. 42.

94. Quoted in *One World* (Monthly Magazine of the World Council of Churches), no. 123 (March 1987), p. 7.

95. *JMP,* 1986, no. 4, p. 44.

96. *JMP,* 1986, no. 5, p. 35.

97. *JMP,* 1987, no. 1, p. 46.

98. *JMP,* 1987, no. 3, p. 41.

99. *JMP,* 1986, no. 6, p. 7.

100. McNamara, "Reducing the Risk," p. 124.

101. *JMP,* 1987, no. 6, p. 34.

102. Text reprinted in *The Illuminator* (Newspaper of the Greek Orthodox Diocese of Pittsburgh), III, no. 25 (August-September 1982), 12.

103. It is not clear whether this support is intended for "absolute pacifists" alone or also for "selective conscientious objectors," who may oppose a particular war at a particular time based on their personal perceptions of its injustice.

104. Text in *The Illuminator,* IV, no. 38 (December 1983), 21. As the special theological consultant who drafted the original text for Bishop Maximos Aghiourgoussis, the diocesan bishop, I include myself among the "guilty," as it were.

105. OCA-M, 1983, pp. 19f.

106. Text in *The Illuminator,* V, no. 46 (October-November 1984), 15.

107. Cf. Charles T. Manatt (chairman, Democratic National Committee), *The 1984 Democratic National Platform* (n.p., n.d.), pp. 47f. The clergy-laity congress oddly omitted from its moral statement any mention of the "nuclear freeze" proposition, which was second only to the SDI controversy as a defense issue that divided Democrat Walter F. Mondale and Republican Ronald Reagan.

108. Text in *Path,* XX, nos. 10-11 (October-November 1984), 10f.

109. "Church's Position on Current Issues," *Orthodox Observer,* LII, no. 975 (September 24, 1986), 4.

110. "Resolution on Environmental/Ecological Crisis," report of Social and Moral Concerns Committee, 30th Biennial Clergy-Laity Congress (Washington, D.C., 1990), p. 3.

111. *UOW,* September 1986, p. 20.

112. K. L. Billingsley, *From Mainline to Sideline: The Social Witness of the National*

Council of Churches (Washington, D.C.: Ethics and Public Policy Center, 1990), p. 40.

113. "Resolution Concerning Follow-Up Action to the Consultation of the Churches on Disarmament," May 9, 1980.

114. *JMP,* 1980, no. 5, pp. 42f.

115. "Resolution on Peacemaking and Ecumenism: A Celebration of the Catholic Bishops' Pastoral Letter," May 13, 1983.

116. See, for example, "Resolution on a Nuclear Weapons Freeze," May 14, 1981, and "Christ Is Our Peace," a joint communiqué with Soviet church representatives issued in August 1980 (text in *JMP,* 1980, no. 10, pp. 25-27).

117. "A Message Concerning Arms Negotiations following the Reagan-Gorbachev Meeting at Reykjavik," November 6, 1986.

118. Text provided by Alan Wisdom of the Institute on Religion and Democracy in Washington, D.C.

119. Text in *Path,* XXIII, nos. 9-10 (September-October 1987), 11.

CHAPTER 7

1. See, for example, Michael Novak, "Moral Clarity in the Nuclear Age," *National Review,* XXXV, no. 6 (April 1, 1983), 365, 368, 370, 390.

2. Paul Ramsey, *Who Speaks For the Church?* (Nashville: Abingdon Press, 1967).

3. Mark R. Amstutz, "Beware of Church Resolutions," *Christianity Today,* XXXIV, no. 8 (May 14, 1990), 10.

4. *LMA,* pp. 90, 92.

5. Vladimir Lossky, *The Mystical Theology of the Eastern Church* (Crestwood, N.Y.: St. Vladimir's Seminary Press, 1976), p. 186.

6. "On the Death Penalty," *TOC,* XXV, nos. 9-10 (September-October 1989), 11.

7. Samuel P. Huntington, "The Clash of Civilizations," *Foreign Affairs,* LXXII, no. 3 (Summer 1993), 22-49, esp. 25 and 31.

8. Irving Kristol, "Russia's Destiny," *Wall Street Journal,* February 11, 1994, p. A12.

9. James H. Billington, "The Case for Orthodoxy," *The New Republic,* May 30, 1994, pp. 24-27.

Index of Names